# Assisted Circulation

Springer
*Berlin*
*Heidelberg*
*New York*
*Barcelona*
*Budapest*
*Hong Kong*
*London*
*Milan*
*Paris*
*Tokyo*

# Assisted Circulation 4

Edited by Felix Unger

With 172 Figures and 58 Tables

Springer

Univ. Prof. Dr. med. h.c. FELIX UNGER
Herzchirurgie Salzburg
Landeskrankenanstalten, Müllner Hauptstr. 48
A-5020 Salzburg, Austria

ISBN-13:978-3-642-79342-4 e-ISBN-13: 978-3-642-79340-0
DOI: 10.1007/978-3-642-79340-0

Library of Congress Catalog Card Number 86-640518.



Typesetting: Best-set Typesetter Ltd., Hong Kong

SPIN: 10481525 23/3130/SPS – 5 4 3 2 1 0 – Printed on acid-free paper

# Preface

It is always a great pleasure editing a book, especially this fourth volume of *Assisted Circulation*. In the last 5 years there has been a dramatic change in the status of assisted circulation and in our understanding of it. The previous volume on assisted circulation was published in 1989. Since then several hundred clinical implantations of pneumatically driven assist blood pumps have been clinically performed, and the technique of bridging has truly become a clinical reality. These results allow a good discussion of long-term device implantation to take place. The first long-term implants (over 200 days) demonstrated the fundamental feasibility of this approach. I am convinced that the next issue of this book in 5 years will contain the first real long-term review of experiences over 1–2 years. The early clinical experience shows dramatically that in certain cardiomyopathies a patient's heart can indeed recover. Verification of this will have a great impact on the whole discussion of heart replacement. The total artificial heart is at present no longer an object of discussion, but further clinical studies on long-term assistance of circulation by means of artificial ventricles will indicate if the artificial heart has a chance for reconsideration.

A great deal of help is necessary in editing such a book, and I want to thank especially my associates R. Schistek and R. Baier as well my secretary C. Stutz. Special thanks go to the Gesellschaft zur Förderung der Herzchirurgie in Salzburg and the Kurt-Polzer-Foundation for support. Hearty thanks also go to Dr. Wieczorek, Dr. Gebhardt, Frau Fingerhuth, and the staff of Springer-Verlag, who have given this fourth volume an attractive format and ensured its accuracy, as usual.

This fourth volume in the series *Assisted Circulation* concentrates on the clinical experience gained in the use of cardiac assist devices, providing both clinical data and experimental ideas. The main unresolved problems in assisted circulation still remain, such as biocompatibility, energy sources, and the driving monitoring components. I would like to express my hopes that the discussion of long-term implantations continues, so that in the fifth edition we can speak about new long-term devices with clinical applications.

Salzburg, January 1995

FELIX UNGER

# Contents

# List of First Named Authors


Aboul-Hosn, W., Sr. R&D Engineer, Interventional Systems Co., 2890 Kilgore Road, Rancho Cordova, CA 95670, USA

Björk, V.O., Professor Emeritus, c/o Frid, Runbergsvagen 8, 19148 Sollentuna, Sweden

Cooley, D.A., Surgeon-in-Chief, Texas Heart Institute, MC 3-258, P.O. Box 20345, Houston, TX 77225-0345, USA

Cooper, D.K.C., Oklahoma Transplantation Institute, Baptist Medical Center, 3300 N.W. Expressway, Oklahoma City, OK 73112, USA

Everts, P.A.M., Department of Cardio-Pulmonary Surgery, Catharina Hospital, P.O. Box 1350, 5602 ZA Eindhoven, The Netherlands

Gattinoni, L., Istituto di Anesthesia e Rianimazione-Ospedale Maggiore, via Francesco Sforza 35, 20122 Milano, Italy

Golding L.A.R., Department of Biomedical Engineering and Applied Therapeutics/Wb 3, The Cleaveland Clinic Foundation, 9500 Euclid Avenue, Cleaveland, OH 44195-5254, USA

Hager, J., I. Universitatsklinik für Chirurgie, Universität Innsbruck, Anichstr. 35, Innsbruck, Austria

Haverich, A., Department of Cardiovascular Surgery, University of Kiel, Arnold Heller Str. 7, 24105 Kiel, Germany

Kantrowitz, A., Clinical Professor of Surgery, Wayne State University School of Medicine, Sinai Hospital of Detroit, 6767 West Outer Drive, Detroit, MI 48235, USA

Kaufmann, R., Helmholtz-Institute for Biomedical Engineering, Pauwelsstrasse 20, 52074 Aachen, Germany

Kolff, W.J., Department of Bioengineering, 2460a Merrill Engineering Bldg. University of Utah, Salt Lake City, UT-84112, USA

Liotta, D., Domingo Liotta Artificial Heart International Foundation, 3 de Febrero 2025, 1428 Buenos Aires, Argentina

Litwak, R.S., Department of Cardiothoracic Surgery, Mount Sinai Medical Center, New York, NY 10029, USA

Loisance, D., Centre de Recherches Chirurgicales Henri Mondor, 8, rue du General Sarrail, 94000 Creteil, France

Moulopoulos, S.D., University of Athens School of Medicine, Department of Clinical Terapeutics, 80, Vas. Sofias – K. Lourou Str., 115 28 Athens, Greece

Nataf, P., Department of Cardiovascular Surgery, Hopital de la Pitié, Paris, France

Ochsner, J., Ochsner Clinic, 1514 Jefferson Highway, New Orleans, LA 70121, USA

Orime Y., C/o Yukihiko Nose, Department of Surgery, Baylor College of Medicine, One Baylore Plaza, Houston, TX 77030, USA

Pearson, G.A., ECMO Fellow, Groby Road Hospital, Groby Road, Leicester UK

Poirier, V., Thermo Cardiosystems Inc., 470 Wildwood Street, P.O. Box 2697, Woburn, MA 01888-2697, USA

Qian, K.X., Institute of Thoracic & Cardiac Surgery, Second Military Medical University, Chang-hai Road 174, Shanghai 200433, China

Rosenberg, G., Division of Cardiothoracic Surgery, Section of Artificial Organs, Department of Surgery, The Pennsylvania State University, The Milton S. Hershey Medical Center, P.O. Box 850, Hershey, PA 17033, USA

Stamatelopoulos, S., Alexandra Hospital, Vas. Sofias Avenue – K. Lourou St., 115 28 Athens, Greece

Steimle, C.N. University of Michigan Medical Center, Section of Thoracic Surgery, TC 2120 Box 0344, 1500 E. Medical Center Drive, Ann Arbor, MI 48109, USA

Stephenson, L.M. Division of Cardiothoracic Surgery, Wayne State University, Harper Professional Building, Suite 228, 3990 John R, Detroit, MI 48201, USA

Unger, F., Herzchirurgie Salzburg, Landeskrankenanstalten, Müllner Hauptstr. 48, 5020 Salzburg, Austria

Vetter, H.O., Department of Cardiac Surgery, University Hospital Grosshadern, Marchionini-Str. 15, 81377 Munich, Germany

Wada, J., Commemorative Heart & Lung Institute, Denki Building N 10F, 1-7 Yuraku-cho 1-Chome, Chiyoda-ku, Tokyo 100, Japan

Watson, J.T., Devices and Technology Branch, Division of Heart and Vascular Disease, National Institutes of Health and National Heart, Lung and Blood Inst., Bethesda, MA 29892, USA

Weiss, W.J., Department of Surgery, Division of Cardiothoracic Surgery, The Pennsylvania State University College of Medicine, The Milton S. Hershey Medical Center, P.O. Box 850, Hershey, PA 17033, USA

Whalen, R.L., Whalen Biomedical Incorporated, 5 Howland Street, Cambridge, MA 02138-1919, USA
Zwischenberger, J.B., Cardiothoracic Surgery, University of Texas Medical Branch, Galveston, TX 77555-0528, USA

# Introduction: The Present Status of Assisted Circulation

It is now 15 years ago that, with the generous help of the publisher, we started the series *Assisted Circulation*. Twenty years ago, experimental research in this field was very intensive and focussed on the total artificial heart, for which Cooley had showed in 1969 the principle feasibility and capability of maintaining normal circulation. In the 25 years since then a great deal of clinical experience has been accumulated, demonstrating today that there are clear indications for assisted circulation using different devices available:

1. There are clear indications for intraaortic balloon pumping.
2. Cardiopulmonary bypass devices in the form of roller pumps or nonpulsatile blood pumps of different shapes are available for patients with cardiac failure. They have been frequently employed throughout the whole world. Nevertheless, practically no literature is available for this group because acute assist devices are implanted in a catastrophic situation.
3. Bridging devices such as left ventricle assist devices are established tools used for heart transplantation. These devices can be considered an indispensible standard in a transplant program.

Based on experience to date, long-term implantation can be considered a possibility, yet it might have an affect on the biological cardiac replacement. Assisted circulation is always indicated when a heart is failing and pharmacological treatment is limited to providing adjunctive support. A number of devices available for assisted circulation have demonstrated their utility for specific purposes:

1. Counterpulsation: intraaortic balloon pumping.
2. Functional heart replacement: ventricular assist devices by means of nonpulsatile or pulsatile blood pumps for partial heart replacement. The pulsatile pumps are driven pneumatically or electromechanically and designed for long-term support. They are used as bridges for heart transplantation. Nonpulsatile blood pumps with open impellers or roller pumps are designed for

weaning off in acute heart failure, such as after open heart surgery, acute myocardial infarction, and shock after PTCA.
3. Cardiomyoplasty: the Latissimus dorsi is used for long-term assistance.
4. Heart replacement: biologic heart replacement by means of transplantation.

To repair or replace a heart is an ancient dream that has come true in part during the past 30 years, with excellent and reliable results. The overall quantity of cardiac surgery has grown enormously, especially due to direct cardiac interventions in acute myocardial infarction. This is reflected by an increasing number of open heart operations worldwide. In 1993 nearly 250000 open heart operations were performed in Europe, of which 60% were coronary cases, 23% valves, 10% congenital problems, 1% cardiac replacement, and 2% aortic aneurysms. This means that in Europe there were 484 operations per million population, as opposed to 300 cases per million population in coronary artery surgery and 343 cases for PTCA.

*Assisted Circulation 4* documents the fantastic progress that has been made in this area over the last 20 years, as was also well illustrated by the volumes 2 and 3. There has been a great transition from an experimental status to clinical routine, providing assisted circulation a clearly defined position in the treatment of heart insufficiency. This volume has eight parts, six of which focus on different forms of assisted circulation: counterpulsation, ventricular assist devices in the clinical use, nonpulsatile blood pumps, biologic assistance, the total artificial heart, and heart transplantation. A new issue, extracorporeal respiratory support, which is clearly related to cardiac assistance, is the focus in another part. In the last part, "Horizons and Future Trends," important investigators attempt to provide a prognosis of future developments. It is always difficult to make a prognosis for a longer time period, expecially in such a complex theme as cardiac assistance. Yet in addition to all the small steps, we also have to observe other techniques, such as genetechnology. As doctors we need visions and dreams that are realistic yet optimistic goals of our endeavors.

F. UNGER

*Previous Volumes*

F. Unger (ed) Assisted circulation. Springer, Berlin Heidelberg New York, 1979
F. Unger (ed) Assisted circulation 2. Springer, Berlin Heidelberg New York, 1984
F. Unger (ed) Assisted circulation 3. Springer, Berlin Heidelberg New York, 1989

# Questions and Predictions

W.J. Kolff

*In 1979*, "Questions and Predictions" concerned what was best: a left ventricular assist device (LVAD) or a total artificial heart (TAH). For those patients a waiting a transplant, the outcome for LVADs or TAHs is about the same, provided one is prepared to use a right ventricular assist device (RVAD) too, when the LVAD alone cannot cope.

*In 1984*, we had the experience with Dr. Barney Clark behind us (December 1982), and the Food and Drug Administration (FDA) had reversed itself. Instead of decreeing that the TAH could be used only in patients who were not candidates for transplantation, the FDA declared that the TAH could be used only as a bridge to transplantation.

*In 1989*, the incidence of thromboemboli in the recipient of a TAH was a real problem. (Recently Dr. Donald B. Olsen pointed out that in 50 consecutive recipients of the Utah-type TAH, from 1990 through part of 1993, not a single incident of thromboembolism has been recorded.)

*In 1989*, we were able to make soft, pliable artificial hearts so that "quick connects" were no longer needed. The intima can avoid thrombosis by making the polyurethane ultrasmooth with dimethyl acetamide (DMAC) [1] and/or coating it with pyrolytic carbon (Sorin Biomedica) or grafting with heparin, as done by Dr. Chisato Nojiri (at Terumo in Japan) or by Dr. Lee-Chien Hsu (of Bentley Laboratories, Division of Baxter Healthcare Corporation): Duraflow, and by others.

Creating a fibrin-coated intima with fused titanium beads or polyurethane fibrils (Thermedics) avoids thrombosis too, at least for the short run, as do Dacron fibrils anchored on polyurethane (R.L. Whalen, Whalen Biomedical Inc., 5 Howland Street, Cambridge Ma 02139).

More and more patients wanted transplantation and were waiting with an artificial heart. Dr. C. Cabrol in Paris, France, had a patient who had been waiting for 620 days. Therefore, I predicted that application of the artificial heart would gradually increase and that *the permanent "TAH" would enter quietly and unannounced through the back door*. This did not happen, as we will see.

*In 1993*, when the FDA forbade the implantation of Symbion Artificial Hearts, the entire TAH program came to a halt. (The reason, as far as we know, was Symbion's failure to keep reliable records.) The Symbion Artificial Heart was the only commercially available TAH. Surgeons used roller pumps, heart-lung machines, LVADs, or nothing at all, and patients died. A nonprofit corporation, Cardio-West Technologies, Inc., became the successor to Symbion, and, slowly, some centers in the United States are receiving permission from the FDA to implant their artificial hearts. They can be sold in Europe, since Cardio-West operates from Canada.

In the meantime, the results of cardiac transplantation have dramatically improved to a 95% survival since the introduction of cyclosporine. I hope that 4 years from now we will be able to report that the high incidence of silent, deadly heart attacks 5 years after transplantation will have subsided. This high after 5-year mortality may perhaps give us a license to apply the TAH with an expected survival time of 5 years, but of course we will strive to do better.

Our greatest problems in 1995 are:

1. To convert the FDA to a supporting agency from being an adversary
2. To obtain specific parts for devices, since certain valves and electrical components cannot be sold for medical devices by order of the manufacturer
3. To obtain materials needed to make elastomeric artificial hearts; silastic from Dow Corning, polyurethane from Dow Chemical, and polyester from DuPont are no longer available for use in devices for human use. All of this (R. Whalen, Whalen Biomedical Inc.; [2]) is induced by fear of liability
4. To obtain enough money for animal implantations

These problems have recently been described in an article entitled "Delays by Recalcitrant FDA, Reluctant NIH and Fearful Industry; the cost in human life, happiness, money and loss of opportunity for American industry" [2].

My own laboratory has concentrated on developing new techniques to make artificial hearts and other blood pumps both quickly and at less cost. We use mainly vacuum forming (VF) and radio-frequency (RF) welding of polyurethane. Indeed, we can "make a heart for you while you wait." We are sending artificial hearts out to other laboratories throughout the world – to Marseilles, Bandung, Beijing, to name a few – to surgeons who are willing to test them in experimental animals.

The ease of manufacturing is important for the development of entirely new devices. One example is our *skeletal muscle and pneumatically powered LVADS* [3–5]. We have combined the muscle-powered pouches (as developed by Dr. Larry Stephenson's group in Detroit, Michigan) with pneumatic power. The pneumatic power can be provided by Datascope Drivers, which are available in most hospitals for intra-aortic balloon pumps. These drivers can maintain a patient's circulation during the 6–8 weeks needed for the skeletal muscles to be trained, and the pumping can start on the operating table. Thus from that moment on, the patient should be out of heart failure. After the 6–8 weeks of training, the muscle power can take over and the pneumatic power is no longer needed; the patient becomes tether free (Fig. 1).

Two Russian physicians, Dr. B.A. Konstantinov and Dr. S.L. Dzemeshkevich, [6] have revived a method to cut off failing ventricles and replace them with *al eless pumping pouches*. There is both a high cut-off and a low cut-off prototype. We prefer the low cut-off, where all four natural valves can be saved [7, 8] (Figs. 2 and 3).

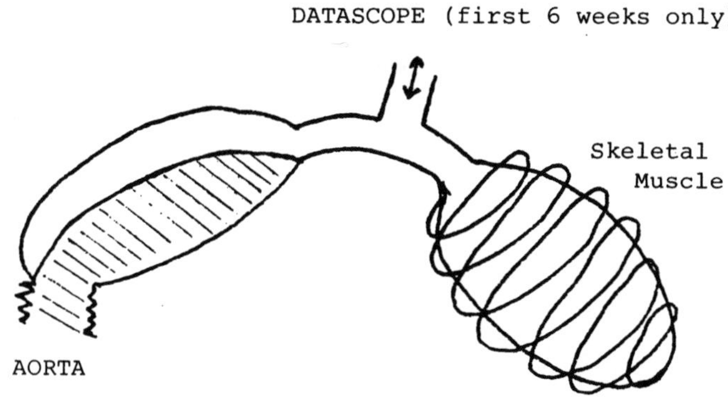


**Fig. 1.** Combination of temporary initial pneumatic power with skeletal muscle power to activate an LVAD. One of the ways in which a skeletal muscle-powered LVAD can work is by counterpulsation in the aorta. Other ways have been described [3–5]

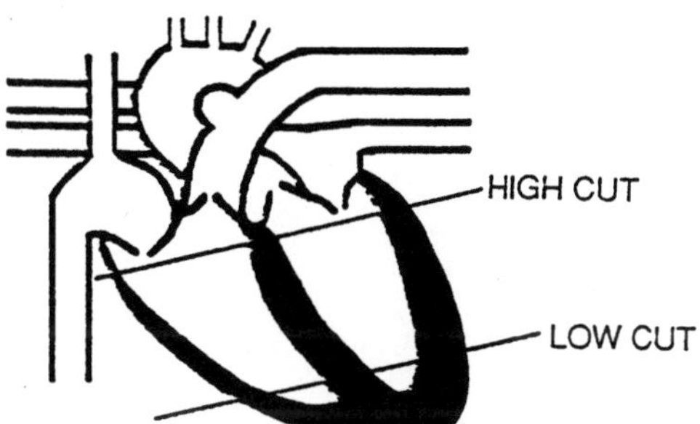


**Fig. 2.** Valveless pulsatile pouches to replace the failing ventricles. The high cut-off requires implantation of artificial mitral and tricuspid valves. The low cut-off saves all four natural valves

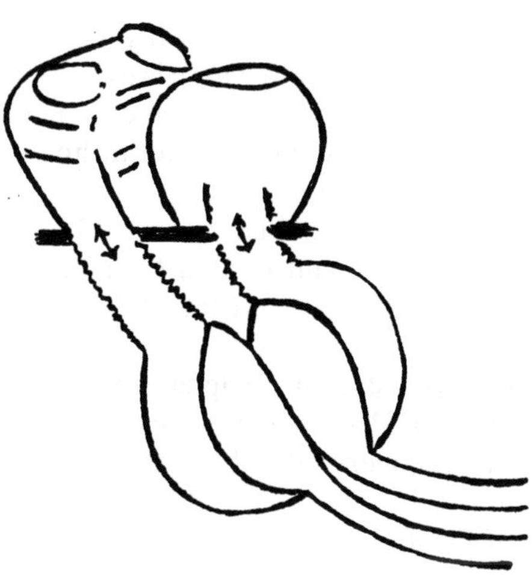

**Fig. 3.** Valveless pulsatile pouches connected to a low cut-off of the failing ventricles located below the diaphragm

*A bedside LVAD with a collapsible atrium* can be adjusted on an i.v. pole so that optimum suction is obtained. When the blood inflow is obstructed, the collapsing atrium chokes off the blood flow and makes suction impossible, automatically preventing the sucking in of air and air embolism (Fig. 4) without the need for electronics. I used these principles in 1949 [9, 10].

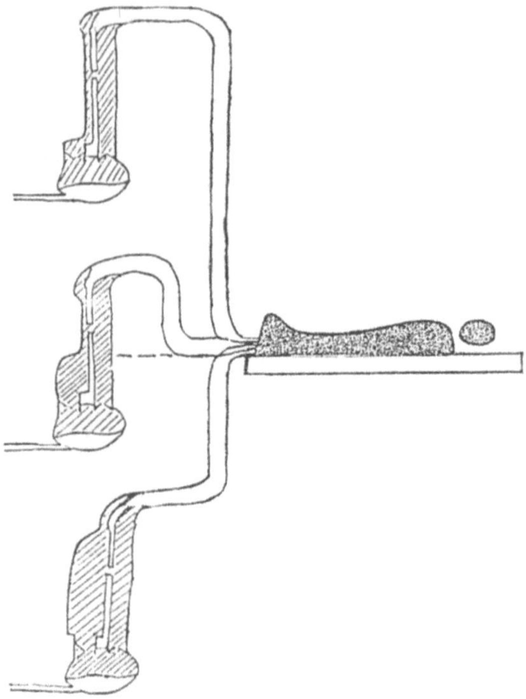

**Fig. 4.** Bedside LVAD with collapsible atrium can be lowered or raised on an i.v. pole. Optimum position: atrium half full

This same pump can be adapted to replace roller pumps or centrifugal pumps for the return of blood from heart1/lung machines or ECMOs. There is extremely little blood damage, no sheared-off particles from the roller pump, and no need for an extra check valve to prevent the retrograde flow in the arterial line of nonocclusive centrifugal pumps which can suck air into the aorta.

Although I remain firmly committed to the total artificial heart, and although I believe that advances in technology will ultimately result in an artificial heart that will excell over any transplant, there is presently a need for alternatives. Patients are dying; they need help now!

I predict that an artificial heart which is able to restore its recipient to a happy existence will be acceptable to the Clinton Health Plan, while, for example, an operation for carcinoma of the pancreas with a recovery rate of less that 5% will not be.

To the many readers of the 4th edition of Dr. Felix Unger's book, I can say, "Let me know what kind of artificial ventricle you need and we can probably make it for you."

## References

1. Yu LS, Versteeg F, Kinoshita M, Yuan B, Bishop D, Kolff WJ (1990) Soft artificial ventricles for infants and adults with or without a clamshell. ASAIO Trans 36:M238–242

2. Kolff WJ (1993) Delays by recalcitrant FDA, reluctant NIH, and fearful industry: the cost in human life, happiness, money, and loss of opportunity for American industry. Artif Organs 17:753–757
3. Kolff WJ, Stephenson LW (1993) Total artificial hearts, LVADS or nothing? Muscle and air-powered LVADS. In: Akutsu T, Koyanagi H (eds) Heart replacement, artificial heart, vol 4. Publ: Springer, Berlin Heidelberg New York, pp 3–11
4. Wilde JCH, van Loon J, Topaz S, Bishop D, Kolff W et al. (1993) Muscle and pneumatic-powered LVADS. Abstr ASAIO 17(6):356
5. Wilde JCH, van Loon J, Bishop ND, Dehlavi Shelton A, Kolff WJ et al. (1995) Muscle and pneumatic-powered, counterpulsating LVADS. Artif Organs: (in press)
6. Konstantinov BA, Dzemeshkevich SL et al. (1991) Total artificial heart without valves: principles of design and implantation technique. Artif Organs 15:369–371
7. van Loon J, Wilde JCH, Topaz S, Bishop D, Kolff WJ (1993) Russian pulsating valve pumps (RPVP). Abstr ASAIO 22:52
8. Van Loon J (1995) The development of a valveless cardiac assist device attached to the ventricular apex. ASAIO J (in press)
9. Kolff WJ, Dubbleman CP (1949) Het kunstmatig hart. Geneesk Gids 1–12
10. Dubbelman CP (1953) Attempts to design an artificial heart-lung apparatus for the human adult. Acta Physiol Pharmacol Neerl 2:1–97

# Part I
# Counterpulsation

# Introduction: Intra-aortic Balloon Pumping as an Established Clinical Method

F. UNGER

By definition, counterpulsation is a method for assisting the heart in series on the basis of the ECG (Fig. 1). The goal is to unload the left ventricle in the ejection phase and to increase the myocardial blood supply in the filling phase of the heart. Due to the fact that counterpulsation works in series for the natural heart, the devices are up to 25% effective and depend on a certain amount of residual minimal circulation. In cases of complete heart deteration or fibrillation, the systems do not work and more capable devices are necessary. Intra-aortic balloon pumping is, at the present time, indicated for:

1. Pump failure after open heart surgery
2. Cardiogenic shock after myocardial infarction
3. Cardiogenic shock in acute heart failure
4. Chronic support for cardiomyopathies

In cases with postoperative heart failure the first step in the cascade of assisted circulation is intra-aortic balloon pumping. This method was reported by Moulopoulos and Kolff in 1962 and Kantrowitz in 1967, and since then has become very well established in clinical use. The basic principle of this technique is to assist the failing heart in series according to the ECG. A balloon built of polyurethane is implanted in the descending aorta via the femoral artery. The balloon is pneumatically driven according to the ECG. In systole the balloon is collapsed, and in the next diastole the balloon is inflated, the expansion creating an increase in diastolic blood pressure. In the next systole the balloon is deflated again, the collapsed balloon creating an area of a lower resistance. In the next balloon inflation phase, in diastole, the flow in the coronary artery is increased up to 60% and the diastolic pressure up to 100%. In the next systole, the balloon collapses again and the less resistance saves the heart energy up to 25%. This is the limit of effective assistance.

There are Complications are reported for up to 10%–25% of the cases. The main complication is kinking of the iliac artery or severe calcification of the abdominal aorta. As a result, another means of access for the balloon to the aorta has been proposed, namely via the chest. Furthermore, a serious breakdown of the circulation in the legs can happen (up to 8%), whereby the balloon has to be removed. Dissection of the aortic wall is another possibility. The most desired effect is the increased flow in the coronary arteries. Timing to achieve proper driving is very important. When the balloon is inflated too early, there is an additional load on the natural heart. An expansion time that is too short should

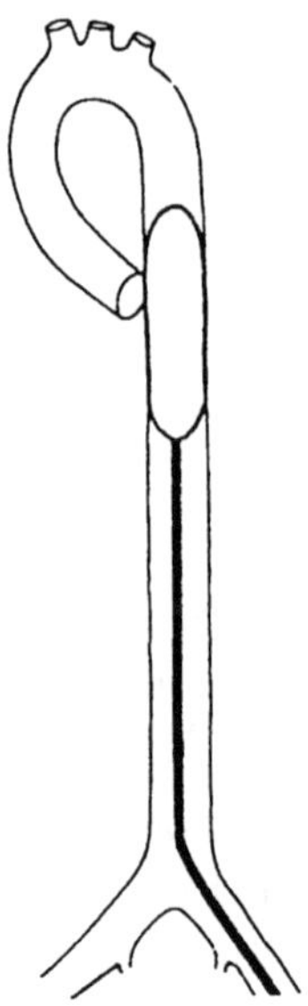

**Fig. 1.** Implantation site of an intra-aortic balloon pump (IABP)

result in a decrease in the coronary artery flow, although I have never observed or recorded it. This phenomenon is like the Flying Dutchman, who was also never seen.

In Salzburg we have seen a proper indication for IABP in only 16 cases in the last 6 years, or in only 0.5% of the total patient population. Out of these 16 cases, six survived (37%, three women and three men). The indication was cardiac failure after coronary bypass grafting, the bypass time was relatively short, and there was a rather short aortic clamping time.

In the group of ten nonsurvivers, nine had coronary heart disease and one underwent a combined procedure (mitral valve replacement and bypass grafting). The bypass time is significant longer than the clamping time.

The intra-aortic balloon pump was designed in the 1970, where 10% of the patients showed problems in weaning off from bypass. Today this problem occurs in at most 1%; in our own cases the incidence of intra-aortic balloon pump use dropped to 0.5%.

This decrease of IABP in clinical use is the result of the skill of the surgeon, the anesthesiologist and the rest of the team. Due to improved operative techniques, especially the cardioplegic solution, and the modern strategy of using nitrates to decrease afterload and also, catecholamines, it is possible to handle cardiac patients much more efficiently than in the 1970s.

This part entitled "Counterpulsation" includes a paper by Kantrowitz, who shows prospects in new techniques and in intraaortic balloon pumping. Moulopoulos, the patron of intra-aortic balloon pumping, focusses on a large volume counterpulsation, and his group on biventricular balloon pumping. Biventricular balloon pumping is sometimes desired in patients with a slight right ventricle failure in consequence to left heart failure.

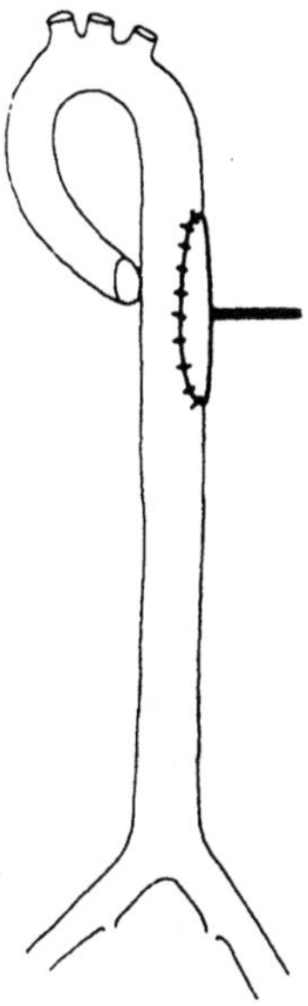

**Fig. 2.** Implantation site of a dynamic aortic patch (DAP)

Balloon pumping is a very well established clinical procedure. Earlier concepts will perhaps have now a chance to be revitalised. The dynamic aortic patch (Fig. 2), the Bash method, external ventricles, and Windkessel ventricles are among the other devices that have been very effective. There has been a renaissance, especially in use of the dynamic aortic patch and the Windkessel ventricle in long-term use, such as in patients with cardiomyopathy. Cardiomyoplasty can be chronic driving source; the energy is sufficient for driving a chronically implanted dynamic aortic patch or an intraaortic balloon pump.

# Intra-aortic Balloon Pumping for Assisted Circulation: New Techniques and New Prospects

A. Kantrowitz, B. Bridgewater, and J. Au

## Introduction

Intra-aortic balloon pumping (IABP) is the most commonly used cardiac assist procedure for temporary support of the failing left ventricle (LV) after acute myocardial infarction and cardiac surgery [1]. The indications, techniques and complications associated with its use have been reviewed extensively [43, 45], but various recent advances are worthy of consideration. This chapter will concentrate on the new uses for the balloon pump, improvements in balloon catheter design intended to minimize associated vascular complications, advances in balloon pump drivers designed to enhance effectiveness and facilitate machine operation, and progress toward a permanent version of the balloon pump (the mechanical auxiliary ventricle) for progressive, refractory chronic heart failure.

## Historical Overview

In 1953, Kantrowitz and Kantrowitz demonstrated that a substantial increase in coronary artery flow resulted from augmenting the arterial pressure pulse of experimental animals during cardiac diastole [49] (Fig. 1). In 1962, Moulopoulos et al. reported studies of counterpulsation by means of a $CO_2$-activated latex balloon placed in the aorta [72]. The year before, Clauss et al. [13] had described the use of an "arterial counterpulsator". In 1966, Kantrowitz and colleagues introduced the forerunner of the IABP used in clinical practice today, a catheter-mounted polyurethane balloon placed in the descending thoracic aorta through a femoral arteriotomy (Fig. 2). The balloon was cycled by admitting pressurized helium into the balloon during diastole through a solenoid valve. The opening and closing of the valve were triggered by a modified oscilloscope that detected the R-wave of the electrocardiogram [97] (Figs. 3 and 4). In animals with induced acute heart failure IABP decreased afterload, as evidenced by a decrease in left ventricular and diastolic pressure of 40% and increases in cardiac output by 50%, in coronary artery blood flow by 100%, and in LV dp/dt by 25% [51, 97]. Myocardial oxygen consumption was also reduced [73, 74].

The initial clinical trial concerning patients with post-infarction cardiogenic shock refractory to maximal pharmacological treatment was reported in 1968 [52] (Fig. 5). This study suggested that IABP could restore patients with that disorder

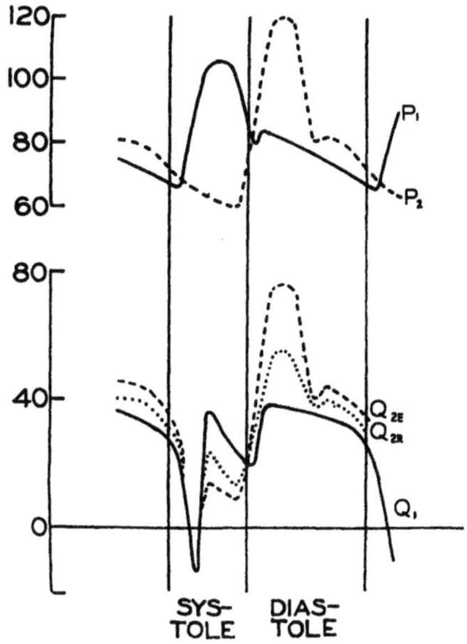


**Fig. 1.** Concept of diastolic augmentation. *Hea y lines* indicate normal aortic pressure ($P_1$) and phasic coronary flow ($Q_1$). *Dashed* and *dotted lines* indicate predicted flows when the anterior descending coronary artery is perfused with pulse pressure out of phase with myocardial systole. $P_2$, Delayed coronary pressure; $Q_{2R}$, calculated flow in presumed rigid coronary system; $Q_{2E}$, calculated flow in presumed elastic coronary system. (Reprinted with permission from [49])

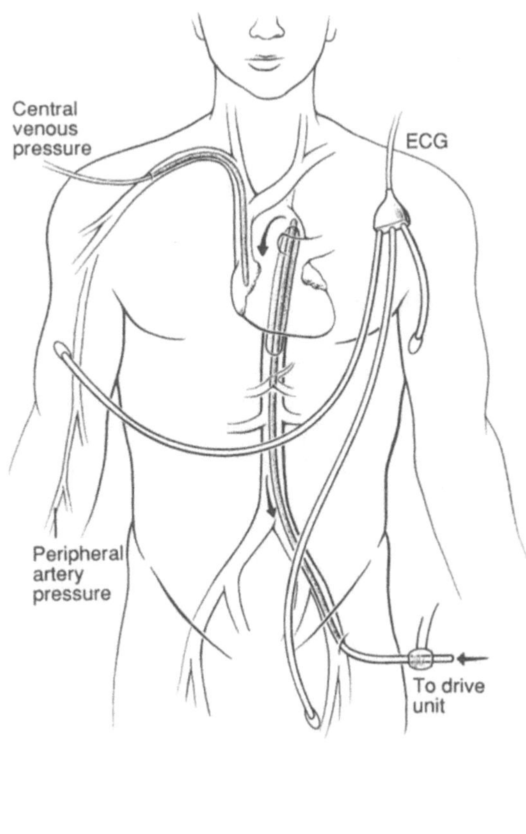


**Fig. 2.** IABP as positioned in initial patients. (Reprinted with permission from [52])

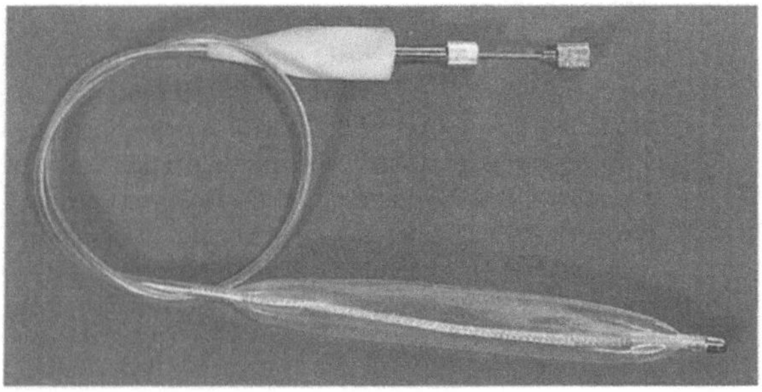

**Fig. 3.** Intra-aortic balloon pump catheter used in initial patients (1967). It was fabricated of polyurethane and exposed to transmembrane pressure of 50 mm Hg during surgery but could withstand 300 mm Hg without undergoing elastic deformation. Markedly higher pressures were required to burst the balloon

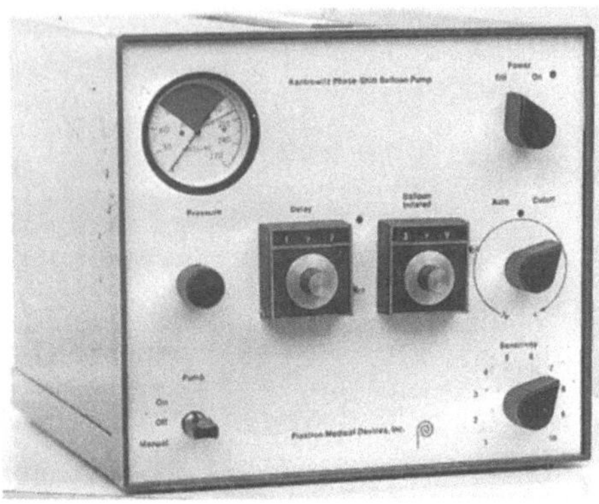

**Fig. 4.** Early control unit used in initial IABP patients

to a satisfactory hemodynamic level and enable many to recover from the shock state. The results of a cooperative clinical trial of IABP in pharmacologically refractory cardiogenic shock after acute myocardial infarction were reported in 1973 [96] and the technique has since been adopted in most cardiac centers, making the balloon pump the only commonly used mechanical device for supporting the failing left ventricle after myocardial infarction and cardiac surgery.

## New Uses for Balloon Pumping

### Percutaneous Transluminal Angioplasty

The established indications for balloon pumping are listed in Table 1. Over the past few years, the indications have been extended, particularly with the rise of percutaneous transluminal coronary angioplasty (PTCA). Various workers have recently published data on the successful use of IABP to support high-risk patients for PTCA [41, 59]. As well as unloading the left ventricle and decreasing

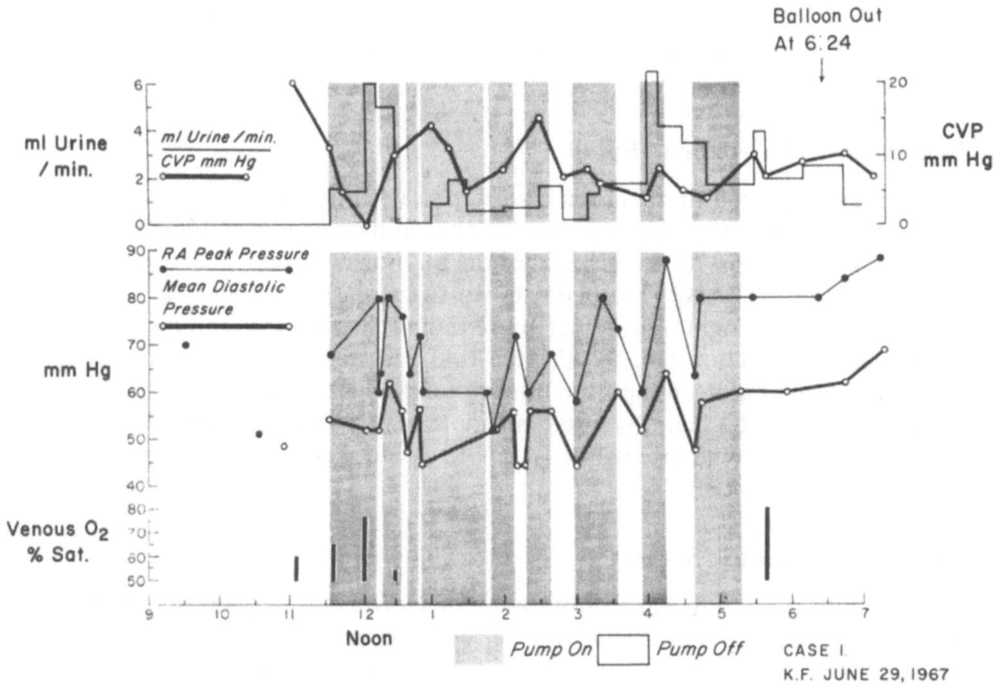


**Fig. 5.** Physiologic data recorded during intra-aortic balloon pumping in the first patient. Note increase in venous oxygen ($O_2$) percentage saturation to normal levels after termination of pumping (low 12:30 p.m. value probably resulted from technical error). Rapid pumping restored urinary output, which had been zero for several hours. (Reprinted with permission from [52])

**Table 1.** Indications for IABP

| |
|---|
| Pump failure after acute MI |
| Pump failure after mechanical complications of acute MI (VSD, etc) |
| Pump failure after onset of acute mitral incompetence |
| Preoperative support for patients awaiting cardiac surgery including transplantation |
| Post-cardiac surgery pump failure, including pump failure after cardiac transplantation |
| Prophylaxis of expected LV failure after cardiac surgery |
| Unstable angina pectoris |
| Failed angioplasty |
| Intraoperative support for patients with cardiac disease undergoing noncardiac surgery |

myocardial oxygen consumption, IABP during PTCA decreases the rate of reocclusion [40, 82]. The mechanisms by which this is mediated are uncertain. Doppler-tipped angioplasty guide wires have been used to study coronary flow before and after angioplasty. IABP was shown to have no effect on blood flow distal to critical stenoses. However, successful angioplasty increases distal coronary blood flow, as demonstrated by increases in parameters of coronary flow such as distal diastolic flow velocity integral, peak diastolic flow velocity, and mean flow velocity [39, 56]. These parameters were further augmented by IABP, and this may be the mechanism by which the decreased reocclusion rate is mediated.

### Pulmonary Artery Balloon Pump

It has been suggested that balloon counterpulsation may be of assistance to the failing right heart after cardiac surgery, either in the aorta in conjunction with a right ventricular assist device [101] or in the pulmonary artery. Pulmonary artery balloon pumping (PABP) has been shown to increase pulmonary artery blood flow and decrease right ventricular preload and afterload in animal models of right ventricular failure [16, 58, 83, 103, 104] and was first described in man in 1980 [68]. Its use has been reported intermittently since then [23, 29, 71, 107]. The mortality tends to be high. In situations more severe than mild right ventricular failure, use of a right ventricular assist device would seem to be more appropriate than recourse to PABP.

### IABP for Noncardiac Surgery

Patients with recent myocardial infarction or known coronary artery disease are at increased risk of perioperative mortality during major noncardiac surgery [18, 34, 66]. The incidence of complications depends on the type of procedure, with emergency vascular, orthopedic, thoracic, and abdominal surgery presenting the highest risks [18, 33, 34]. Various researchers have suggested the use of prophylactic IABP in patients undergoing such operations [10, 14, 24, 28, 36, 70, 102]. Their reports present data on a variety of noncardiac operations in patients with cardiac disease; although the numbers are small and the groups heterogeneous, IABP seems to have been of benefit for selected patients. A decision analysis, weighted for the risk of life-threatening complications against the risk of serious vascular complications and based on a study of 13 of these case reports, suggested that the patients who would benefit most from prophylactic IABP are those whose preoperative assessment places them at very high risk of perioperative complications (i.e., patients in Goldman class IV or Detsky class II undergoing major surgical procedures) [28].

### Balloon Pumping in Pediatric Patients

Technical problems are associated with the use of the balloon pump in pediatric patients: smaller balloons are necessary and must be accurately related to the patient's size; balloon catheters of small caliber are required to prevent ischemic sequelae in narrow-diameter femoral arteries; and sophisticated driving units are essential to provide satisfactory augmentation in the face of the tachycardia usually present in infants. It has also been suggested that the elasticity of the aorta in young children can contribute to poor augmentation. The first reported use was in 1980 [89] in a series of 14 children, with successful balloon counterpulsation achieved in eight. No child under 5 years survived, but, with the advent of smaller balloons, satisfactory support has been achieved in infants as small as 2 kg at heart rates up to 200 bpm [17, 84, 111, 112, 114]. IABP is now a useful addition to conventional medical treatment of cardiogenic shock in children.

## Post-infarction Cardiogenic Shock–Improved Survival

The first large trial of the use of IABP for cardiogenic shock unresponsive to pharmacological treatment following acute myocardial infarction was, as noted, reported in 1973. Shock was reversed in the majority of the 87 patients treated although only 16% survived to leave the hospital [96]. Similar results were reported by Dunkman [20]. Since then, various workers have reported survival rates between 15% and 46%, the differences presumably reflecting patient selection and variations in the technique of IABP and its adjunctive management [31, 44, 80, 93, 105, 113]. Nevertheless, cardiogenic shock following myocardial infarction has remained a highly lethal condition, and there is no consensus in the literature as to whether IABP should be used as a salvage procedure in this condition. Recent advances in the management of acute myocardial infarction, however, including reperfusion by thrombolysis, angioplasty, or emergency surgery, and reports of improved survival following early treatment with angiotensin-converting enzyme inhibitors [3, 85] suggest that the role of IABP in the management of patients with refractory heart failure following myocardial infarction should be reevaluated. Can prognosis be improved for that group of patients who previously were weaned from IABP but died before leaving the hospital?

Recently, Waksman et al. studied 45 patients with cardiogenic shock after acute myocardial infarction [113]. IABP was possible in 24 and performed in 20. Twenty-one other patients with similar disease were not able to undergo IABP during the same time period. Early revascularization was performed in 16 of the 20 IABP patients. In the entire IABP group, in-hospital and 1-year survivals were, respectively, 46% and 38%, compared with 19% and 10% in the group in which there was no access to the balloon pump. These data were prospectively collected. However, data from randomly chosen subjects that confirm these findings have yet to be reported, and numerous other avenues of treatment remain unexplored. What seems certain is that IABP offers the best available treatment for cardiogenic shock after acute myocardial infarction and, when combined with other recent advances in care, may yet offer important improvements in short- and long-term survival.

## IABP in Unstable Angina

IABP can be an effective treatment of unstable angina. Initiation of IABP usually causes rapid reversal of myocardial ischemia and associated relief of pain [6, 90], and it has been suggested that if symptoms fail to resolve, the accuracy of the diagnosis of unstable angina should be questioned. Most patients with unstable angina will respond to conventional therapies of rest and medications, but use of the IABP should be considered for the small percentage of patients with refractory, unstable angina, usually as a bridge to other therapies such as coronary artery bypass surgery or angioplasty [115]. This indication for IABP has recently been endorsed by the Agency for Health Care Policy and Research in their clinical guideline for the treatment of unstable angina [2].

## Initiation of IABP

The primary considerations in selecting a balloon pump for a given patient are that its stroke volume match that of the failing left ventricle as closely as possible, and that, when inflated, it not occlude the aorta; in addition, as discussed below, catheter length should be matched to the patient's height.

The displacement volume of most balloon pumps is close to that of the failing LV (i.e., 30–40 ml), and their inflated diameter is just less than that of the aorta (i.e., 16–18 mm). In patients with a narrow aorta, a smaller balloon should be used. The techniques of balloon pump insertion have been described extensively [45]. Insertion into the femoral artery, either percutaneously or by surgical cutdown, remains the technique of choice. When the femoral route is contraindicated, transthoracic insertion [37, 88] or use of the subclavian artery [81] should be considered. The presence of prosthetic graft material in the aortoiliac system had been cited as a contraindication to IABP, but successful cases have recently been reported [61, 75].

## Complications

The overall incidence of IABP complications ranges from 12% to 41% [5, 9, 22, 32, 35, 53, 62, 64, 65, 67, 78]; the majority are vascular, including both acute limb ischemia and long-term ischemic sequelae [27], and infectious [53]. Numerous other complications of IABP occur less frequently [45] (Table 2). It is important to note that the rate of major complications is only 4–9%.

Several studies have compared complication rates following surgical and percutaneous routes of insertion, and most, but not all, have reported a higher incidence of vascular complications with the percutaneous technique [4, 15, 19, 22, 30, 53, 60, 63, 86, 98]. It has been suggested that the surgical technique is more suitable for those patients at highest risk of vascular complications [69], i.e., those of female sex, the obese, and those wi th diminished or absent femoral pulses or known peripheral vascular disease. If the IABP was inserted percutaneously in a patient with a bleeding diathesis or hemorrhagic or ischemic complications, it may be advisable to remove it by direct surgical cut down [91].

Deeper appreciation of the vascular risks of percutaneous femoral balloon pump insertions has led to the recent development of fenestrated balloon sheaths, which allow blood flow through the sheath to the distal vessels [95]. This technique is associated with a lower incidence of vascular complications than were earlier methods using conventional sheaths [116]. Balloon pumps which can be inserted without the use of a sheath have also been produced; they may reduce the frequency of complications involving ischemia following percutaneous insertion [77, 87, 110].

**Table 2.** Complications of IABP

| |
|---|
| Acute vascular complications |
| Loss of distal pulse |
| Pain |
| Thrombosis |
| Embolism |
| Amputation |
| Aortic dissection |
| Iliac artery laceration |
| Delayed vascular complications |
| Arterial stenosis |
| Claudication |
| Foot drop |
| False aneurysm |
| Infectious complications |
| Local infection |
| Graft infection |
| Septicemia |
| Other |
| Excessive would bleeding |
| Disseminated intravascular coagulation |
| Gastrointestinal/genitourinary bleeding |
| IABP rupture |
| IABP perforation |
| Gas embolism |
| Small bowel infarction |
| Late paraplegia |
| Neurological abnormalities of the leg |

Position of the balloon in the descending thoracic aorta has generally been confirmed by chest X-ray, but transesophageal Doppler echocardiography [54, 57, 109] is beginning to be used to make this determination. The exact position of the balloon is important; positioning the distal end in the upper abdominal aorta may cause significant impairment of renal perfusion or even renal artery occlusion [106], but superior mesenteric flow continues unaffected [100]. The size of the balloon pump (both as to volume and as to length) should therefore be chosen with respect to patient height. It has been suggested that transesophageal echocardiography can assist in balloon positioning and optimization of timing, as well as in prediction of the optimal time for weaning from the balloon [55, 99, 109].

## Balloon Timing and New Developments in Drive Units

To achieve maximal hemodynamic benefits of IABP, the timing of balloon inflation and deflation must be precise (Fig. 6). Inappropriate timing can lead to reduced effectiveness of assistance [45]. Helium is used as the drive gas because of its low viscosity. Agreement is general that inflation should begin immediately after the appearance of the dicrotic notch on the central aortic blood pressure waveform, whereas most authors accept the fact that deflation should occur at the

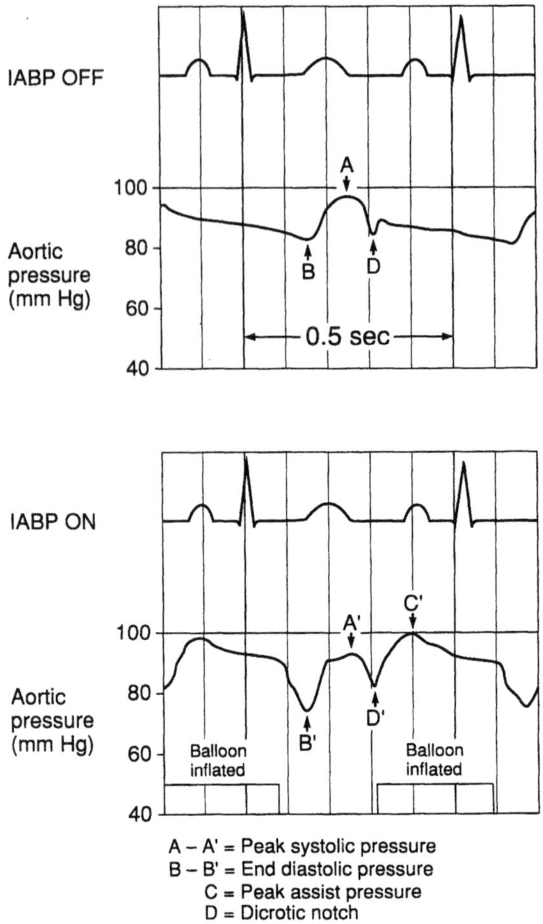


**Fig. 6.** Idealized waveforms showing timing of IABP inflation. (Reprinted with permission from [45])

end of diastole [43, 45]. It has been pointed out that the precise timing and rate of deflation may vary according to whether the intent is to maximize ventricular unloading or coronary artery flow [43]. For effective diastolic augmentation during every heart beat, the patient should have a regular rhythm, and balloon timing should be adjusted by a trained operator to maximize both coronary flow and reduction in LV afterload.

Most commercially available drive units can trigger from 60 to 200 beats per minute (bpm), but at rates greater than 120 bpm the balloon stroke volume is reduced and the hemodynamic benefits are decreased [21]. Some workers have suggested that in patients with tachyarrhythmias a better effect is seen with balloon inflation on every second beat [94], but others believe that this practice reduces already suboptimal augmentation still further [45]. Occasional premature beats do not decrease the benefits of assistance, but in atrial fibrillation with a fast ventricular response it is generally not possible to maintain effective augmentation, even with the continuous intervention of a skilled operator.

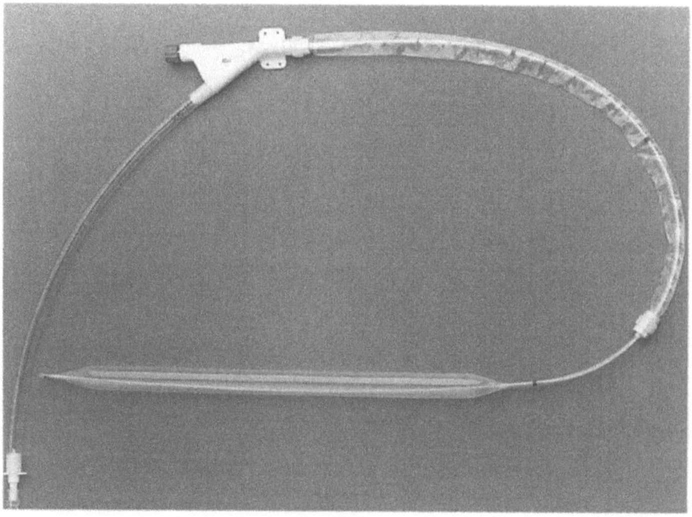

**Fig. 7.** Representative current intraaortic balloon pump catheter: the Boston Scientific 9 Fr features unibody construction. (Courtesy of Cardiac Assist, Boston Scientific Corporation)

Balloon pump drive units and catheters are now offered by several manufacturers (Fig. 7). As compared with early (1970s) drivers, contemporary units offer sophisticated new features; one third-generation drive unit provides "closed-loop" control, with complete automation of balloon timing even in various cardiac arrhythmias, as discussed below. Makers of second-generation drivers with some automated features are Bard Cardiopulmonary Division of C.R. Bard, Inc., Datascope, Kontron Instruments, and St. Jude Medical Cardiac Assist Division (Figs. 8–11).

Generally, the design of second-generation drivers presumes that the time intervals between the occurrence of the QRS complex and aortic valve opening – the systolic time intervals – are a function of heart rate. At the initiation of IABP, the console operator selects time delays appropriate to the patient's current heart rate and enters them into the drive unit's circuitry. When the patient's heart rate changes, the console resets the time delays. It does so on the basis of a built-in "function curve", which contains averaged data from large numbers of patients that provide estimates of the systolic time intervals for each of the heart rates likely to be encountered in the clinical setting. Manual adjustment is still necessary to achieve maximal augmentation whenever the patient's heart rate changes significantly or an arrhythmia comes into play.

A third-generation IABP (Fig. 12) has been developed by Aisin Human Systems[1] and L. VAD Technology, Inc.[2] (the laboratory of Adrian Kantrowitz). This machine has dual modes: the standard IABP panel and the fully automated. The fully automated mode allows the timing of balloon inflation and deflation, as well as other parameters such as balloon volume to be adjusted beat by beat, so as to maximize the hemodynamic efficacy of each balloon inflation cycle. This

[1] Kariya City, Japan

[2] Auburn Hills, MI, USA

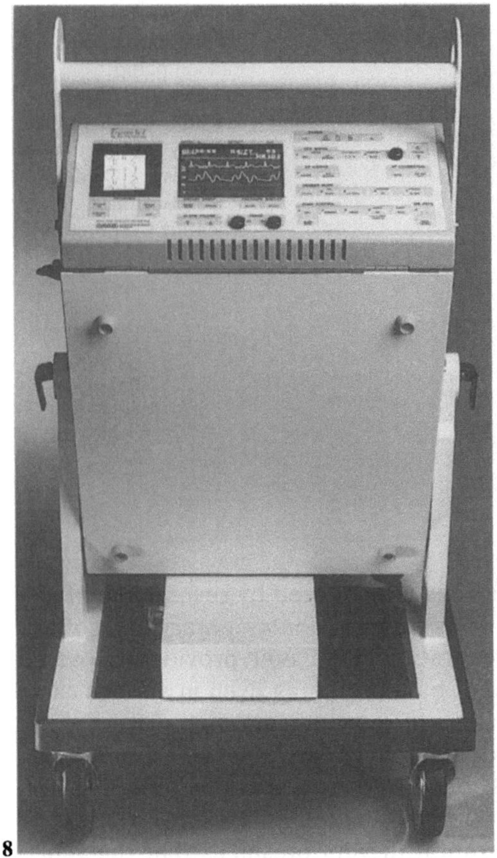

8

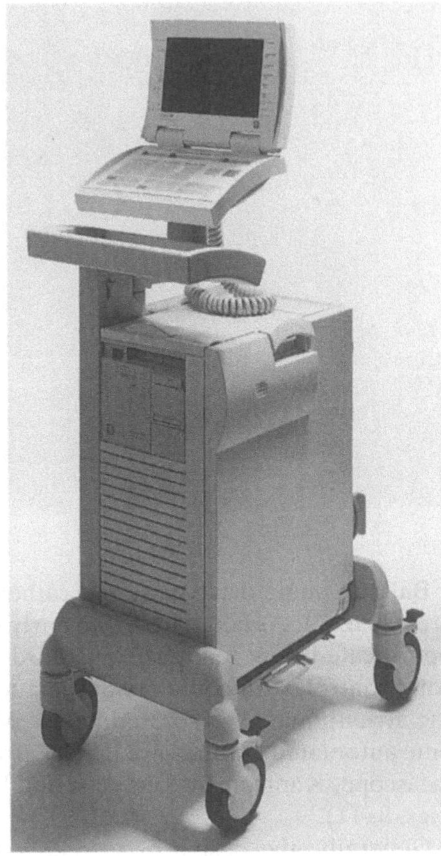

9

**Fig. 8.** Bard TransAct System with handles for bed mounting. (Courtesy of Bard Cardiopulmonary Division, C.R. Bard, Inc.)

**Fig. 9.** Datascope System 97 for bedside and transport use. (Courtesy of Datascope Corp.)

new system comprises a polyurethane balloon mounted on a catheter incorporating ECG electrodes, a pressure sensor which is advanced to the tip of the balloon catheter as soon as it has been placed in the descending thoracic aorta, and a computerized drive unit with a single control button for pumping [46]. Accurately timed IABP begins within a few seconds after placement of the pressure sensor. The driver is capable of executing volume weaning over an operator-selected interval ranging from 12 min to 24 h. This driver has been shown to respond to tachyarrhythmias at rates of up to 200 bpm in animals [12, 46].

In a clinical trial of an investigational configuration of the Aisin-L. VAD driver to examine its efficacy in delivering diastolic augmentation in the clinical setting, it was used to counterpulsate ten patients with symptomatic coronary artery disease (three with hemodynamic instability during catheterization, two undergoing high-risk PTCA, four with angina post infarction and preoperative support, and one with cardiogenic shock) [46] (Figs. 13 and 14). Every 60 min assistance was interrupted for 4 s.

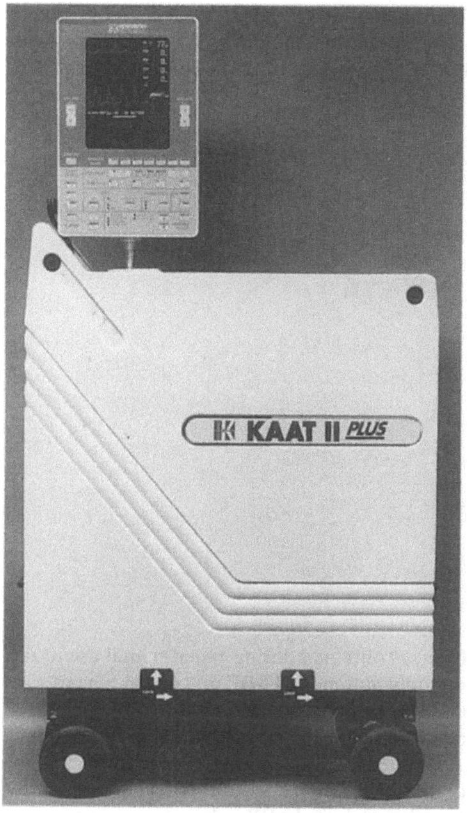


10

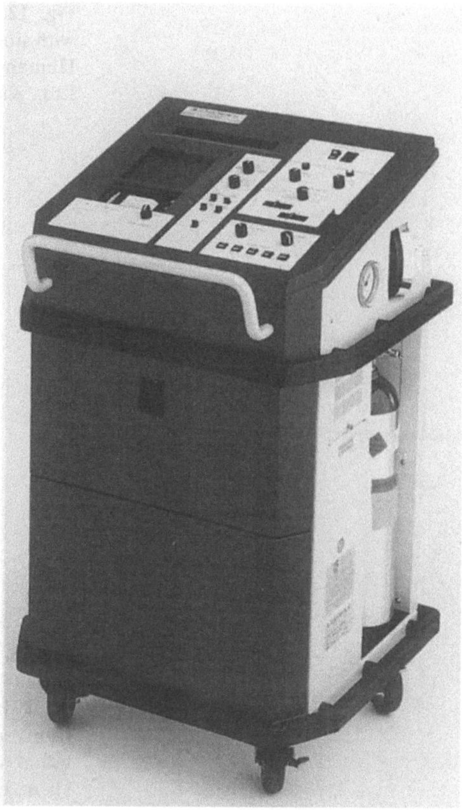

11

**Fig. 10.** Kontron Instruments KAAT II Plus Drive Unit for hospital and transport use. (Courtesy of Kontron Instruments, Inc.)
**Fig. 11.** St. Jude Medical Model 700 IABP Control System. (Courtesy of St. Jude Medical, Cardiac Assist Division)

The last augmented and the first unassisted heart beats in each sequence were compared to assess counterpulsation effects on hemodynamic parameters, and assisted aortic pressure waveforms were analyzed to determine the accuracy of balloon inflation and deflation. The driver delivered the expected hemodynamic benefits of diastolic augmentation. Evaluation of all of the hourly recordings, totalling 186 (180 with complete data), showed that inflation began within 20 ms of the dicrotic notch 99% of the time; the correlation coefficient was 0.941 out of a theoretical maximum of 0.958. Deflation always straddled the first half of ventricular ejection; it began 48 ± 21 ms before opening of the aortic valve and was complete almost at the midpoint of ventricular ejection.

Another study [76] compared the commercial version of the Aisin-L. VAD driver, Corart BP-1, with a second-generation driver in patients with "severe" coronary artery disease. The Corart BP-1 unit inflated and deflated the balloon more rapidly than the conventional unit, afforded a longer period of balloon inflation, and provided better systolic unloading, as judged on the basis of end-systolic myocardial wall stress and mean circumferential shortening velocity. A

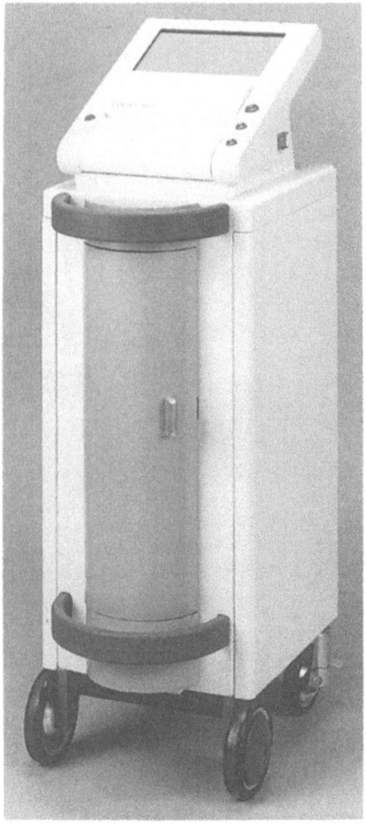

**Fig. 12.** Third-generation fully automatic IABP system with single control button, the Corart BP-1, made by Aisin Human Systems. (Courtesy of Aisin Human Systems Co. Ltd., Kariya City, Japan)

**Fig. 13.** Tracings obtained during experimental use of the closed-loop, fully automatic IABP in a dog at a heart rate of 197 bpm. The symbols indicate features of the waveforms as detected by the drive unit. Note that full augmentation was obtained even at this rate. (Paper speed 50 mm/s); ▲, End diastole; ▼, peak systole; ▽, peak assist pressure; ♠, dicrotic notch; ↑, IABP inflation

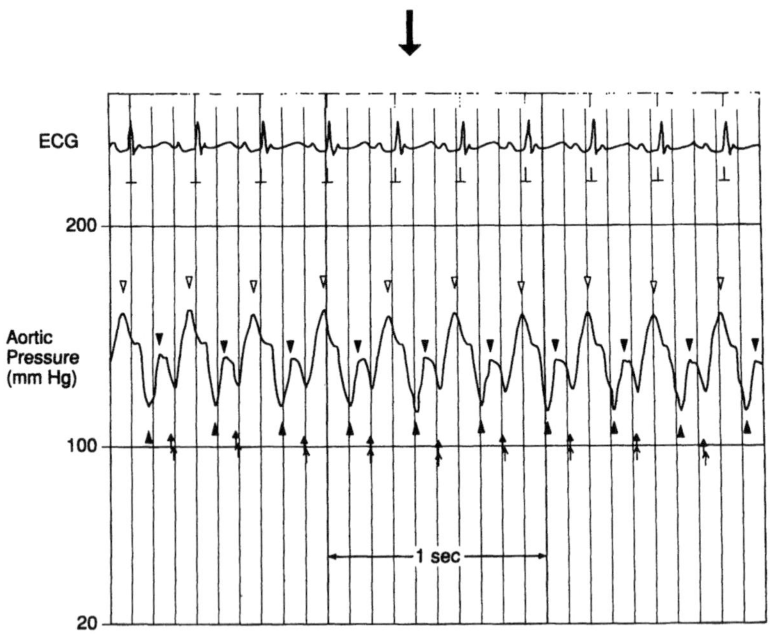

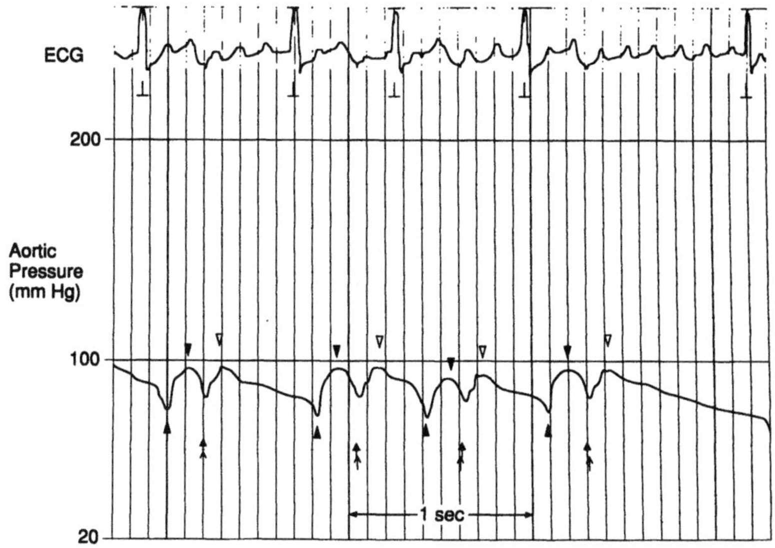


**Fig. 14.** Tracings obtained during experimental use of the closed-loop, fully automatic IABP in a dog in atrial flutter. Note that the timing of augmentation is adjusted automatically on each beat, even though R-R intervals vary widely (paper speed 50 mm/s). (Reprinted with permission from [46])

mock circulation study [92] confirmed that the design of the automated, third-generation driver made possible a greater degree of systolic unloading than a second-generation driver can achieve. Nishimura et al. [79] used the third-generation driver in seven cardiac patients. Balloon inflation was found to begin within 0–5 ms of the dicrotic notch in 99% of the heart beats sampled, averaging 2.3 ms; deflation began within 0–5 ms after the R-wave. The authors concluded that closed-loop control of the balloon pump provided stable timing, and that during automated weaning there is a straight-line reduction of augmentation with time. In a separate study, Tanaka et al. [108] confirmed the clinical efficacy of the Corart BP-1 driver. Further clinical studies of this closed-loop driver are being carried out in Japan, where it is also being used routinely, and additional clinical trials are planned for the USA.

## Prospects for Long-term Counterpulsation

Whereas the short-term use of IABP has been well accepted for the indications described above, long-term use is less well established. Freed et al. [26] described 27 patients in whom balloon pumping had been continued for over 1 month; 17 (60%) survived to leave the hospital. Of these, some had surgical correction of their cardiac defect and good long-term survival, but seven of the early survivors who had a history of congestive cardiac failure were dead by 6 months after discharge, one due to a cerebrovascular accident and six of congestive cardiac failure [26]. These patients had myocardial function incompatible with long-term survival, despite modern pharmacological treatment. It has been estimated that up to 100000 new patients fall into this category each year [38].

The available therapeutic options for this category of patient are cardiac transplantation, which is donor limited and carries numerous contraindications at present, or some other form of treatment which inputs energy into the cardiovascular system. Recently, advances have been made in permanently implantable ventricular assist devices, skeletal muscle ventricles, and cardiomyoplasty. The latter two are covered in depth elsewhere in this book; here we report progress with a mechanical auxiliary ventricle (MAV) [117].

Our goals in developing this system were to take advantage of the demonstrated simplicity and reliability of IABP in providing counterpulsation to create a reliable assist system that could meet the needs of a substantial proportion of patients with CHF. We envisaged the MAV as one of a family of permanent left ventricular assist systems. Left ventricular assist systems which functioned in parallel with the natural heart and incorporated two valves in the blood pump would find application in patients who require a maximal assist device output. Such systems must possess 100% reliability, inasmuch as interruption of their action significantly increases the risk of activating the hemostatic mechanisms. The MAV, in contrast, could find use in patients with some functioning LV myocardium. Although larger (60 cc) in stroke volume than the balloon pump, the MAV replicates its hemodynamic actions. Therefore, the benefits of MAV implantation and activation could be predicted from the candidate's response to IABP. There are several other MAV advantages that clinicians might wish to take into account in choosing an assist system: the ability to discontinue support at will without risk to the patient from low flow or stasis of blood in artificial conduits (when inactivated, the MAV pumping chamber collapses, then having the shape and function of a passive graft in the wall of the aorta), and a design that (a) minimizes the exposure of the patient's vascular system to artificial material and (b) does not compress adjacent bodily structures.

Early work on this configuration of the MAV began in 1968 [48]. The prosthesis comprised an avalvular pumping bladder incorporated in a Dacron velour graft which was sutured into the wall of the aorta in the same location as the IABP. An air tube led from the lateral aspect of the pumping chamber to a percutaneous access device (PAD) implanted in the vicinity of the umbilicus. An external tube led to a modified IABP driver. Experimental studies established that the MAV delivered effective counterpulsation comparable or superior to that provided by the IABP. Between 1971 and 1976, a clinical trial of the MAV system was conducted in three patients with chronic heart failure for whom all nonsurgical options had been exhausted [7, 48, 50]. Hemodynamic benefits were observed in all three patients. One patient was discharged from the hospital and enjoyed markedly improved cardiac function for several weeks, with relief of his congestive failure. An infection originating in proximity to the PAD triggered the sequence of events that led to his death.

Since these experiences, the problem of long-term stable percutaneous access has been overcome by the development of a novel PAD in a collaboration between our surgical research group and colleagues at the University of Michigan

School of Public Health. In this PAD, the Lexan device-tissue interface is rendered nanoporous by nuclear bombardment and incubated with fibroblasts from the prospective host, which gradually coat the device and extend cell processes into the nanopores. After implantation, the fibroblasts on the device coalesce

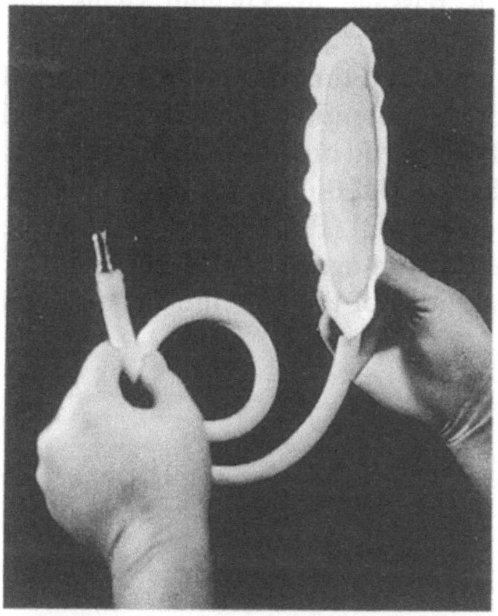

**Fig. 15.** The mechanical auxiliary ventricle, a simple pumping bladder of unilayer construction with no valves, is implanted in the descending thoracic aorta

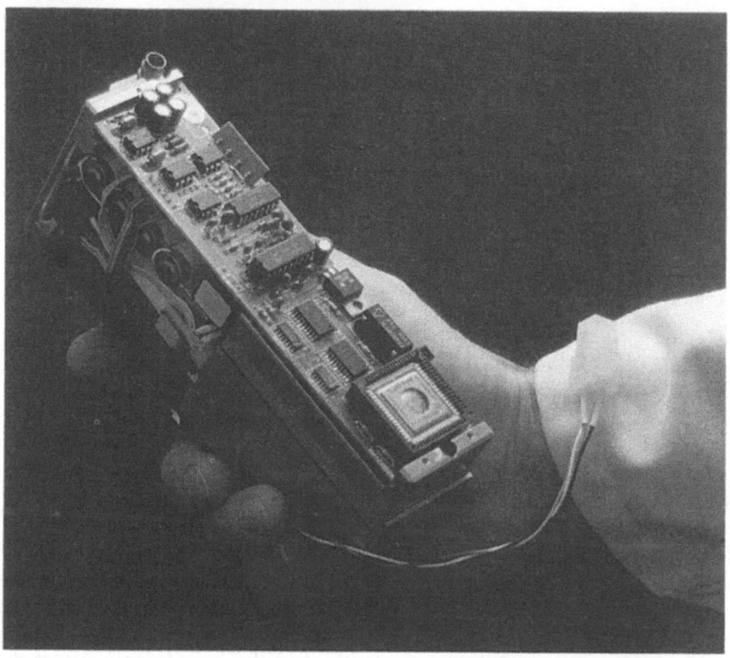

**Fig. 16.** Drive unit for the mechanical auxiliary ventricle, which can be vest mounted or attached to a belt. Current weight with batteries is about 2 kg

with host fibroblasts to create a biological barrier to reduce the risk of infection and epithelial cell migration. A large flange firmly attaches the PAD to the dermis, causing the PAD and surrounding tissues to move as a unit in response to applied forces, and thus protecting the critically important junction between device and host [8, 11, 25]. PADs based on this design have been demonstrated to provide reliable long-term percutaneous passage in Yucatan swine and Holstein calves.

A more subtle problem was detected for the first time in the MAV clinical studies carried out in the 1970s, that of slight but potentially consequential fluid migration to the extravascular space behind the aortic prosthesis. This difficulty has been overcome by using the impermeable material Biomer for the wall of the pumping chamber and a unilayer construction [42, 43] (Fig. 15). In addition, the MAV drive units have been redesigned to take advantage of new technologies. A line-powered driver has essentially the capabilities of the new third-generation

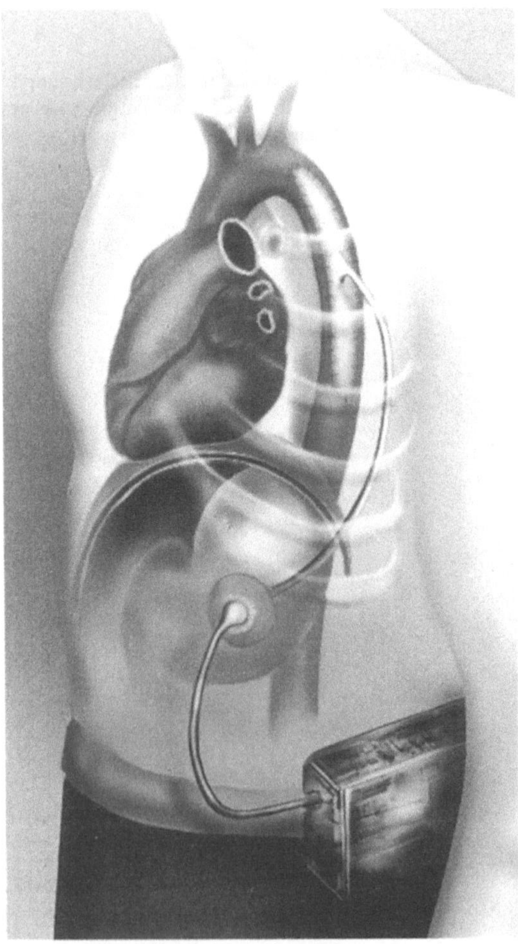

**Fig. 17.** The mechanical auxiliary ventricle has two implantable components. The blood pump, which can be used intermittently, and the percutaneous access device. The patient can detach the connector to the external drive unit when the blood pump is passive

IABP driver described above. A wearable, belt-mounted unit has been further miniaturized, now weighing about 1 kg, with its batteries about 2 kg (Fig. 16).

The redesigned MAV system was tested by long-term implantation in four normal male calves, with intermittent assist device activation (generally, for 2 h in the morning and 2 h in the afternoon on 5 weekdays). Pumping was continued in three animals for 22, 26, and 60 weeks, and a fourth animal was still alive at 80 weeks; no medications were given during these periods. A panel of laboratory data was collected every 2 weeks in each animal. By 5–16 weeks after initiation of pumping, all laboratory parameters were normal except for the total protein level. In particular, there was no laboratory evidence of erythrocyte hemolysis, infection, or thrombus formation; histologic studies confirmed the latter two findings. Thus, despite many instances of activating and deactivating the MAV system (as many as 800 "restarts" in one animal) no activation of the hemostatic mechanisms was detected and the animals remained infection free. These observations suggest strongly that the difficulties noted in the earlier clinical trials have been overcome, and that the MAV system may provide an effective approach to long-term diastolic augmentation in selected patients with chronic congestive failure [47]. Currently, preparations for clinical assessment of the new MAV[3] system are in progress (Fig. 17).

## References


1. ACC/AHA Task Force (1991) Guidelines and indications for coronary artery bypass surgery. A report of the American College of Cardiology/American Heart Association Task Force on assessment of diagnostic and therapeutic cardiovascular procedures (Subcommittee on Coronary Artery Bypass Graft Surgery). J Am Coll Cardiol 17:543–589
2. Agency for Health Care Policy and Research (AHCPR), US Department of Health and Human Services Agency for Health Care Policy and Research (1994) Unstable angina diagnosis and Management, clinical practice guideline no 10. National Heart, Lung and Blood Institute, p 71
3. AIRE (Acute Infarction Ramipril Efficacy) study investigators (1993) Effect of ramipril on mortality and morbidity of survivors of acute myocardial infarction with clinical evidence of heart failure. Lancet 342:821–828
4. Alcan KE, Stertzer SH, Wallsh E, Franzone AJ, Bruno MS, DePasquale NN (1983) Comparison of wire-guided percutaneous insertion and conventional surgical insertion of intra-aortic balloon pumps in 151 patients. Am J Med 75:24–28
5. Alvarez JM, Gates R, Rowe D, Brady PW (1992) Complications from intraaortic balloon counterpulsation: a review of 303 cardiac surgical patients. Eur J Cardiothorac Surg 6:530–535
6. Aroesty AM, Weintraub RM, Paulin S, O'Grady SP (1979) Medically refractory unstable angina pectoris. II. Hemodynamic and angiographic effects of intraaortic balloon counterpulsation. Am J Cardiol 43:883–888
7. Baechler CA, Barnhart MI, Schraut W, Kantrowitz A (1973) Studies on the dynamic aortic patch and the aorta in clinical trials. Proceedings of the Scanning Electron Microscopy Workshop. Research Institute, Chicago, pp 443–449
8. Bar-Lev A, Freed PS, Mandell G, Cardona R, Vaughan F, Bernstam L, Bernstein I, Kantrowitz A (1987) Long-term percutaneous access device. In: Advances in continuous ambulatory peritoneal dialysis. Proceedings of the seventh annual CAPD Conference, Kansas City, Missouri, February 1987. Perit Dial Bull 81–87


[3] Cardiovad, L. VAD Technology, Inc., Auburn Hills, MI, USA

9. Beckman CB, Geha AS, Hammon GL, Baue AE (1977) Results and complications of intraaortic balloon counterpulsation. Ann Thorac Surg 24:550–559
10. Bonchek LI, Olinger GN (1979) Intra-aortic balloon counterpulsation for cardiac support during non-cardiac operations. J Thorac Cardiovasc Surg 78:147–149
11. Cardona RR, Kantrowitz A (1990) Autologous fibroblast coating used to enhance percutaneous access device longevity. American College of Surgeons, Michigan Chapter, p 29 (abstr)
12. Cardona RR, Rios C, Freed PS, Gage KP, Bar-Lev A, Keller D, Suzuki A, Kantrowitz A, Hayakawa K, Takano T (1992) Experimental models for studies of a closed-loop, fully automatic intraaortic balloon pump. Cardiovascular Science and Technology Conference, Washington DC
13. Clauss RH, Birtwell WC, Albertal G, Lunzer S, Taylor WJ, Fosberg AM, Harken DE (1961) Assisted circulation. I. The arterial counterpulsator. J Thorac Cardiovasc Surg 41:447–458
14. Cohen SI, Weintraub RM (1975) A new application of counterpulsation: safer laparotomy after recent myocardial infarction. Arch Surg 110:116–117
15. Curtis JJ, Boland M, Bliss D, Walls J, Boley T, Schmaltz R, Flaker G, Anderson SK (1988) Intraaortic balloon cardiac assist: complication rates for the surgical and percutaneous insertion techniques. Am Surg 54:142–147
16. de la Riviere AB, Haasler G, Malm JR, Bregman D (1983) Mechanical assistance of the pulmonary circulation after right ventricular exclusion. J Thorac Cardiovasc Surg 85:809–813
17. del Nido PJ, Swan PR, Benson LN, Bohn D, Charlton MC, Coles JG, Trusler GA, Williams WG (1988) Successful use of intraaortic balloon pumping in a 2-kilogram infant. Ann Thorac Surg 46:574–576
18. Detsky AS, Abrams HB, McLaughlin JR, Drucker DJ, Sasson Z, Johnson N et al. (1986) Predicting cardiac complications in patients undergoing non-cardiac surgery. J Gen Intern Med 1:211–219
19. Di Lello F, Mullen DC, Flemma RJ, Anderson AJJ, Kleinman LH, Werner PH (1988) Results of intraaortic balloon pumping after cardiac surgery: experience with the Percor balloon catheter. Ann Thorac Surg 46:442–446
20. Dunkman WB, Leinback RC, Buckley MJ, Mundth ED, Kantrowitz AR, Austen WG, Sanders CA (1972) Clinical and hemodynamic results of intraaortic balloon pumping and surgery for cardiogenic shock. Circulation 46:465–477
21. ECRI (Emergency Care Research Institute) (1987) Health devices. Intraaortic balloon pumps. Plymouth Pa Meeting 16:135–176
22. Eltchaninoff H, Dimas AP, Whitlow PL (1993) Complications associated with percutaneous placement and use of intraaortic balloon counterpulsation. Am J Cardiol 71:328–332
23. Flege JB, Wright CB, Reisinger TJ (1984) Successful balloon counterpulsation for right ventricular failure. Ann Thorac Surg 37:167–168
24. Foster ED, Olsson CA, Rutenberg AM, Berger RL (1976) Mechanical circulatory assistance with intra-aortic balloon counterpulsation for major abdominal surgery. Ann Surg 183:73–76
25. Freed PS, Wasfie T, Bar-Lev A, Hagiwara K, Vemuri D, Vaughan F, Bernstam L, Gray R, Bernstein I, Kantrowtiz A (1985) Long-term percutaneous access device. Trans Am Soc Artif Organs 31:230–234
26. Freed PS, Wasfie T, Zado B, Kantrowitz A (1988) Intraaortic balloon pumping for prolonged circulatory support. Am J Cardiol 61:554–557
27. Funk M, Ford CF, Foell DW, Bonini S, Sexton DL, Ostfeld AM, Cabin HS (1992) Frequency of long-term lower limb ischaemia associated with intraaortic balloon pump use. Am J Cardiol 70:1195–1199
28. Georgeson S, Coombs T, Eckman MH (1992) Prophylactic use of the intraaortic balloon pump in high-risk cardiac patients undergoing noncardiac surgery: a decision analytical view. Am J Med 92:665–678
29. Gold JP, Shemin RJ, DiSesa VJ, Cohn L, Collins JJ Jr (1985) Balloon pump support of the failing right heart. Clin Cardiol 8:599–602
30. Goldberg MJ, Rubenfire M, Kantrowitz A, Goodman G, Freed PS, Hallen L, Reimann P (1987) Intraaortic balloon pump insertion: a randomized study comparing percutaneous and surgical techniques. J Am Coll Cardiol 9:515–523

31. Goldberger M, Tabak SW, Prediman SK (1986) Clinical experience with intra-aortic balloon counterpulsation in 112 consecutive patients. Am Heart J 111:497–502
32. Goldman BS, Hill TJ, Rosenthal GA, Scully HE, Weisel RD, Baird RJ (1982) Complications associated with use of the intra-aortic balloon pump. Can J Surg 25:153–156
33. Goldman L (1987) Multifactorial index of cardiac risk in noncardiac surgery: ten-year status report. J Cardiothorac Anesth 1:237–244
34. Goldman L, Caldera DL, Nussbaum SR, Southwick FS, Krogstad D, Murray B et al. (1977) Cardiac risk factors and complications in non-cardiac surgery. N Engl J Med 297:845–850
35. Gottlieb SO, Brinker JA, Borkon AM, Kallman CH, Potter A, Gott VL, Baughman KL (1984) Identification of patients at high risk for complications of intraaortic balloon counterpulsation: a multivariate risk factor analysis. Am J Cardiol 53:1135–1139
36. Grotz RL, Yeston NS (1989) Intra-aortic balloon counterpulsation in high-risk cardiac patients undergoing noncardiac surgery. Surgery 106:1–5
37. Hazelrigg SR, Auer JE, Seifert PE (1992) Experience in 100 transthoracic balloon pumps. Ann Thorac Surg 54:528–532
38. Helmus MN, Citrin DB (1987) Cardiovascular implants. In: Spectrum: diagnostics, medical equipment and supplies, and ophthalmics products and technologies. Arthur D Little Decision resources, Cambridge, MA, pp 2–72
39. Ishihara M, Sato H, Tateishi H, Kawagoe T, Muraoka Y, Yoshimura M (1992) Effects of intra-aortic balloon pumping on coronary hemodynamics after coronary angioplasty in patients with acute myocardial infarction. Am Heart J 124:1133–1138
40. Ishihara M, Sato H, Tateishi H, Uchida T, Dote K (1991) Intraaortic balloon pumping as the postangioplasty strategy in acute myocardial infarction. Am Heart J 122:385–389
41. Kahn JK, Rutherford BD, McConahay DR, Johnson WL, Giorgi LV, Hartzler GO (1990) Supported "high-risk" coronary angioplasty using intra-aortic balloon pump counterpulsation. J Am Coll Cardiol 15:1151–1155
42. Kantrowitz A (1988) In-series temporary and permanent cardiac assistance. In: Kantrowitz A (ed) ASAIO primers in artificial organs, no 3: ventricular assist devices. Lippincott, Philadelphia, pp 77–96
43. Kantrowitz A (1989) Intra-aortic balloon pumping: clinical aspects and prospects. In: Unger F (ed) Assisted circulation III. Springer, Berlin Heidelberg New York, pp 52–73
44. Kantrowitz A (1977) The physiologic bases of in-series cardiac assistance and the clinical application of intra-aortic devices. In: Davila JC (ed) 2nd Henry Ford Hospital International Symposium on Cardiac Surgery. Appleton-Century-Croft, New York, pp 640–643
45. Kantrowitz A, Cardona RR, Au J, Freed PS (1994) Intra-aortic balloon pumping in congestive heart failure. In: Hosenpud JD et al. (eds) Congestive heart failure. Springer, Berlin Heidelberg New York
46. Kantrowitz A, Freed PS, Cardona RR, Gage K, Marinescu GN, Westveld AH, Litch B, Suzuki A, Hayakawa H, Takano T, Rios CE, Rubenfire M (1992) Initial clinical trial of a closed-loop, fully automatic intra-aortic balloon pump. ASAIO J 38:M617–621
47. Kantrowitz A, Freed PS, Cardona RR, Zhou Y, Rios CE, Mandell G, DeDecker P, Piontkowski J, Kuhn W, Riddle J, Hassouna H, Wilson D (1993) Hematologic effects of repeated interruption during long-term left ventricular assistance. Proceedings of the Association for the Advancement of Medical Instrumentation, Cardiovascular Science and Technology Conference, Washington DC, 10–12 Dec, p 158
48. Kantrowitz A, Freed PS, Wasfie T, Kozlowski J, Rubenfire M (1985) Permanent cardiac assistance in chronic congestive failure by means of mechanical auxiliary ventricle. In: Chang TMS et al. (eds) Hemoperfusion and artificial organs. Academic, Beijing, pp 149–169
49. Kantrowitz A, Kantrowitz A (1953) Experimental augmentation of coronary flow by retardation of the arterial pressure pulse. Surgery 34:678–687
50. Kantrowitz A, Krakauer J, Rubenfire M, Jaron D, Freed PS, Welkowitz W, Cascade P, Wajszczuk WJ, Lipsius M, Ciborski M, Phillips SJ, Hayden MT (1972) Initial clinical experience with a new permanent mechanical auxiliary ventricle: the dynamic aortic patch. Trans Am Soc Artif Intern Organs 18:159–167
51. Kantrowitz A, Krakauer JS, Zorzi G, Rubenfire M, Freed PS, Phillips S, Lipsius M, Titone C, Cascade P, Jaron D (1971) Current status of intraaortic balloon pump and initial

clinical experience with aortic patch mechanical auxiliary ventricle. Transplant Proc 3:1459–1472
52. Kantrowitz A, Tjonneland S, Freed PS, Phillips SJ, Butner AN, Sherman JL Jr (1968) Initial clinical experience with intraaortic balloon pumping in cardiogenic shock. JAMA 203:135–140
53. Kantrowitz A, Wasfie T, Freed PS, Rubenfire M, Wajszczuk W, Schork MA (1986) Intraaortic balloon pumping 1967 through 1982: analysis of complications in 733 patients. Am J Cardiol 57:976–983
54. Kaplan LJ, Langan N, Sokil AB, Whitman GJ (1992) Safe intraaortic balloon pump placement through the ascending aorta using transoesophageal untrasound. Ann Thorac Surg 54:374–375
55. Katz ES, Tunick PA, Kronzon I (1992) Observations of coronary flow augmentation and balloon function during intraaortic balloon counterpulsation using transoesophageal echocardiography. Am J Cardiol 69:1635–1639
56. Kern MJ, Aguirre F, Back R, Donohue T, Siegal R, Segal J (1993) Augmentation of coronary blood flow by intraaortic balloon pumping in patients after coronary angioplasty. Circulation 87:500–511
57. Koyanagi T, Endo M, Hashimoto A, Koyanagi H, Kondo I, Nomura M, Fujita M (1992) Intraoperative introduction of intra-aortic balloon catheter guided by transoesophageal echocardiography. Kyobu Geka 45:305–307
58. Kralios AC, Zwart HHJ, Moulopoulos SD, Collan R, Kawn-Gett CS, Kolff WJ (1970) Intrapulmonary artery balloon pumping. Assistance of the right ventricle. J Thorac Cariovasc Surg 60:215–232
59. Kreidieh I, Davies DW, Lim R, Nathan AW, Dymond DS, Banim SO (1992) High-risk coronary angioplasty with elective intra-aortic balloon pump support. Int J Cardiol 35:147–152
60. Kvilekval KH, Masosn RA, Newton GB, Angnostopoulos CE, Vlay SC, Giron F (1991) Complications of percutaneous intra-aortic balloon pump use in patients with peripheral vascular disease. Arch Surg 126:621–623
61. LaMuraglia GM, Vlahakes GJ, Moncure AC, Brewster DC, Buckley MJ, Daggett WM, Palacios I, Cambria R, Akins CW, Torchiana DF (1991) The safety of intraaortic balloon pump catheter insertion through suprainguinal prosthetic vascular bypass grafts. J Vasc Surg 13:830–837
62. Lefemine AA, Kosowsky B, Madoff I, Black H, Lewis M (1977) Results and complications of intraaortic balloon pumping in surgical and medical patients. Am J Cardiol 40:416–420
63. Lorente P, Gourgon R, Beaufils P, Masquet C, Rosengarten M, Azancot I, Slama R (1980) Multivariate statistical evaluation of intraaortic counterpulsation in pump failure complicating acute myocardial infarction. Am J Cardiol 46:124–134
64. McEnamy MT, Kay HR, Buckley MJ et al. (1978) Clinical experience with intra-aortic balloon pumping in 728 patients. Circulation 58[Suppl 1]:I-124–132
65. Mackenzie DJ, Wagner WH, Kulber DA, Treiman RL, Cossman DV, Foran RF, Cohem JL, Levin PM (1992) Vascular complications of the intra-aortic balloon pump. Am J Surg 164:517–521
66. Mahar LJ, Sreen PA, Tinjer JH, Vlietstra RE, Smith HC, Pluth JR (1978) Perioperative myocardial infarction in patients with cornoary artery disease with and without aorto-coronary bypass grafter. J Thorac Cardiovasc Surg 76:533–537
67. Makhoul RG, Cole CW, McCann RL (1993) Vascular complications of the intra-aortic balloon pump: an anlysis of 436 patients. Am Surg 59:564–568
68. Miller DC, Moreno-Cabral RJ, Stinson EB, Shinn JA, Shumway NE (1980) Pulmonary artery balloon counterpulsation for acute right ventricular failure. J Thorac Cardiovasc Surg 80:760–763
69. Miller JS, Dodson TF, Salam AA, Smith RS (1992) Vascular complications following intra-aortic balloon pump insertion. Am Surg 58:232–238
70. Miller MG, Hall SV (1975) Intra-aortic balloon counterpulsation in a high-risk cardiac patient undergoing emergency gastrectomy. Anesthesiology 42:103–105

71. Moran JM, Opravil M, Gorman AJ, Rastegar H, Meyers SN, Michaelis LL (1984) Pulmonary artery balloon counterpulsation for right ventricular failure. II. Clinical experience. Ann Thorac Surg 38:254–259
72. Moulopoulos SD, Topaz SR, Kolff WJ (1962) Extracorporeal assistance to the circulation and intraaortic balloon pumping. Trans Am Soc Artif Intern Organs 8:85–89
73. Mueller H, Ayres SM, Conklin EF, Giannelli S Jr, Mazzara JT, Grace WT, Nealon TF Jr (1971) The effects of intraaortic counterpulsation on cardiac performance and metabolism in shock associated with accute myocardial infarction. J Clin Invest 50:1885–1900
74. Mueller H, Ayres SM, Giannelli S, Conklin EF, Mazzara JT, Grace WJ (1972) Effect of isoproterenol, l-norepinephrine, and intraaortic counterpulsation on hemodynamics and myocardial metabolism in shock following acute myocardial infarction. Circulation 45:335–351
75. Nagata M, Tashiro T, Tanaka K, Haruta Y, Todo K (1991) Intragraft balloon pumping – a clinical case report. Nippon Kyobe Geka Gakkai Zasshi 39:2251–2254
76. Nakatani H, Nakano K, Nishida H, Kitamura M, Hashimoto A, Endo M, Koyanagi H (1993) Excellent systolic unloading effect of a new IABP driving unit. American Society of Artificial Internal Organs, 39th Annual Meeting, New Orleans, April 29–May 1, p 42 (abstr)
77. Nash IS, Lorell BH, Fishman RF, Baim DS Donahue C, Diver DJ (1991) A new technique for sheathless percutaneous intraaortic balloon catheter insertion. Cathet Cardiovasc Diagn 23:57–60
78. Naunheim KS, Swartz MT, Pennington DG, Fiore AC, McBride LR, Peigh PS, Barnett MG, Vacar KJ, Kaiser GC, Willman VL (1992) Intraaortic balloon pumping in patients requiring cardiac operations. Risk analysis and long-term follow-up. J Thorac Cardiovasc Surg 104:1654–1660
79. Nishimura M, Nakano S, Kaneko M, Miyamoto Y, Kadoba K, Kawada H, Chang J, Amemiya A, Sato S, Matsuda H (1992) Seven experiences using the new IABP Corart BP-1: a study of the balloon operation timing and auto-weaning feature of the system in automatic mode. Japanese Society for Artificial Organs, 30th Annual Meeting, Tokyo, 5–6 Nov 1992, p 62 (abstr)
80. O'Rourke MF, Change VP, Windsor HM et al. (1975) Acute severe cardiac failure complicating myocardial infarction. Experience with 100 petients referred for consideration of mechanical left ventricular assistance. Br Heart J 36:169–181
81. Ogino H, Yamazato A, Hanada M, Makayama S (1993) Introduction of intra-aortic balloon pumping catheter throught left subclavian artery guided by trans-oesophageal echocardiography. Kyobu Geka 46:858–861
82. Ohman EM, Califf RM, George BS, Quigley PJ, Kereiakes DJ, Harrelson-Woodlief L, Candela RJ, Flanagan C, Stack RS, Topol EJ (1991) The use of intra-aortic balloon pumping as an adjunct to reperfusion therapy in acute myocardial infarction (TAMI) study group. Am Heart J 121:895–901
83. Opravil M, Gorman AJ, Krejcie TC, Michaelis LL, Moran JM (1984) Pulmonary artery balloon counterpulsation for right ventricular failure. I. Experimental results. Ann Thorac Surg 38:242–253
84. Park JK, Hsu DT, Gersony WM (1993) Intraaortic balloon pump management of refractory congestive heart failure in children. Paediatr Cardiol 14:19–22
85. Pfeffer MA, Braunwald E, Moye LA, Basta J, Brown EJ Jr et al. on behalf of the SAVE investigators (1992) Effect of captopril on mortality and morbidity in patients with left ventricular dysfunction after myocadial infarction. N Engl J Med 327:669–677
86. Pelletier LC, Pomar JL, Bosch X, Galinanes M, Hebert Y (1986) Complications of circulatory assistance with intra-aortic balloon pumping: a comparison of surgical and percutaneous techniques. J Heart Transplant 5:138–142
87. Phillips SJ, Tannenbaum M, Zeff RH, Iannone LA, Ghali M, Kongtahworn C (1992) Sheatheless insertion of the percutaneous intra-aortic balloon pump: an alternate method. Ann Thorac Surg 53:162
88. Pinkard J, Utley JR, Leyland SA, Morgan M, Johnson H (1993) Relative risk of aortic and femoral insertion of intraaortic balloon pump after coronary artery bypass grafting procedures. J Thorac Cardiovasc Surg 105:721–728

89. Pollock JC, Charlton MC, Williams WG, Edmonds JR, Trusler GA (1980) Intraaortic balloon pumping in children. Ann Thorac Surg 29:522–528
90. Rankin JS, Newton JR, Califf RM, Jones RH, Wechsler AS, Oldham HN, Wolfe WG, Lowe JE (1984) Clinical characteristics and current management of medically refractory unstable angina. Ann Surg 200:457–465
91. Rohrer MJ, Sullivan CA, McLaughlin DJ, Cutler BS (1992) A prospective randomised study comparing surgical and percutaneous removal of intraaortic balloon pump. J Thorac Cardiovasc Surg 103:569–572
92. Sakamoto T, Arai H, Suzuki Akio, Kazama S, Suzuki Akira, Shoji Y (1992) Optimum setting of systolic unloading for IABP and increased benefits: review of conventional driving method and fundamentals. Japanese Society for Artificial Organs, 30th Annual Meeting, Tokyo, 5–6 Nov 1992, p 62 (abstr)
93. Sanfelippo PM, Baker NH, Ewy GH, Moore PJ, Thomas JW, Brahos GJ, McVicker RF (1986) Experience with intraaortic balloon counterpulsation. Ann Thorac Surg 41:36–41
94. Satler LF, Rackley CE (1986) Assessment of adequate circulatory assist during intra-aortic balloon counterpulsation. Cardiovasc Clin 16:141–149
95. Satoh H, Kobayashi T, Hiraishi T, Sakarai M, Fudemotot Y, Kaneko Y, Nakano S, Matsuda H (1992) New side-holed sheath for intraaortic balloon pumping to maintain limb perfusion. Ann Thorac Surg 54:794–796
96. Scheidt S, Wilner G, Mueller H, Summers D, Lesch M, Wolff G, Krakauer J, Rubenfire M, Fleming P, Noon G, Oldham N, Killip T, Kantrowitz A (1973) Intraaortic balloon pumping in cardiogenic shock. Report of a co-operative clinical trial. N Engl J Med 288:979–984
97. Schilt W, Freed PS, Khalil G, Kantrowitz A (1967) Temporary non-surgical intraarterial cardiac assistance. Trans Am Soc Artif Intern Organs 13:322–327
98. Shahian DM, Neptune WB, Ellis FH Jr, Maggs PR (1983) Intraaortic balloon pump morbidity: a comparative analysis of risk factors between percutaneous and surgical techniques. Ann Thorac Surg 36:644–653
99. Shimamoto H, Kawazoe K, Kito H, Fujita T, Shomamoto Y. Does juxtamesenteric placement on intraaortic balloon interrupt superior mesenteric flow? Clin Cardiol 15:285–290
100. Shimamoto H, Kawazoe K, Kito K, Oohara K, Kosakai Y, Kito H, Fujita T (1992) Effects of intra-aortic balloon pumping on mitral flow dynamics in patients with coronary bypass operations. Am Heart J 123:1229–1236
101. Shimizu T, Sasaki H, Kaneto T, Akutsu T (1991) Management of post-operative biventricular failure by means of a right ventricular assist device and an intraaortic balloon pump. ASAIO Trans 37:M339–340
102. Siu SC, Kowalchuk GJ, Welty FK, Benotti PN, Lewis SM (1991) Intraaortic balloon counterpulsation in the high-risk cardiac patient undergoing urgent noncardiac surgery. Chest 99:1342–1345
103. Spence PA, Weisel RD, Easdown J, Jabr AK, Yap V, Salerno TA (1985) The hemodynamic effects and mechanism of action of pulmonary artery balloon counterpulsation in the treatment of right ventricular failure during left heart bypass. Ann Thorac Surg 39:329–335
104. Spotnitz HM, Berman MA, Reis RL, Epstein SE (1971) The effects of synchronized counterpulsation of the pulmonary artery on right ventricular hemodynamics. J Thorac Cariovasc Surg 61:167–174
105. Sturm JT, McGee MG, Fuhrman TM, Davis GL, Turner SA, Edelman SK, Norman JC (1980) Treatment of postoperative low output syndrome with intraaortic balloon pumping: experience with 419 patients. Am J Cardiol 45:1033–1036
106. Swartz MT, Sakamoto T, Arai H, Reedy JE, Salenas L, Yuda T, Standeven JW, Pennington DG (1992) Effects of intraaortic balloon position on renal artery blood flow. Ann Thorac Surg 53:604–610
107. Symbas PN, McKeown PP, Santora Ah, Vlasis SE (1985) Pulmonary artery balloon counterpulsation for treatment of intraoperative right ventricular failure. Ann Thorac Surg 39:437–440
108. Tanaka K, Takano T, Suzuki A, Iyedokoro T, Sugimoto T, Tomita Y, Kojima J, Takayama M, Hayakawa H (1992) Development of fully automatic intraaortic balloon pumping (super bal-

loon pump) with catheter tip electrocardiogram and arterial pressure sensor. Japanese Society for Artificial Organs, 30th Annual Meeting, Tokyo, Nov 5–6, p 63 (abstr)

109. Tatar H, Cicek S, Demirkilic U, Suer H, Ozturk O (1993) Exact positioning of intraaortic balloon catheter. Eur J Cardiothorac Surg 7:52–53
110. Tatar H, Demirkilic U, Ozal E, Suer H, Aslan M, Ozturk OY (1993) Vascular complications of intraaortic balloon pumping: unsheathed versus sheathed insertion. Ann Thorac Surg 55:1518–1521
111. Veasy LG, Blalock RC, Orth JL, Boucek MM (1983) Intra-aortic balloon pumping in infants and children. Circulation 68:1095–1100
112. Veasy LG, Webster HF, McGough EC (1986) Intra-aortic balloon pumping: adaptation for pediatric use. Crit Care Clin 2:237–249
113. Waksman R, Weiss AT, Gotsman MS, Hasing Y (1993) Intra-aortic balloon counterpulsation improves survival in cardiogenic shock complicating acute myocardial infarction. Eur Heart J 14:71–74
114. Webster H, Veasy LG (1985) Intra-aortic balloon pumping in children. Heart Lung 14:548–555
115. White LD, Lee TH, Cook EF, Weisberg MC, Ronan GW, Brand DA, Goldman L (1990) Comparison of the natural history of new onset and exacerbated chronic ischemic heart disease. J Am Coll Cardiol 16:304–310
116. Yaminishi H, Watanabe S, Nishinaka T, Hayashi K, Minami M, Abe H, Aoki T, Kawai Y, Kishino K, Ota S (1993) A new device: a fenestrated sheath for IABP, which reduces the incidence of ischaemia in the lower limbs. Kakyu To Junkan 41:769–772
117. Ruggiero R, Niinami H, Hooper TL, Pochettino A, Hammond RL, Lu H, Spanta AD, Nakajima H, Nakajima H, Mannon JD, Acker MA, Bridges CR, Anderson DR, Colson M, Kantrowitz A, Salmons S, Stephenson LW (1991) Skeletal muscle ventricles for cardiac assistance. Basic Appl Mycol 1(2):129–137

# Large-volume Counterpulsation

S.D. Moulopoulos

The intriguing principle of "counterpulsation" [1] introduced the possibility of affecting the circulation by separately interfering with the two cardiac cycles, systolic and diastolic. It derived from the observation that myocardial oxygen consumption depends on the myocardial time-tension index [2]. If, therefore, pressure during ventricular ejection could be reduced, oxygen consumption could also be reduced, provided mean arterial perfusion pressure was maintained at the same level. This principle has been used in the only method of assistance to gain acceptance as a standard clinical therapy, intra-aortic balloon pumping [3].

The quantitative characteristics of the system were designed on the basis of negative rather than positive requirements. They are not determined on the basis of how much assistance the particular patient needs in his present condition. They are determined by factors such as the length and diameter of the aorta, or the limitation of the air conduction catheter size; it must be small enough to be easily introduced through the small femoral artery and large enough to allow fast inflation and deflation of the balloon. Balloons with displacement volumes of 20–60 ml have been manufactured and used clinically, depending on the above criteria.

Interestingly enough, many authors have tried to describe the hemodynamic effects of intra-aortic balloon pumping without taking into consideration the volume of counterpulsation. It is generally accepted [4] anyway that counterpulsation with common-sized balloons is not effective in severe cases of shock and, more specifically, when systolic aortic pressure is below 60–70 mm Hg.

In this paper experimental and clinical data are reported to determine the importance of volume in counterpulsation, to help explain the ineffectiveness of balloon pumping in severe cases, and to suggest possible expanded indications for counterpulsation devices.

## Material and Methods

### Intra-aortic Counterpulsation

A canine model of cardiogenic shock with ligated branches of the coronary arteries and, in some experiments, with propranolol administration was used. In 29 animals (20–30 kg body wt) two balloons were inserted into the aorta, one of 30 ml through the left subclavian artery or the brachiocephalic trunk and one of 15 ml through the femoral artery.

Three modes of operation of the balloons were applied: (a) the small balloon alone, (b) the large balloon alone, and (c) both balloons. Pumping for each mode lasted 20 min and the sequence was changed for each experiment.

Aortic flow and coronary artery flow were measured with an electromagnetic flowmeter probe placed around the ascending aorta and the left main coronary artery, and left ventricular and aortic pressure were also recorded before pumping, during the 20 min of pumping, and 10 min after pumping had stopped.

### Para-aortic Counterpulsation

In the same experimental model as described above, a valveless air chamber [5] was connected with the help of a Dacron graft to the ascending aorta in 12 animals (body weight 17–25 kg). The pneumatic chamber had a maximal volume of 100 ml and was driven from the R-wave of the electrocardiogram, using a common counterpulsation system. The same measurements as above were made before and during pumping, except for coronary flow recordings.

With repeated propranolol injections, and in some experiments with ligation of more arteries, several degrees of shock severity were attained, with systolic arterial pressures over 70 mm Hg, 30–70 mm Hg, or less than 30 mm Hg.

### Para-aortic plus Intra-aortic Pumping

In the same cardiogenic shock model the simultaneous operation of the para-aortic pump and one intra-aortic balloon was tried. The balloon had a volume of 20 ml.

The same measurements were made before and during pumping with the para-aortic devices and the intra-aortic balloon operating together for 10 min.

### Clinical Observations

In three patients with terminal heart failure due to cardiomyopathy, maximal medical treatment was used. When this was unsuccessful, the intra-aortic balloon was inserted, and it improved the patients' condition for 2, 11, and 10 days. Following these time periods the condition of the patients deteriorated, with a systolic aortic pressure of <50 mm Hg. In this condition of intractable cardiogenic shock, the para-aortic, valveless pneumatic pump was connected to the ascending aorta [5]. The para-aortic pump was functional for periods of up to 54 days. In two of the patients intra-aortic and para-aortic pumps operated together.

## Results

### Intra-aortic Counterpulsation

The larger the counterpulsation volume with the intra-aortic balloons, the higher was the increase in aortic flow, coronary artery flow, and aortic pressure during

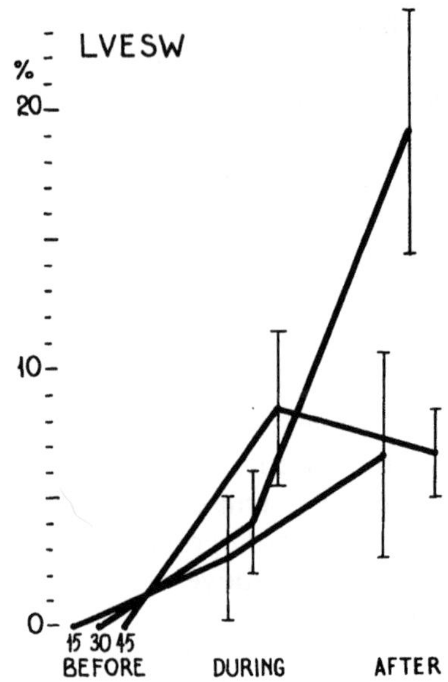


**Fig. 1.** Percent change of left ventricular end-systolic work during and after counterpulsation with 15-; 30-; and 45-ml balloons. Note that the largest favourable change following termination of assistance is seen with the 30-ml balloon, despite the fact that during assistance the 45-ml balloon shows the best results

pumping ($p > 0.001$). Left ventricular end-diastolic pressure decreased significantly ($p > 0.01$).

Following termination of assistance there was no significant change from the control value for the 15-ml balloon. A significant change from the control values in all parameters, except the left ventricular end-diastolic pressure, was observed for the 30- and 45-ml balloons. However, the increase was significantly larger with the 30-ml balloon (Fig. 1) than with the 45-ml ($p < 0.01$ for stroke volume and $p < 0.05$ for systolic pressure).

## Para-aortic Counterpulsation

The application of para-aortic counterpulsation had a favourable effect on all parameters during pumping, provided systolic aortic pressure was over 70 mm Hg or between 30 and 70 mm Hg. It was ineffective, i.e. there was no significant change in any parameter, when systolic aortic pressure was less than 30 mm Hg.

Endocardial viability ratio increased during para-aortic pumping by 91.5 ± 90.1% when pumping was applied to animals with systolic aortic pressure above 70 mm Hg. When the same pressure was between 30 and 70 mm Hg before pumping, the increase observed was 349.2 ± 320.2%.

## Para-aortic plus Intra-aortic Pumping

The simultaneous operation of the para-aortic pumping chamber and intraaortic balloon pumping improved all parameters in animals with a systolic aortic pressure above 70 mm Hg or between 30 and 70 mm Hg. It did not change significantly any parameter in animals with a systolic aortic pressure below 30 mm Hg.

In animals with systolic aortic pressure above 70 mm Hg simultaneous pumping induced a change in the endocardial viability ratio by 136.8 ± 93.5% (versus

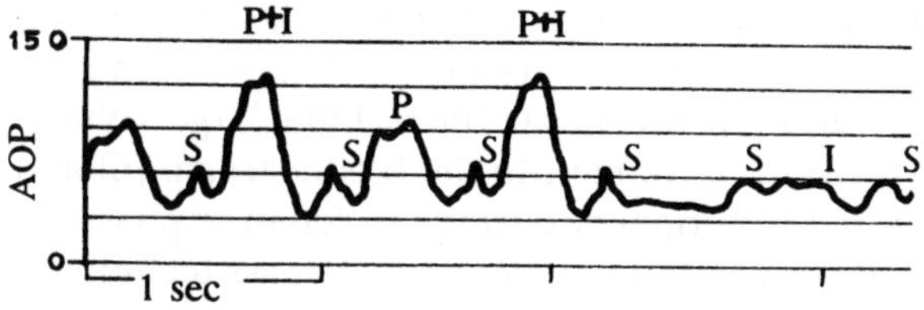


**Fig. 2.** Aortic pressure of a patient in heart failure. *S*, Pressure waves produced by his own heart; *I*, pressure wave produced by intra-aortic balloon pumping; *P*, pressure wave produced by para-aortic pump systole; *P + I*, pressure waves produced by combined pumping of para-aortic device and intra-aortic balloon. Scale is in mm Hg

91.5 ± 90.1% for simple para-aortic pumping). In animals with systolic aortic pressure between 30 and 70 mm Hg the change was 406.1 ± 345.5% (versus 349.2 ± 320.2% for para-aortic pumping).

### Clinical Observations

Three patients in intractable cardiogenic shock, in whom intra-aortic balloon pumping had been ineffective, survived with a para-aortic pump for 6, 54 days, and 9 days, respectively. In one patient the operation of a 40-ml intra-aortic balloon pump increased systolic aortic pressure from 50 to 60 mm Hg, while para-aortic pumping alone, with an estimated volume of 80 ml, increased the pressure to 90 mm Hg and combined of intra-aortic balloon and para-aortic pumping increased the pressure to 120 mm Hg (Fig. 2). In another patient with a systolic aortic pressure of 50 mm Hg, the intra-aortic balloon pumping was ineffective and the para-aortic pump increased pressure to 90–110 mm Hg.

## Discussion

The data mentioned in this report, in accordance with existing clinical experience, indicate the limits of counterpulsation as it can be applied with the techniques in common use. The larger the volume of intra-aortic balloon pumping, the higher was stroke index and stroke work and the lower left ventricular end-diastolic pressure, during pumping.

It is clear from the results of the second group of experiments that a larger volume of counterpulsation could be effective in severe cases of cardiogenic shock, where the intra-aortic balloon alone was ineffective.

The large-volume para-aortic pump [5] was effective in shock models with a systolic pressure of 30–70 mm Hg. This was more evident with the combination of para-aortic pumps and intra-aortic balloon. It was also seen in the small number of clinical cases, where a large-volume para-aortic pump alone or together with an intra-aortic balloon reversed a heart failure condition with a systolic aortic pressure of 50 mm Hg.

The data show, therefore, that large-volume assistance may improve the circulation more than small-volume assistance and may be helpful in cases where counterpulsation with common-sized intra-aortic balloons is not.

How can large-volume assistance help, where lower volume assistance cannot? This may be attributed not only to lower resistance to the left ventricle achieved by large-volume counterpulsation, but also to the fact that large-volume counterpulsation imparts faster forward movement to the blood stream [6] and probably thus lessens backflow from the periphery during the deflation phase. In this way, counterpulsation may help in conditions where only bypass techniques have been effective up to now.

There is little doubt that large volume counterpulsation, achieved with whatever devices, may be effective during pumping and can thus be useful as a bridge to transplantation. The question remains which volume of assistance is more beneficial if the heart is going to survive and recover from shock without being replaced by a transplant or by an artificial heart.

Out data [7] indicate that, following termination of assistance, a better left ventricular performance is seen not when the volume of counterpulsation was the highest during assistance, but when assistance took over 25–30% of the ventricle's work. This was measured more accurately in left ventricular bypass experiments [8]. It is not very clear how one can estimate the equivalent effect of intra-aortic balloon pumping. It was found, for example [4], that pulmonary wedge pressure was reduced during balloon pumping from $20 \pm 2$ to $15 \pm 2$ mm Hg, and in another series from $22 \pm 5$ to $17 \pm 2$ mm Hg. If this represents approximately a 25% reduction in the preload of the left ventricle, it may be that balloon pumping achieves optimal assistance for the heart to recover with the balloon volume commonly in use.

## The Future of Counterpulsation

Although counterpulsation is the most widely applied assistance technique, its use has been limited mainly to specific cases of cardiogenic shock for temporary assistance. It was proven ineffective in cases of severe shock with aortic systolic pressures below 60–70 mm Hg. It was also proven ineffective when tried for longer periods of time in cases of left ventricular failure. It has not been useful as a bridge-to-transplant technique, since it cannot usually support a failing circulation for periods longer than a few days; for a device to be considered for bridging, a period of effective operation for over 30 days is needed.

Newer techniques to apply counterpulsation, such as the para-aortic pump, have indicated for the first time the possibility of assisting severe shock cases or cases of left ventricular failure for longer periods. Since in the experimental situations mentioned in this report and in the few clinical cases no difference was seen between the use of the para-aortic pump and that of the intra-aortic balloon except in the volume of counterpulsation, it is suggested that the use of counterpulsation can be effectively expanded by applying large-volume techniques.

Among these techniques, the surgical implantation of the para-aortic pump seems promising. The use of larger volume balloons (up to 100 ml) may be feasible by elongating the balloons to the limits of the aorta length and/or by increasing the diameter of the balloons. Tapering of a long balloon may be necessary to exploit the space available from the aortic arch to the bifurcation of the aorta. The need for larger catheters may be an acceptable disadvantage, if one could thereby avoid bypass techniques requiring surgical implantation and thoracotomy.

In conclusion, counterpulsation techniques may be used in the future not only for temporary circulatory system support, but also for longer periods of assistance as the less invasive (not requiring thoracotomy) bridge-to-transplant method. What may be more important, however, is the possibility of using larger volume intra-aortic balloons in cases of severe shock, where common-sized balloons are ineffective.

## References

1. Clauss R, Birtwell C, Albertal G, Lunzer S, Taylor W, Fosberg A, Harken D (1961) Assisted circulation. I. The arterial counterpulsator. J Thorac Cardiovasc Surg 41:447
2. Welch G, Sarnoff S, Braunwald E, Stainsby W, Case R, Macruz R (1958) The influence of cardiac output, aortic pressure and heart rate on myocardial oxygen utilization. Surg Forum 8:294
3. Moulopoulos S, Topaz S, Kolff W (1962) Diastolic balloon pumping (with carbon dioxide) in the aorta: a mechanical assistance to the failing circulation. Am Heart J 62:669
4. Moulopoulos S (1983) Mechanical cardiac assistance. In: Hurst A (ed) Clinical assays on the heart. McGraw-Hill, New York, p 233
5. Nanas J, Poyadjis A, Charitos C, Nanas S, Kontoyannis D, Anastasiou M, Alevizakos N, Voudris V, Moulopoulos S (1990) Additional salutary hemodynamic effects of the combined use of the paraaortic counterpulsation device and intraaortic balloon pump versus a paraaortic counterpulsation device alone. ASAIO Trans 36:505
6. Wiggers C (1939) Physiology in health and disease. Lea and Febiger, Philadelphia
7. Moulopoulos S, Stamatelopoulos S, Plassaras G, Sideris D, Hassapoyannis C (1976) A nomogram for optimal assistance by intraaortic balloon pumping. Abstracts of the 7th European Congress on Cardiology, Amsterdam, vol 1, p 708
8. Moulopoulos S, Anthopoulos L, Stamatelopoulos S, Boufas D (1973) Optimal changes in stroke work during left ventricular bypass. J Appl Physiol 24:12

# Optimal Conditions of Biventricular Balloon Pumping During Ventricular Fibrillation in the Experimental Animal

S. Stamatelopoulos, N. Zakopoulos, N. Saridakis, J. Kanakakis,
S. Stefanou, A. Gougoulakis, and S. Moulopoulos

It is possible to maintain the circulation in the experimental animal during cardiac arrest for several hours, by means of a catheter-mounted balloon introduced into the left ventricle and driven by an external pump [1–4]. An optimal relationship between left ventricular geometry and capacity on the one hand and intraventricular balloon shape and volume on the other appears to exist [3]. The selection of an optimal balloon shape and volume is not always easy, despite the use of echocardiography prior to its insertion [4]. Thus, additional pumping into the aorta may be needed [4].

In the case of severe myocardial pump failure, some authors [5] support the use of biventricular assist devices as more effective than ventricular devices assisting only the left ventricle. Others [6] indicate that if the reduced right ventricular function and the increased pulmonary vascular resistance respond – to a certain extent – to drugs, then a left ventricular assist device may be enough to support the circulation. In the case of cardiac arrest, it is not very clear how left ventricular assistance alone, for instance, by left intraventricular balloon pumping [1], can maintain a sufficient circulation with a nonfunctioning right ventricle. This experimental study examines the optimal conditions for adding a right intraventricular balloon pump to improve the efficacy of the left intraventricular balloon pump. The additional effect of right intraventricular balloon pumping on the function curve of the left intraventricular balloon pump is investigated.

## Methods

### Experimental Set-up

Sixteen anaesthetized, open-chest dogs, weighing 18–26 kg, were used in these experiments. A catheter-mounted pear-shaped balloon [1, 3] was introduced into the left ventricle either via the left subclavian artery or via the apex of the heart. The end-diastolic volume of the left ventricle was measured by echocardiography prior to balloon insertion, and balloons with a capacity, in full expansion, equal to that volume were used. A catheter-mounted balloon having a volume equal to 60% of the one inserted into the left ventricle was introduced into the right ventricle via the right subclavian vein. Two electrically connected pumps were used to drive the balloons, as shown in Fig. 1. An optimal [1] pump rate of 75–80 bpm was used. Other pumping characteristics have been described in detail

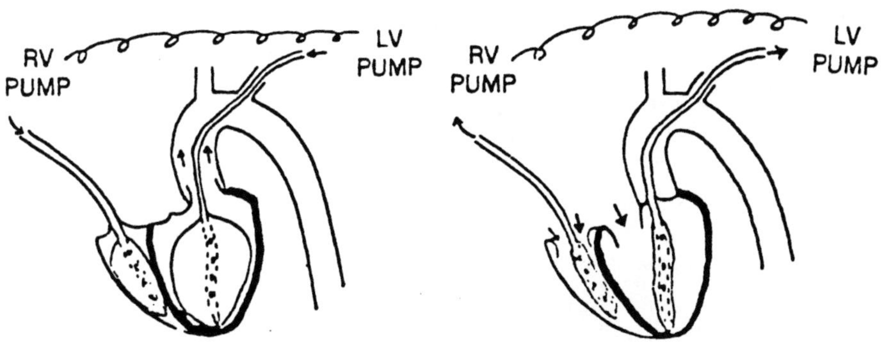


**Fig. 1.** The experimental setup. The right ventricular (*RV PUMP*) and left ventricular (*LV PUMP*) pumps are electrically connected. Both balloons are inflated *left* and deflated *right*

elsewhere [1]. The flow in the ascending aorta and the pressures in the right ventricle, the left atrium and the aorta were recorded using, respectively, the probe of an electronic flowmeter and catheters inserted via the right carotid artery, the right external jugular vein and the left auricle. The central venous pressure was measured by a catheter introduced into the inferior vena cava via the left femoral vein.

### Experimental Protocol

Left intraventricular (LV) balloon pumping was initiated and the central venous pressure was raised to 15 cm $H_2O$ by means of intravenous fluid infusion, as soon as ventricular fibrillation was induced by DC current. Periods (up to 10 min) of LV balloon pumping were interchanged with simultaneous right and left intraventricular (RV + LV) balloon pumping. Several delays between right and left intraventricular balloon expansion were tested. Continuous recordings of the above-mentioned haemodynamic parameters were made under both types of pumping while the heart was fibrillating. Some experiments were carried out under electromechanical dissociation, since ventricular fibrillation was automatically converted to an irregular ventricular electrical rate without mechanical response after several minutes of pumping. Statistical evaluation was by Student's *t*-test. All values are provided as mean ± standard error.

## Results

LV balloon pumping was interchanged with RV + LV balloon pumping in 33 instances in the 16 animals in cardiac arrest (ventricular fibrillation or electromechanical dissociation with mechanical arrest). The 16 experimental animals were classified into two groups on the basis of the systolic AP level maintained – during cardiac arrest – by LV pumping alone: group A consisted of six animals with systolic AP $\geq$ 100 mm Hg and group B of ten animals with systolic AP < 100 mm Hg under LV pumping alone.

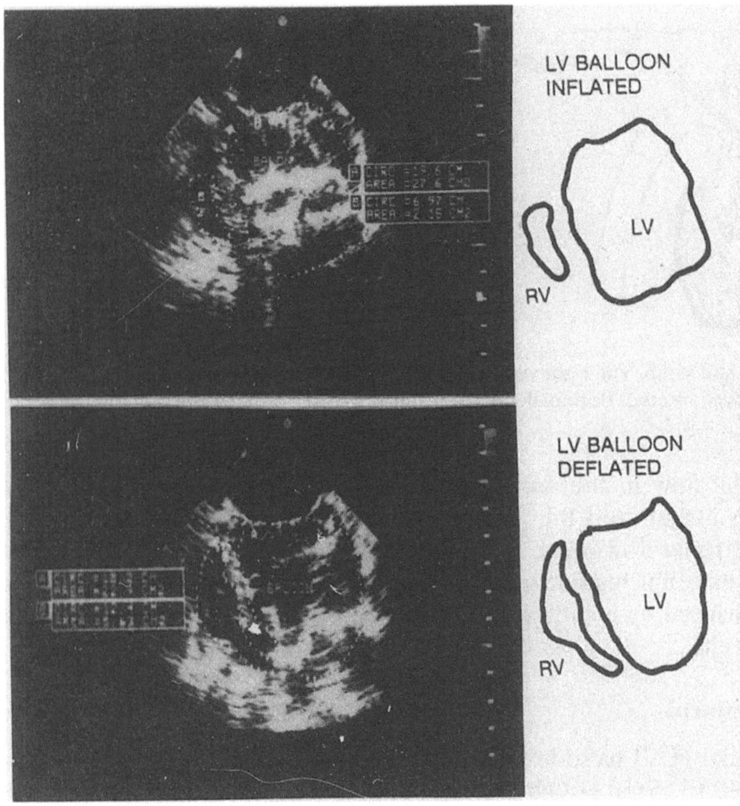


**Fig. 2.** Two-dimensional echocardiography (transoesophageal examination) during pumping by a single balloon into the left ventricle. Right ventricular dimensions decrease (*above*) during left intraventricular balloon inflation, due to rightward shifting of the intraventricular septum, and increase (*below*) during left intraventricular balloon deflation. Thus, biventricular pumping was performed in group A (see text) animals by a single balloon inserted into the left ventricle

Transoesophageal echocardiography in group A indicated (Fig. 2) a rightward shifting of the intraventricular septum during expansion of the LV balloon. The right ventricular cavity was markedly (Fig. 2) reduced during inflation and increased in size during deflation of the LV balloon. Thus, simultaneous left and right ventricular pumping was performed in this group of animals by means of a single balloon into the left ventricle. This phenomenon was less marked in group B.

In group A, RV + LV balloon pumping was interchanged (Figs. 3 and 4) with LV balloon pumping alone in 16 instances. As shown in Table 1, the addition of RV balloon pumping to the already functioning LV balloon pump resulted in a significant decrease in central venous pressure and in a significant increase in systolic right ventricular and mean left atrial pressures, but these effects were not followed by an increase in flow and pressure in the ascending aorta. When RV pumping was carried out for several minutes pulmonary oedema was initiated. The oedema subsided after discontinuation of RV balloon pumping.

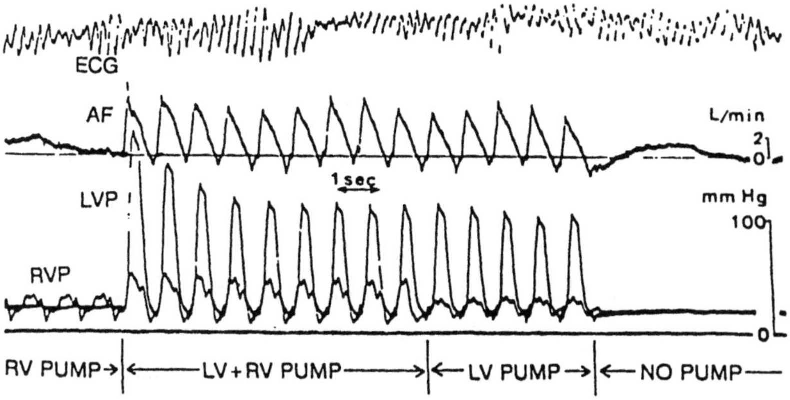


**Fig. 3.** Simultaneous tracings of flow in the ascending aorta (*AF*) and pressure into the left (*LVP*) and right (*RVP*) ventricle in an animal of group A during ventricular fibrillation, as indicated by the electrocardiogram (*ECG*). The effect of pumping by a single right intraventricular balloon (*RV PUMP*), by balloons into both ventricles (*LV + RV PUMP*) and by a single left intraventricular balloon (*LV PUMP*) is indicated. Both balloons remain deflated (*NO PUMP*) at the end of the tracing

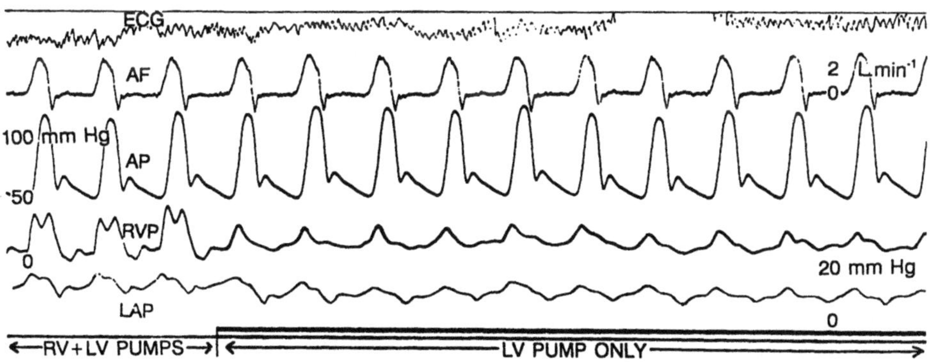


**Fig. 4.** Simultaneous tracings of flow in the ascending aorta (*AF*) and pressures into the aorta (*AP*), the right ventricle (*RVP*) and the left atrium (*LAP*) in an animal of group A during ventricular fibrillation, as indicated by the electrocardiogram (*ECG*). Balloons into both ventricles are pumped at the left part of the panel (*RV + LV PUMPS*). Discontinuation of the right intraventricular balloon pump (*LV PUMP ONLY*, *right*) is followed by an immediate reduction in RVP and LAP but no change in AF and AP

In group B, where the systolic aortic pressure could not be raised above 100 mm Hg by a single balloon into the left ventricle, RV + LV balloon pumping was interchanged (Figs. 5 and 6) with LV balloon pumping alone in 17 instances. As shown in Table 2, the addition of RV to LV balloon pumping increased significantly the pressure in the right ventricle and the pressure and flow in the aorta, although no significant change had been noted (Table 2, Fig. 5) in mean left atrial pressure. It also induced a significant decrease in central venous pressure. Epicardial echocardiography in this group of animals indicated (Fig. 7) a leftward

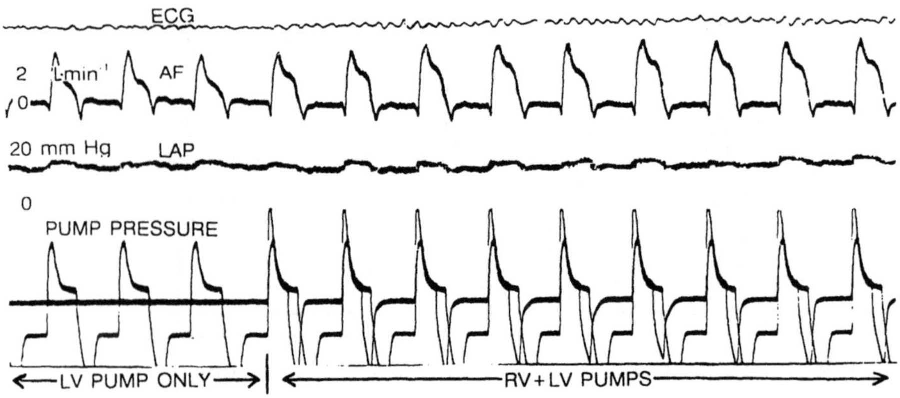


**Fig. 5.** Simultaneous tracings of flow in the ascending aorta (*AF*), pressure into the left atrium (*LAP*) and pressures of both external pumps (*PUMP PRESSURE*), driving the balloons into the left and right ventricle, in an animal of group B during ventricular fibrillation, as indicated by the electrocardiogram (*ECG*). Pumping by a single left intraventricular balloon is indicated on the *left* (*LV PUMP ONLY*). The addition of right intraventricular balloon pumping (*RV + LV PUMPS*) is followed by an immediate increase in AF but no change in LAP

**Table 1.** Mean values ± standard error of aortic flow (A*F*), systolic aortic pressure (*Syst. AP*), systolic right ventricular pressure (*Syst. RVP*), mean left atrial pressure (*Mean LAP*) and central venous pressure (*CVP*) in group-A animals under right plus left intraventricular pumping (*RV + LV*) and left intraventricular pumping alone (*LV alone*). In all animals of this group the systolic aortic pressure maintained by left intraventricular pumping alone was well above 100 mm Hg

| Variable | RV + LV | LV alone | |
|---|---|---|---|
| AF ($ml \cdot kg^{-1} \cdot min^{-2}$) | 81.1 ± 3.1 | 81.1 ± 2.0 | N.S. |
| Syst. AP (mm Hg) | 117.3 ± 4.3 | 109.8 ± 2.0 | N.S. |
| Syst. RVP (mm Hg) | 28.8 ± 2.5 | 16.2 ± 1.2 | $p < 0.001$ |
| Mean LAP (mm Hg) | 18.5 ± 0.6 | 11.2 ± 0.8 | $p < 0.001$ |
| CVP (mm Hg) | 14.0 ± 0.5 | 16.2 ± 0.6 | $p < 0.01$ |

shifting of the intraventricular septum when the RV balloon was inflated while the LV balloon was starting to collapse. Thus, additional pumping into the left ventricle was performed through the intraventricular septum: An immediate – following the initiation of RV pumping – increase in stroke volume of the LV balloon pumping was noted (Figs. 5 and 6). An optimal delay of 127 ± 2.7 (mean ± SEM) ms between LV balloon and RV balloon expansion was determined to obtain a maximal LV pump stroke volume (Fig. 8).

Function curves of the LV balloon pump were obtained by loading the circulation both under RV + LV balloon pumping and under LV balloon pumping alone. The addition of RV balloon pumping to the already operating LV balloon pump in group A seemed (left, Fig. 9) to add a plateau to the initial function curve, by increasing the mean left atrial pressure without further increasing the

**Table 2.** Mean values ± standard error of aortic flow (*AF*), systolic aortic pressure (*Syst. AP*), systolic right ventricular pressure (*Syst. RVP*), mean left atrial pressure (*Mean LAP*) and central venous pressure (*CVP*) in group-B animals under right plus left intraventricular pumping (*RV + LV*) and left intraventricular pumping alone (*LV alone*). In all animals of this group the systolic aortic pressure maintained by left intraventricular pumping alone was below 100 mmHg

| Variable | RV + LV | LV alone | |
|---|---|---|---|
| AF ($ml \cdot kg^{-1} \cdot min^{-2}$) | 72.0 ± 3.9 | 56.8 ± 2.6 | $p < 0.005$ |
| Syst. AP (mm Hg) | 108.8 ± 3.5 | 81.0 ± 2.6 | $p < 0.001$ |
| Syst. RVP (mm Hg) | 22.0 ± 2.1 | 16.5 ± 0.6 | $p < 0.05$ |
| Mean LAP (mm Hg) | 17.3 ± 1.4 | 15.0 ± 1.0 | N.S. |
| CVP (mm Hg) | 15.9 ± 0.6 | 21.0 ± 0.5 | $p < 0.001$ |

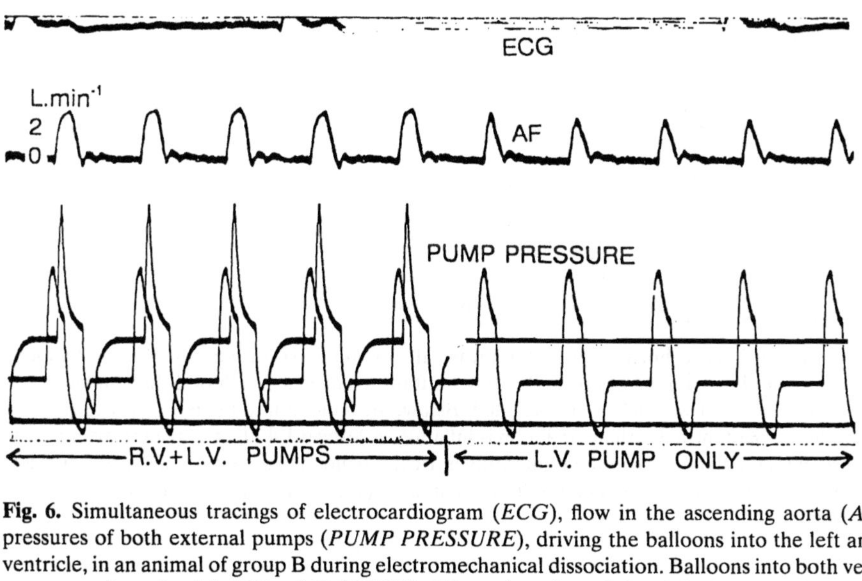


**Fig. 6.** Simultaneous tracings of electrocardiogram (*ECG*), flow in the ascending aorta (*AF*) and pressures of both external pumps (*PUMP PRESSURE*), driving the balloons into the left and right ventricle, in an animal of group B during electromechanical dissociation. Balloons into both ventricles are pumped on the *left* (*RV + LV PUMPS*). Discontinuation of the right intraventricular balloon pump (*LV PUMP ONLY*, *right*) is followed by an immediate decrease in AF

aortic flow. Simultaneous RV + LV balloon pumping in group B (right, Fig. 9) shifted the function curve of LV balloon pump to the left by inducing a higher aortic flow for the same mean left atrial pressure.

## Discussion

We have shown [3] that the closest the shape and volume of the balloon to the shape and volume of the left ventricle, the highest the efficacy of left intraventricular balloon pumping during cardiac arrest. Larger or smaller

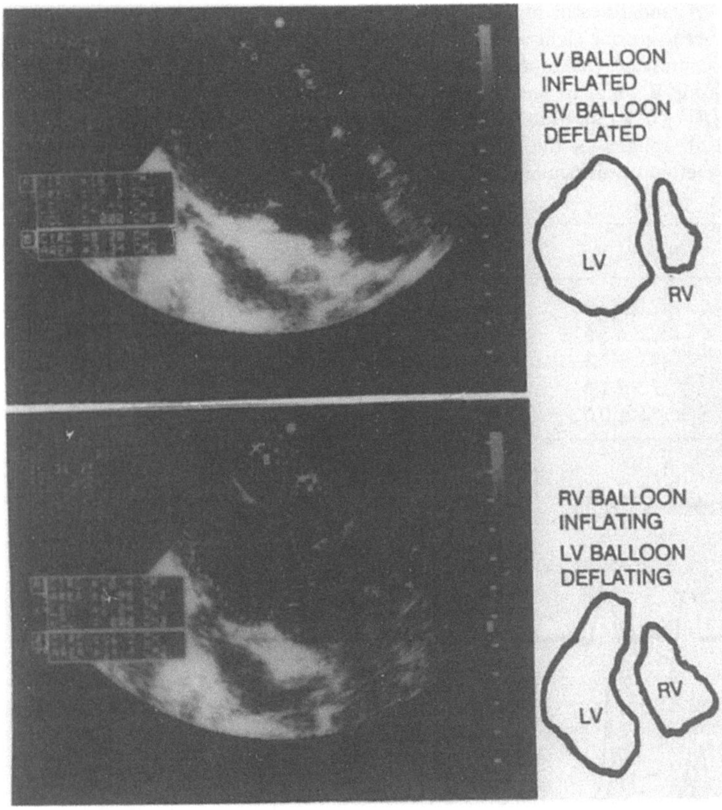


**Fig. 7.** Two-dimensional echocardiography (epicardial examination) during pumping by balloons into both ventricles in an animal of group B. *Above*, left intraventricular balloon is fully inflated, but the balloon into the right ventricle is still deflated. *Below*, the balloon into the left ventricle starts to deflate, while the right intraventricular balloon is inflating. A leftward shifting of the intraventricular septum is seen (*below*), induced by the right intraventricular balloon expansion. Thus, additional left ventricular pumping was performed in this group of animals (see text) by the second balloon into the right ventricle

balloons, or balloons not properly "fitting" in expansion to the geometry of the fibrillating left ventricle, are associated with a lower aortic flow. The findings of this experimental study indicate that optimal left intraventricular pumping – as judged by its ability to maintain a systolic aortic pressure above 100 mmHg during cardiac arrest – is associated with a rightward shifting of the intraventricular septum during balloon expansion. Thus, a balloon "well fitting" in expansion to the geometry of the left ventricle may result in simultaneous pumping into both ventricles. This explains how animals in ventricular fibrillation can survive for over 10 h [1] by left intraventricular balloon pumping alone.

The findings presented here indicate that although the addition of right intraventricular pumping increased the inflow to the left ventricle (by decreasing central venous pressure and increasing both the systolic right ventricular and

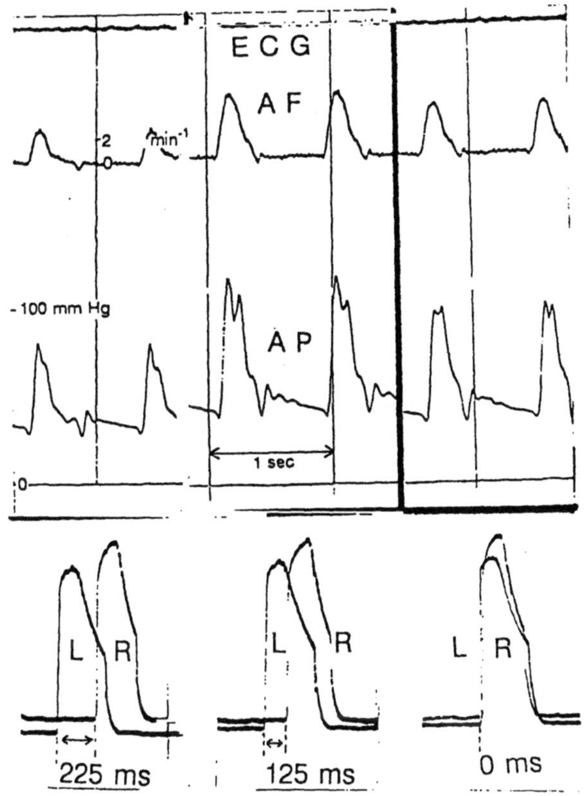


**Fig. 8.** Simultaneous tracings of electrocardiogram (*ECG*, indicating ventricular fibrillation), aortic pressure (*AP*) and pressures of both external pumps driving the left (*L*) and right (*R*) intraventricular balloons in an animal of group B. The delay between the two pumps was 225 ms in the *left*, 125 ms in the *middle* and 0 ms in the *right* tracing. An optimal aortic pressure and flow was obtained in this animal with a delay of 125 ms

**Fig. 9.** Function curves obtained by plotting aortic flow against mean left atrial pressure during different volume loads of the circulation. *Full circles* indicate operation of left intraventricular balloon only, *empty circles* operation of left plus right intraventricular balloons. The function curves on the *left* are obtained from an animal of group A and the ones on the *right* from an animal of group B

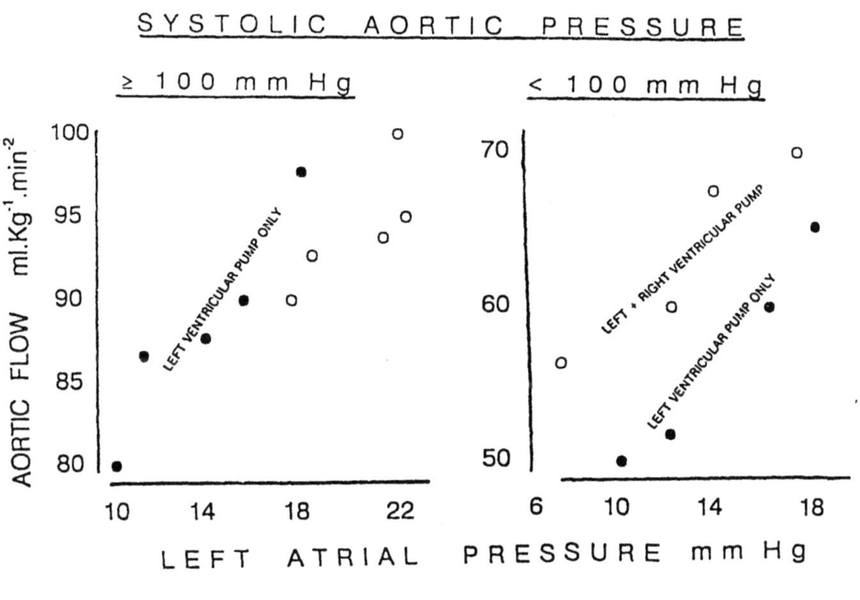

mean left atrial pressures), it did not add any further increase in the output of the left ventricular pump. Apparently, the increase in left atrial pressure induced by adding right intraventricular balloon pumping to an already optimal left intraventricular balloon pumping exceeds the limitations of the latter pump, concerning its capability to increase its output in response to a rise in preload. Indeed, the operation of the left intraventricular balloon pump was shifted to the plateau of its function curve, as shown in these experiments. Pulmonary oedema was noted to occur if biventricular pumping continued under these circumstances.

In the case of ineffective left intraventricular balloon pumping due to a nonoptimal (balloon/left ventricular cavity) relationship, the findings indicated a beneficial effect of additional right intraventricular balloon pumping. An increase was noted in both aortic flow and pressure for the same left atrial pressure. Again, it is not easily understood how the output of the left intraventricular pump could be raised by additional right intraventricular balloon pumping without an increase in its preload (left atrial pressure). This is probably explained if one considers that two ways of interaction between right and left intraventricular pumps may exist, one by increasing the preload of the left intraventricular pump and the other by mechanical interaction, namely optimizing "left ventricular" output by additional pumping through the intraventricular septum. Indeed an "inotropic" effect of right intraventricular balloon pumping on the left intraventricular pump appears to exist: Inflation of the right balloon a few milliseconds after inflation of the left balloon results in additional left ventricular pumping by shifting the intraventricular septum to the left. This is indicated both by echocardiography (Fig. 7) and by the fact that a prompt – within one beat – increase was noted (Figs. 5 and 6) in aortic flow after initiation of right intraventricular pumping, that is, before any increase in left atrial pressure was attained. Due to this "inotropic" effect, the operation of the left intraventricular balloon pump was shifted (Fig. 9, right) to a better function curve when right balloon pumping was added. Thus, the combined effect of the left intraventricular balloon expansion and the leftward shifting of the intraventricular septum induced by expansion of the right balloon effectively manipulated the increased left ventricular inflow: Aortic flow increased without any significant change in left atrial pressure.

Before summarizing the results of this study, it must be stressed that left intraventricular pumping by means of a catheter-mounted balloon is a method intended to be used as a bridge to transplantation or to the implantation of a more permanent assist device following intractable cardiac arrest. Its main advantage is the possibility of rapid application. The balloon can be inserted, via a peripheral artery, at the patient's bed. The use of a second catheter-mounted balloon introduced into the right ventricle may render this potentially simple method a more complicated procedure. Thus, the results may be summarized as follows: If optimal left intraventricular balloon pumping alone applied during cardiac arrest can maintain a systolic aortic pressure of at least 100 mm Hg, the addition of right intraventricular balloon pumping may not further improve pressure and flow in the circulatory system. If left intraventricular balloon pumping alone is unable to increase systolic aortic pressure to the level of 100 mm Hg, the addition of right intraventricular balloon pumping may improve aortic pressure and flow via a positive "inotropic" effect by means of additional pumping through the intraventricular septum.

## References

1. Moulopoulos S, Stamatelopoulos S, Zakopoulos N, Saridakis N, Adractas A, Stefanou S, Kanakakis J (1989) Intraventricular plus intra-aortic balloon pumping during intractable cardiac arrest. Circulation 80[Suppl III]:III-167–III-173
2. Stamatelopoulos S, Zakopoulos N, Saridakis N, Kanakakis J, Stefanou S, Adractas A, Kokkolakis N, Abraamides A, Moulopoulos S (1989) Left and right intraventricular balloon pumping in cardiac arrest. Eur Heart J 10[Suppl]:347 (abstr)
3. Stamatelopoulos S, Zakopoulos N, Toumanides S, Saridakis S, Stefanou S, Myrianthefs M, Moulopoulos S (1990) Left intraventricular balloon pumping: optimization of balloon shape and pumping characteristics. ASAIO, p 62 (abstr)
4. Stamatelopoulos S, Zakopoulos N, Saridakis N, Stefanou S, Adractas A, Kanakakis J, Vinieratos N, Zoumis G, Gougoulakis A, Moulopoulos S (1993) Catecholamine infusion versus intraaortic counterpulsation at the initial phase of left intraventricular balloon pumping in the fibrillating animal heart. Int J Artif Organs 16:86–90
5. Shuman TA, Palazzo RS, Jaquis RBD, Harper BD, Bargilai B, Cox JL, Koutsoukos NT, Wareing TH (1991) A model of right ventricular failure after global myocardial ischemia and mechanical left ventricular support. ASAIO Trans 37:M213
6. Bennink GBWE, Noda H, Duncan JM, Frazier OH (1992) Clinical evaluation of right ventricular function in patients with left ventricular assist device (LVAD). Int J Artif Organs 16:109–113

# Part II
# Ventricular Assist Devices

# Introduction: Clinical Reality

F. UNGER

Ventricular assist devices were first designed 30 years ago, at a time when open heart surgery posed a real challenge and the early postoperative mortality was near 10%. The designs of the pulsatile devices have not changed very much, being basically membrane pumps available in the form of a sac (Portner) or a moving diaphragm (Pierce, Unger, Frazier, Whalen) (Table 1). The driving source is either pneumatic or electromechanical via a tube through the skin. In the electromechanical driving mode, the incorporated devices need a compliance chamber. Furthermore, nonpulsatile blood pumps are also available.

In this part specific emphasis is given to pulsatile artificial ventricles, which can be implanted or left paracorporeal. The devices are implanted between the left ventricule and the aorta (Fig. 1). The atrial aortic bypass concept is not in use anymore, since it does not provide the desired efficiency.

Left ventricular assist devices support the failing left ventricle in parallel to the heart up to 100%. The basic requirement is a working right ventricle. If the right ventricle also fails, an additional assist device, such as an RVAD, is mandatory (BVAD) (Fig. 2).

Access for LVAD to the left ventricle can be achieved via the apex (Fig. 1a, d) or transatrially (Fig. 1a, a–c). For permanent implantation or for bridging, transapical cannulation is preferable. The arterial return is then to the ascending (Fig. 1b, c) or descending aorta. If the ventricles are temporary and paracorporeal, the ascending aorta is used for arterial access.

The pumps in clinical use are designed primarily for temporary support. They show excellent performance. The main indication for their clinical use is bridging toward transplantation. The main requirement is that the patient meet an indication for transplantation. Figure 3 depicts the indications for cardiac assistance. The devices described in this part are too expensive for postoperative use, especially when in the acute phase of wean off problems the future indication for a transplantation is not forseen. Ventricular assist devices have been used in 36% of the cases of cardiac assistance, and of these patients 68% later received a transplant and 46% survived (see Table 2). Regarding the increasing survival rates, ventricular assist devices are an indispensible tool in any heart transplant program. The improving clinical experience today enables us to plan long-term implantation of these devices. Initial experience is now being gathered.

All the ventricular assist devices described in this part are pulsatile artificial heart chambers (Portner, Pierce, Frazier, Whalen) driven pneumatically or mechanically. The only indication for using these devices, which are commercially

**Table 1.** Blood pumps

| | |
|---|---|
| Axis symmetrical | Bernhard<br>Frazier |
| Diaphragm | Jarvik, Pierce<br>Ellipsoid<br>Berlin, Moskow<br>Vienna<br>Japan National Cardiovascular Center blood pump<br>Thomas Engineering |
| Sac type | Atsumi (CORAT)<br>Lepayre<br>Portner<br>Abiomed |
| Impeller | Biomedicus<br>Hager<br>Schistek<br>Wampler |

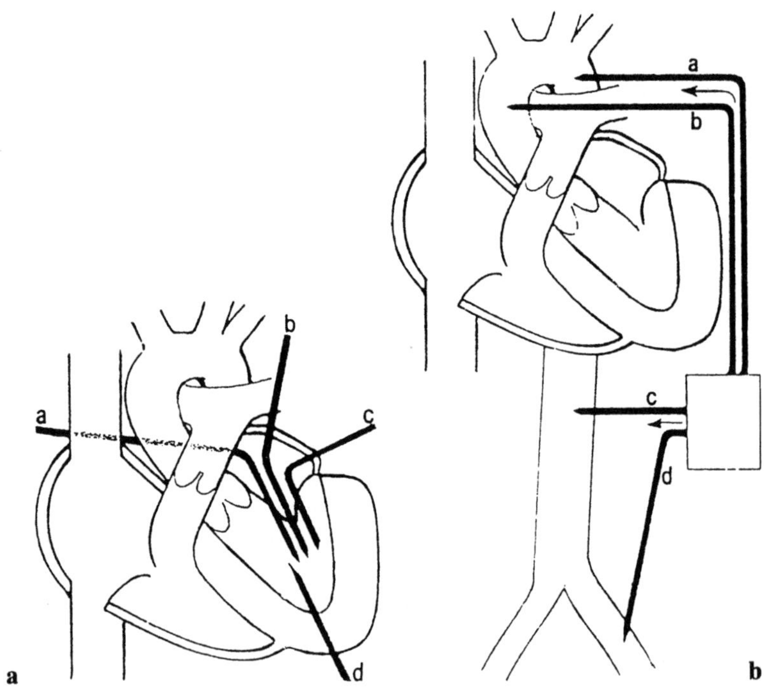


**Fig. 1.** **a** Ventricular cannulation. *a–c* Transmitral: via the right pulmonary vein (*a*), the roof (*b*), and the left appendage (*c*). *d* Transapical. **b** Arterial return to the thoracic aorta (*a*), ascending aorta (*b*), abdominal aorta (*c*), and femoral artery

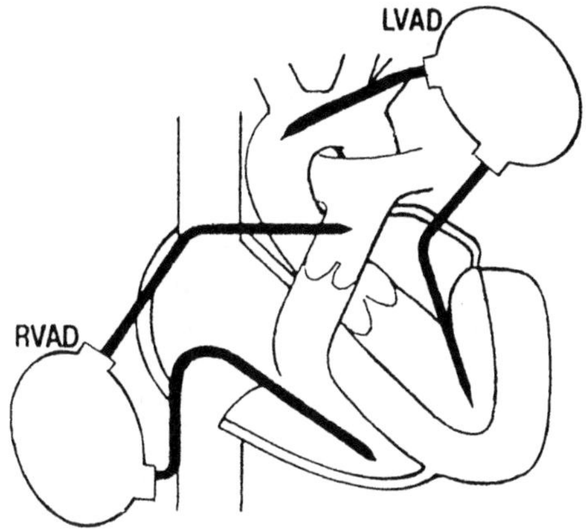


**Fig. 2.** Biventricular assist device (BVAD). *LVAD*, left ventricular assist device. *RVAD*, right ventricular assist device

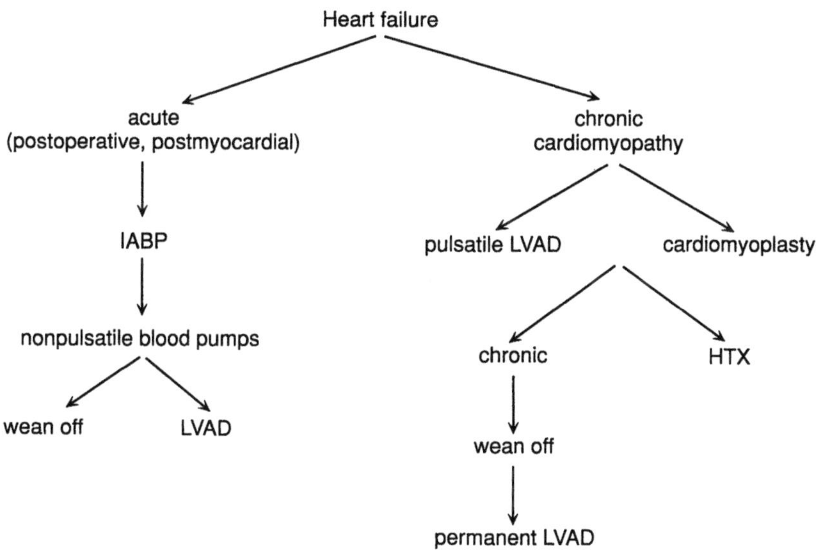


**Fig. 3.** Schematic description of treatment for cardiac failure after failure of all possible pharmacologic support

available (Baxter, Thoratex, Heart Mate) but very expensive, for left ventricular assistance is for bridging toward transplantation. Biventricular assist devices (BAVD) are indicated when left ventricular assist devices are not working properly due to additional right heart failure (Fig. 2). A biventricular assist device (BVAD) is a functional heart replacement.

In this section Loisance and Vetter et al. report on the Novacor system, a bridging device which can be used up to 40 days. The Novacor system has transapical access to the left ventricle, and blood is returned in the abdominal aorta. The pump is driven pneumatically or electrically by a pusher plate driving system. The Novocor system allows a very reliable postoperative course, and based on these excellent clinical results this device may remain the device of

**Table 2.** Indications for use of ventricular assist devices in 900 patients from 1962 to 1994

| Indication | Proportion of total patients | Result | Comment |
|---|---|---|---|
| Postoperative cardiac failure | 62% | 30% weaned off, 11% died | nonpulsatile pump intra-aortic balloon pump roller pump |
| Bridging | 36% | 68% transplantation, 46% survived | Implantable assist devices preferable (total artificial heart?) |
| Long-term support | – | – | intra-aortic balloon pump |
| Cardiomyoplasty | – | – | left ventricular assist device (mechanical) |

choice for long-term use. The Heart Mate is another electrically driven pusher plate pump. When electromagnetically driven, both pumps need a compliance chamber. Frazier reports on his clinical results and compares the pneumatic and electrical driving modes.

The Abiomed system is designed for the use in postoperative heart failure. Everts et al. report on their experience in weaning off. Whalen reports on a new bladder pump, focussing especially on costs. Weiss et al. report on clinical experience using the Thoratec ventricular assist device. This device, designed by Pierce, is mainly implanted paracorporeally as LVAD or BVAD. He shows the feasibility for a long-term implantation, whereby in these experiments devices are implanted over 100 days. A specific aim is to drive this device electrically for permanent implantation. The Novocor, Heart Mate, and Thoratec devices as well as the Berlin heart, are the devices most frequently used clinically. Further study of all these devices is necessary to achieve long-term use. In my opinion, the pumps must be redesigned to improve efficacy. The energy loss is too high, a fact which was not problematic in the pneumatic extracorporeal driving mode. A redesigned blood pump should have a myoplastic biologic driving source. I am pretty sure that in the next volume in this series there will be a specific chapter dedicated to chronic implants.

# Mechanical Circulatory Support at Henri Mondor Hospital: Indications for the Use of Different Devices

D. Loisance, P.H. Deleuze, J.P. Mazzucotelli, and M.L. Hillion

## Introduction

At Henri Mondor Hospital, the application of mechanical circulatory support (MCS) has, for many years, been a major interest. After a long period of experimental research, our first clinical use of MCS, as a bridge to transplantation, was in 1986. An ECMO system, in place for 12 h, allowed cardiac transplantation in a patient who could not be weaned from cardiopulmonary bypass [1]. Since then we have progressed, first using the Jarvik in 1987 [2], then the Hemopump in 1989, the Novacor LVAS in 1991, and implanting the first wearable Novacor in the spring of 1993 [3].

This activity is the result of a strategic decision made under circumstances which are probably shared by most surgical departments. Our main objective has been to develop protocols for patient and device selection, taking into account our relative lack of experience in the technological development of the systems, the large number of patients in cardiogenic shock who are referred to us, our well-integrated medical and surgical services, and economic and ethical considerations. As a result of these factors we have developed a dual approach: first an evaluation of the optimal method of patient selection, integrating both pharmacological progress (the pharmacological bridge) and the benefits and limitations of the various MCS systems (the mechanical bridge) [4]; second a strategy, based on experience, for device selection.

Previous papers have described and discussed the various aspects of our patient selection strategy [4, 5]. This paper gives an analysis of our results with mechanical bridges and, based on this, our opinion on device selection.

## Clinical Material

Our clinical experience comprises 58 patients. Two cases of bridge to transplantation, with prolonged extracorporeal circulation, and 17 cases of prophylactic implantation of the Hemopump in patients undergoing high-risk PTCA are excluded. Thus, this report is based upon the results achieved with 39 patients.

From 1987 to November 20, 1993, these 39 patients were selected from 84 patients referred in cardiogenic shock, from several causes, for urgent transplantation and/or MCS. Patients were selected according to the previously described protocol [4]; briefly, there had to be no contra-indication to transplantation and no response to medical therapy comprising optimal oxygenation and fluid balance and maximum i.v. sympathomimetic and phosphodiesterase inhibitor support. This group includes all patients treated by MCS despite the major changes that have occurred over this period [4]. There has been a trend towards earlier implantation since 1991.

The characteristics of these patients are: mean age 48 ± 10 years (21–67), 36 male and three female. Cardiogenic shock resulted from recent (< 3 weeks) AMI ($n$ = 13), dilated, idiopathic cardiomyopathy ($n$ = 10), ischemic cardiomyopathy ($n$ = 2), post-partum cardiomyopathy ($n$ = 1), myocardial failure immediately after cardiopulmonary bypass ($n$ = 9), and problems related to a transplanted heart in four, either early in three (graft failure) or late (rejection) in one. The total duration of assistance was 280 days, with an average of 7.3 days (0.5–59) per patient (Table 1). The annual frequency of MCS is given in Fig. 1. These figures demonstrate our recognition of the limitations of the pharmacological bridge since 1991 [5].

We have used MCS as either a bridge to recovery or a bridge to transplantation. MCS as a bridge to recovery was used in those patients who could not be

**Table 1.** Systems used and time on assistance

| Simple systems (CF, HP) | | | Complex system | | |
|---|---|---|---|---|---|
| | *n* | Mean duration (days) | | *n* | Mean duration (days) |
| Left VAD | 8 | 3.4 (2–7) | Left pneumatic Symbion | 1 | 3 |
| Right VAD | 3 | 2 (1–5) | Bi-VAD Symbion | 2 | 6 (1–12) |
| Bi-VAD | 1 | 1 | Bi-VAD Nippon Zeon | 11 | 10 (1–32) |
| Hemopump | 3 | 2 (1–3) | Left VAD Novacor[a] | 6 | 25 (8–58) |
| | | | Jarvik | 4 | 3.5 (1–7) |
| | 15 | | | 24 | |

*CF*, Centrifugal pump; *HP*, Hemopump
[a] One Novacor patient is still on device.

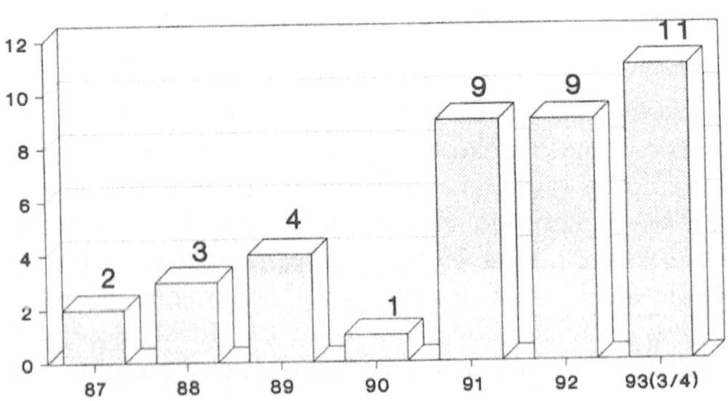


**Fig. 1.** Annual frequency of mechanical circulatory support among 39 patients studied

weaned from CPB ($n = 9$) and in three of the four cases of failure post transplantation (those with graft failure). In these circumstances, the system used was a left ventricular assist with a centrifugal pump in five, an left intraventricular assist in three, a right ventricular assist with a centrifugal pump in three, and biventricular support with a Nippon-Zeon in one. The systems used as a bridge to transplantation are listed in Table 1.

## Results

The results for the entire group are as follows: one patient is waiting with a device (a wearable Novacor). Fourteen patients died during support. Twenty-four either were weaned from assistance ($n = 5$) or underwent transplantation ($n = 19$). Of those weaned from support, two died in hospital after weaning and three are long-term survivors. Of those who received transplants, ten died in the first month and nine were discharged and are alive and well. The longest survivor has a follow-up of 5 years.

The causes of death during assistance are: multiple organ failure in eight, primary loss of vascular tone in two, bleeding in one, thromboembolism and a disseminated coagulopathy in one, pulmonary hypertension in one, and further myocardial infarction in one patient rehabilitated with a LVAD Novacor.

The cause of death in the two patients who died after weaning was severe neurological injury, which is likely to have been due to a prolonged period of resuscitation prior to the implantation. In the transplant group ($n = 9$) the cause of death was infection in two, persistent and irreversible multiple organ failure in five, acute graft failure in one, and a coagulopathy, present at the time of implantation, with multiple embolic events in one.

We have experienced a learning curve with both patient and device selection. Prior to 1991 we achieved two survivors in nine cases; from 1992 on we have a 61% overall survival among 13 patients with AMI or dilated cardiomyopathy.

An analysis of the results by the device used is given in Table 2 for patients in both the bridge-to-weaning and bridge-to-transplantation groups. An analysis of the results according to etiology of the cardiogenic shock is given in Table 3. The age of the patient is, in our experience, critical; we have no survivors among patients older than 55 years of age but a 70% success rate among those under 55 years.

## Comments

The systems available in our institution have permitted an evaluation of the indications for use of each. The Hemopump intraventricular system, in both 21F and 14F configurations, is not indicated in patients with cardiogenic shock; no survivors have been obtained in our experience. This contrasts with the efficacy of the Hemopump used as prophylactic support in patients undergoing high-risk procedures such as PTCA, when satisfactory results are obtained in most cases

**Table 2.** Systems used and overall results, expressed as number of patients either transplanted (*Htx*) or weaned from mechanical circulation

| System | (*n*) | Weaned or Htx (*n*) |
|---|---|---|
| Right VAD CF | 3 | 0 |
| Left VAD | | |
| Hemopump | 3 | 0 |
| Centrifugal | 8 | 6 |
| Pneumatic | 1 | 1 |
| Novacor | 6[a] | 2 |
| Bi-VAD | | |
| Centrifugal | 1 | 1 |
| Pneumatic (NZ+S) | 13 | 11 |
| Jarvik TAH | 4 | 2 |
| Total | 39 | 23 |

*NZ*, Nippon Zeon; *S*, Symbion; *CF*, centrifugal pump
[a] One patient was still on device at the time of the study.

**Table 3.** Results according to etiology of cardiogenic shock

| | *n* | System | | Htx or weaned | LT survivor |
|---|---|---|---|---|---|
| AMI | 13 | LVAD CF | 3 | 3 | 2 |
| | | LVAD pneumatic | 1 | 1 | 1 |
| | | LVAD Novacor | 2 | 0 | 0 |
| | | Bi-VAD pneumatic | 4 | 4 | 2 |
| | | Jarvik TAH | 3 | 1 | 1 |
| | | | 13 | 9 | 6 |
| DC | 13 | LVAD CF | – | – | – |
| | | LVAD Novacor | 4 | 1 | 1 |
| | | Bi-VAD CF | 1 | – | – |
| | | Bi-VAD pneumatic | 8 | 7 | 5 |
| | | | 13 | 8 | 6 |

*AMI*, Acute myocardial infarction; *DC*, dilated cardiomyopathy; *CF*, centrifugal pump; *Htx*, transplanted; *LT*, long-term

[6]. This difference may be related to the maximum flow of 3–3.5 l/min obtained with the Hemopump, which is inadequate to support a patient in severe cardiogenic shock. In addition, the Hemopump system does not appear to allow safe assistance for more than a few days. In two of our cases where the Hemopump was used as a bridge to recovery, the clinical situation was initially good but rapidly deteriorated due to bleeding and hemolysis.

The best results have been obtained with external bi-VADs and mostly with the Nippon Zeon. All of these devices were implanted without the use of CPB, and the duration of assistance has been quite short: the longest period is 32 days, and the mean is 10 days. The good results in terms of suitability for transplantation and overall success are related to our policy of giving the bridge cases maximum priority for transplantation. This policy may need to be reconsidered, however, in view of the shortage of donor organs and the less than optimal transplantation success rate that it has produced.

Furthermore, over this period the benefits of full rehabilitation that a period of prolonged assistance provides have become established and obtainable with an implantable device [3]. Given the donor organ shortage, it is essential that patients requiring bridge to transplantation be in the best possible condition. The period of support provided by an external VAD is often not adequate to achieve this.

Our experience with the Novacor Baxter LVAS has been both frustating and encouraging. In four cases, the benefits given by the implanted system have been spectacular. Nevertheless, one patient ultimately died because of further myocardial infarction, one as a result of graft failure after 40 days of assistance, one with increased pulmonary vascular resistance and one with a pre-existing, undetected heparin-induced thrombocytopenia. Our experience with this small group of patients clearly points out the current limitations of the system: right ventricular dysfunction due to recurrence or extension of the ischemic process to the right side, elevated pulmonary vascular resistance, and problems present before the implantation or, as in our patient, arising during and following CPB. As a result of this experience we prefer to use this system in patients who are not in a desperate condition at the time of implantation.

Our current indications for a Jarvik implantation are restricted to large patients who, at the time of implantation, are not in a pre-lethal condition, but who have thrombosis in one or both ventricles and a ventricular septal rupture. These narrow criteria account for our infrequent use of this device.

The indications for use of the various systems are now clearer than they were some years ago. Systems using centrifugal pumps or external pneumatic devices are most suitable in situations where the major objective of treatment is resuscitation. The choice between these two systems is made on the basis of the patient's age, the aetiology of the cardiogenic shock and the likelihood of recovery from this. In both system types the authorized safe period of support is nevertheless limited to a few days for centrifugal pumps and a few weeks for external pneumatic VADs. Our experience in the present situation of organ shortage clearly shows that the emotional pressure related to waiting for an organ is not relieved and that deterioration of the patient's condition while on support, usually due to infection, creates a difficult situation for the medical and nursing staff. Our experience with these devices is not unique; in the various registries and in-house reports, the number of patients who are bridged for more than 3 months with external VADs is small [7].

For patients who deteriorate while on the transplant list or initially respond favorably to intensive medical therapy, semi-elective implantation of a Novacor gives the best chance of long-term support, active rehabilitation, and improvement in the general clinical condition. The rehabilitation process is easily accepted by both patient and medical staff, and the easy adaptation of the patient to this new mode of living (4 h autonomy with the wearable batteries) gives us hope for prolonged implantation (months) and discharge from hospital to a half-way house or even the individual's home [8]. Finally, the technique allows evaluation of the problems of definitive, permanent implantations.

## References

1. Loisance D, Hillion ML, Deleuze PH, Tavolaro O, Heurtematte Y, Castaigne A, Cachera JP (1987) Extracorporeal circulation with membrane oxygenation as a bridge to transplantation in cardiac surgical patients. Transplant Proc 9:3786–3788
2. Loisance D, Deleuze PH, Kawasaki K, Hillion ML, Binhas M, Heurtematte PH, Tavolaro O, Leandri J, Cachera JP (1987) Total artificial heart bridge to retransplantation. J Heart Transplant 6:281–285
3. Loisance D, Deleuze PH, Mazzucotelli JP, Le Besnerais P, Dubois Rande JL, Cachera JP (1994) The first clinical implantation of the wearable Baxter Novacor ventricular assist system. Ann Thorac Surg (in press)
4. Loisance D, Dubois Rande JL, Deleuze PH, Hillion ML, Duval AM, Tavolaro O, Romano P, Castaigne A, Tarral A, Cachera JP (1989) Pharmacological bridge to cardiac transplantation. Eur J Cardiothorac Surg 3:196–202
5. Loisance D, Benvenuti C, Leclerc A, Houel R, Deleuze PH, Tarral A, Lebrun TH, Sailly JC (1993) The pharmacological bridge to cardiac transplantation. The current limitations. Ann Thorac Surg 55:310–313
6. Shiiya N, Zelinsky R, Deleuze PH, Loisance D (1992) Changes in hemodynamics and coronary blood flow during left ventricular assistance with the Hemopump. Ann Thorac Surg 53:1074–1079
7. Thoratec, in House Report 1993
8. Dew AM, Kormos RL, Roth LH, Armitage JM, Pristal JM, Harris RC, Capretta C, Griffith BP (1993) Life quality in the era of bridging to cardiac transplantation. Bridge patients in an out-patient setting. ASAIO J 20:145–152

# Use of the Novacor Left Ventricular Assist System as a Bridge to Cardiac Transplantation: First Experience with Long-term Patients on the Wearable System

H.O. Vetter, H.G. Kaulbach, M. Haller, T. Hummel, C. Schmitz,
O. Dwvald, P. Brenner, E. Kreuzer, P. Überfuhr, and B. Reichart

## Introduction

During the past decade, cardiac transplantation has become an accepted method in clinical therapy for end-stage heart disease. However, donor shortage is still responsible for a high percentage of patients dying while awaiting heart transplantation. Therefore, electrically powered ventricular assist devices [1] and pneumatically driven artificial hearts [2] were used in clinical programs to rescue critically ill cardiac transplant candidates.

As patients do not qualify for a higher priority on the waiting list during circulatory assistance, and as the average waiting time for a donor heart has increased during the past few years, this situtation resulted in prolonged periods of mechanical circulatory support. Because the incidence of thromboembolism remains a major threat to the chronically supported patients, anticoagulation protocols as well as changes in device design are very important factors for the outcome of such patients [3]. Since 1993 the controller of the Novacor left ventricular assist system (LVAS) was miniaturized and can be worn on a belt, thereby allowing a higher degree of mobility and quality of life.

## Material and Methods

### Device

The Novacor N100 LVAS (Novacor Division, Baxter Healthcare Corp., Oakland/CA, USA) is an electromagnetically actuated, totally implantable pump which consists of a seamless one-piece smooth polyurethane sac that is bonded to symmetrically opposed dual pusher plates. The housing is a light-weight shell, incorporating bovine-pericardial valve fittings and an energy converter. Via a percutaneous lead the pump unit is connected to an extracorporeal control console or controller (Fig. 1). Inflow and outflow Dacron grafts connect the pump to the left ventricular apex and to the ascending aorta, both traversing the diaphragm. A maximal stroke volume of 70 ml can provide a pump output of up to 10 l/min, and operating in synchronous counterpulsation cardiac rates of up to 240 beats/min can be achieved [4].

The new "wearable" Novacor LVAS (N100P) has a substantially smaller controller unit which can be worn on a belt or within a shoulder bag (Fig. 2). It allows untethered operation if two DC power sources are connected (Fig. 1).

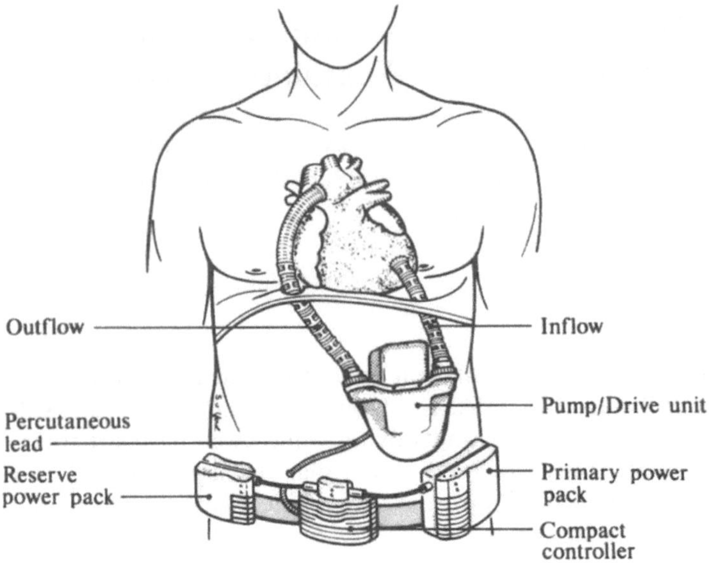


**Fig. 1.** The wearable Novacor left ventricular assist system

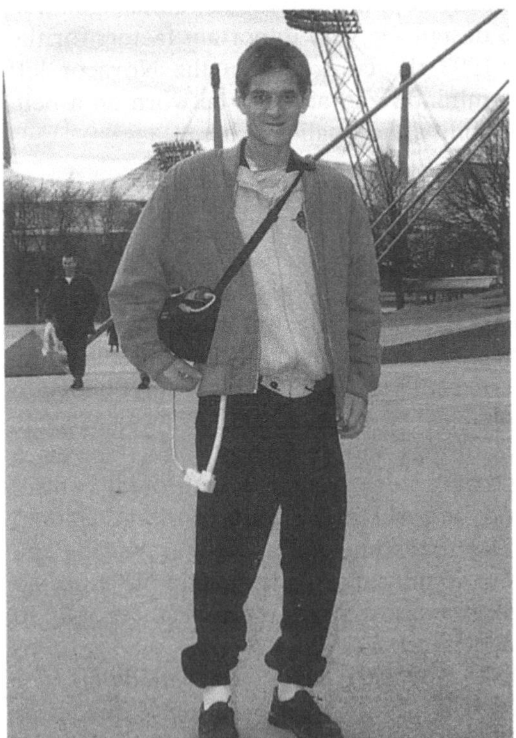

**Fig. 2.** A patient, 105 days after implantation of the wearable Novacor LVAS, during a trip to the Olympic Park in Munich

With both batteries, the patient is fully mobile for up to 5 h, independent of either AC power or console monitor. This is a major step in getting the patients out of bed in order to improve quality of life during mechanical circulatory support.

## Patients

Between February 1992 and April 1994, the Novacor LVAS was implanted in eight patients as a bridge to cardiac transplantation. The last four patients were supported with the wearable system. One patient had been supported for a total of 122 days. Underlying diseases were dilated cardiomyopathy in five patients, end-stage ischemic heart disease in two patients, and acute myocarditis in another. Two patients were supported by intra-aortic balloon counterpulsation prior to Novacor implantation. The mean age of the patients at the time of implantation was 31.6 ± 12.9 years (range 16–49 years). The body surface area was 1.83 ± 0.10 $m^2$ on average, ranging from 1.72 to 1.98 $m^2$.

Despite inotropic and vasodilator support, the clinical status and hemodynamics of all patients were deteriorating. Preoperative data of left and right heart function are given in Table 1. Cardiac output and parameters of right heart function were evaluated by means of a rapid-response thermodilution catheter. Among the eight patients, right ventricular ejection fraction was only 4% in two and 13%, 15%, and 16% in one patient each. Renal function was reduced, with oliguria or even anuria in two patients; mean serum creatinine measured 1.50 ± 0.54 mg/dl. Total bilirubin was 2.11 ± 1.51 mg/dl on average, and the mean value of serum glutamic-oxaloacetic transaminase was 198 ± 246 mg/dl (range 70–660 mg/dl) prior to Novacor implantation.

Patient selection was based on the following criteria: (a) accepted transplant candidate; (b) age between 15 and 65 years; (c) body surface area between 1.5

**Table 1.** Hemodynamic data of patients prior to implantation of the Novacor left ventricular assist system

| Patient no. | CVP (mmHg) | MPAP (mmHg) | RVEF (%) | PCWP (mmHg) | MAP (mmHg) | CI (l/min/$m^2$) |
|---|---|---|---|---|---|---|
| 1 | 34 | 58 | 4 | 30 | 66 | 1.0 |
| 2 | 7 | 36 | 13 | 24 | 52 | 2.0 |
| 3 | 28 | 46 | – | 34 | 70 | 1.3 |
| 4 | 14 | 33 | 15 | 25 | 65 | 1.5 |
| 5 | 5 | 29 | 30 | 22 | 72 | 2.0 |
| 6 | 20 | 41 | 4 | 28 | 74 | 2.2 |
| 7 | 20 | 40 | 16 | 30 | 70 | 1.8 |
| 8 | 17 | 48 | 28 | 30 | 90 | 2.0 |
| Mean | 18 | 41 | 16 | 27 | 70 | 1.7 |
| SD | ±9.8 | ±9.2 | ±10.3 | ±4.5 | ±10.6 | ±0.4 |

*CVP*, Central venous pressure; *MPAP*, mean pulmonary artery pressure; *RVEF*, right ventricular ejection fraction; *PCWP*, pulmonary capillary wedge pressure; *MAP*, mean arterial pressure; *CI*, cardiac index; *SD*, standard deviation

and 2.5 $m^2$; (d) NYHA classification class III–IV; (e) cardiac index <2.0 l/min/$m^2$ and mean arterial pressure <65 mmHg or pulmonary capillary wedge pressure >18 mmHg; (f) level of inotropic drug support or use of intra-aortic balloon counterpulsation. As contraindications we considered irreversible end organ dysfunction, sepsis, pulmonary parenchymal disease, peripheral vascular disease, neurological deficits, and coagulopathy or malignancies.

**Surgical Technique**

The implantation technique suggested by Oyer et al. [5] was modified in various steps in order to minimize bleeding and other procedure-related complications (Table 2). The patient's heart was exposed through a median sternotomy. In all cases the original outflow graft (Dacron, not preclotted) of the pump system was replaced by a preclotted vascular graft (Vascutek, Vascutek, Renfrewshire, Scotland), while the inflow graft was preclotted with fibrin glue (Tissucol, Immuno, Vienna, Austria). A pocket was then prepared in the left upper quadrant of the abdominal wall, anterior to the posterior rectus muscle sheath. Cardiopulmonary bypass was instituted by cannulating the ascending aorta for arterial perfusion and the superior and inferior vena cava for venous return. A vent was placed inside the left ventricular cavity via the right upper pulmonary vein. After anastomosing the outflow graft to the ascending aorta, cardiopulmonary bypass was started for insertion of the left ventricular apical conduit. The aorta was cross-clamped and the heart arrested using either Bretschneider solution or blood cardioplegia according to Buckberg [6]. After the anastomosis was finished at the left ventricular apex, the heart, the pump, and the grafts were carefully evacuated of air and continuous pumping was begun. In order to prevent adhesions the outflow graft was covered with a sheath of polytetrafluoroethylene (GoreTex Surgical Membrane, W.L. Gore and Assoc., Putzbrunn, Germany). The abdominal fascia was extended by a resorbable mesh (Vicryl mesh) in six patients to provide suitable space to accommodate the pump.

**Anticoagulation**

The perioperative anticoagulation management consisted of 2 million units of aprotinin and regular heparinization (300 IU/kg body wt.) for cardiopulmonary bypass. Systemic heparinization was fully antagonized with protamine sulfate at the end of cardiopulmonary bypass.

Postoperatively, the following tests were frequently used to monitor anticoagulation therapy: activated partial thromboplastin time (aPTT), prothombin time after Quick (PT), platelet count, fibrinogen, activated coagulation time (ACT), antithrombin III, α-haptoglobin, and hemopexin-S. For evaluation of platelet function a specific test – "bleeding time ex vivo" – after Kratzer and Born [7] was applied (Thrombostat 4000, Baxter, Unterschleissheim, Germany).

In the postoperative phase we administered 60% dextran solution as soon as platelet function returned to normal. Intravenous administration of heparin was started when the aPTT was less than 50 s or the ACT was less than 140 s.

**Table 2.** Important facts for the management of the surgical procedure, postoperative mobilization, anticoagulation, and for prophylaxis of infections

| | Surgical procedure and mobilization | Anticoagulation | Prophylaxis for infection |
|---|---|---|---|
| Perioperative | Cardiopulmonary bypass | 2 million units aprotinin | Intensive skin cleaning: chlorhexidine (Phisohex) |
| | Cardioplegic arrest (Bretschneider/blood cardioplegia) | Protamine sulfate | Antibiotic prophylaxis: Vancomycin 500 mg i.v. |
| | Preclotted outflow graft (Vascutek) | | Mupirocin nasal |
| | Fibrin glue | | Bowel decontamination |
| | PTFE (Surgical Membrane) | | |
| | Vicryl mesh for pocket | | |
| Postoperative | Wound dressing of the extension cable: betadine | *Early:* | Vancomycin 500 mg/day |
| | | If bleeding time ex vivo normal: dextran 60% at 20 ml/h | Imipenem 1.5–2.0 mg/day |
| | *Mobilization:* | After bleeding stops: heparin i.v. (aPTT 60–80 s) | Removal of i.v. lines and urine catheter as soon as possible |
| | Physical training | *Late:* | |
| | Psychological support | Heparin (aPTT 60–80 s) s.c. *or* phenprocoumon (INR 3.0–4.5) ASA 100 mg/day<br>Dipyridamole 225 mg/day | |

*aPTT*, Activated partial thromboplatin time; *ASA*, acetyl salicyl acid; *INR*, international normalized ratio

Heparinization was considered sufficient if aPTT ranged between 60 and 80 s. Once the patients were mobilized, we changed to oral phenprocoumon (Marcumar) – maintaining the PT level at an INR of 3.0–4.5 [8] – or to heparin subcutaneously. After our first long-term patient (patient 5) had a thromboembolic complication we added acetylsalicylic acid (ASA) 100 mg/day and dipyridamole 225 mg/day. Antithrombin III was substituted when levels fell below 80%. The current protocol for anticoagulation in the early and chronic phase of patients during mechanical circulatory support is summarized in Table 2.

### Postoperative Recovery

Three patients were transferred from the intensive care unit to the regular ward. A program for physical activities was initiated. Patients were mobilized and were finally able to walk to the hospital park and shopping area. Accompanied by the LVAS operators, the patients were taken on trips to sightseeing areas in the town (Fig. 2). Psychological support was provided by a daily schedule that included physical activities, games (e.g., chess), and visits from relatives and medical students involved in the clinical study.

### Statistics

Data are given as mean values ± standard deviation (SD). The chi-square test was used to calculate significant differences between groups; Fisher's exact test was used in small sample sizes. Yates' correction for continuity was performed. A *p*-value of 0.05 was taken as the level of significance.

## Results

### Hemodynamic Data

The hemodynamic situation was improved significantly after implantation of the left ventricular assist system (Figs. 3 and 4). Mean arterial pressure increased

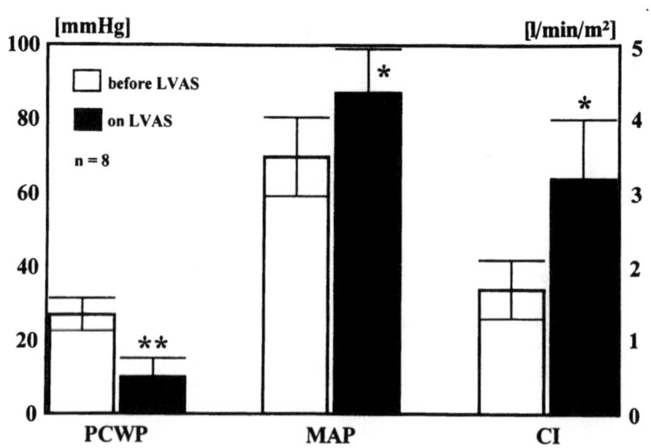


**Fig. 3.** Left heart function of patients before and 24 h after implantation of the Novacor left ventricular assist system (LVAS). PCWP, Pulmonary capillary wedge pressure; MAP, mean arterial pressure; CI, cardiac index; *, $p < 0.05$; **, $p < 0.01$

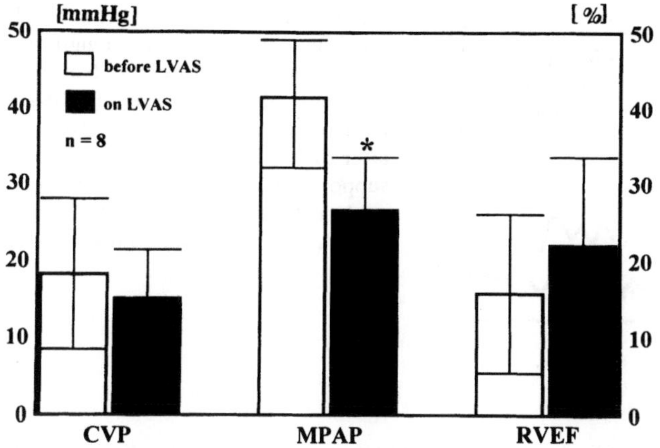


**Fig. 4.** Right heart function of patients before and 24 h after implantation of the Novacor left ventricular assist system (LVAS). CVP, central venous pressure; MPAP, mean pulmonary artery pressure; RVEF, right ventricular ejection fraction; *, $p < 0.05$

from 70 ± 11 mmHg on average to 87 ± 13 mmHg ($p < 0.05$). The cardiac index was calculated as 1.71 ± 0.42 l/min/m² before Novacor implantation and rose to 3.23 ± 0.74 l/min/m² on average 24 h after mechanical circulatory support ($p < 0.01$). Average pulmonary capillary wedge pressure was 27.1 ± 4.4 mmHg (range 22–34 mmHg) preoperatively and decreased to 9.9 ± 5.2 mmHg on average postoperatively, ranging from 4–13 mmHg ($p < 0.05$).

Parameters of the right heart function were significantly deteriorated in six cases preoperatively. Central venous pressure was 18.1 ± 9.8 mmHg on average before Novacor implantation and was measured at 15.0 ± 6.3 mmHg during left ventricular support (n.s.). Mean pulmonary artery pressure decreased from 41 ± 9 mmHg on average preoperatively to a mean value of 27 ± 6 mmHg postoperatively ($p < 0.05$). Calculation of right ventricular ejection fraction was performed in seven patients; the mean value was reduced preoperatively at 16.7 ± 10.3% (range 4–30%) and increased during mechanical left ventricular support to 22.0 ± 11.6% (range 10–45%). However, this increase was not statistically significant. There was no significant difference in heart rate pre- and postoperatively; it averaged 120 ± 17 beats/min and 117 ± 7 beats/min, respectively. Mean values of these parameters did not differ significantly when evaluated immediately before heart transplantation was performed. In the long-term patients who were supported for more than 20 days, hepatic and renal functions were improved before transplantation (Fig. 5).

## Complications

Perioperatively, all patients were treated prophylactically with a combination of antibiotics (vancomycin and piperacillin). Chest tubes, drains, and central venous lines were removed as soon as possible to minimize the risk of infection (Table 2). Only documented infections were treated. One patient accquired a serious pulmonary infection caused by *Legionella bozemanii*. He was treated succesfully with erythromycin, ciprofloxacin, and fluconasol.

A tendency to prolonged bleeding was observed in most of the patients (Table 3). Surgical intervention was neccesary in five patients; three of them had a cardiac tamponade within the first postoperative week, and in two long-term

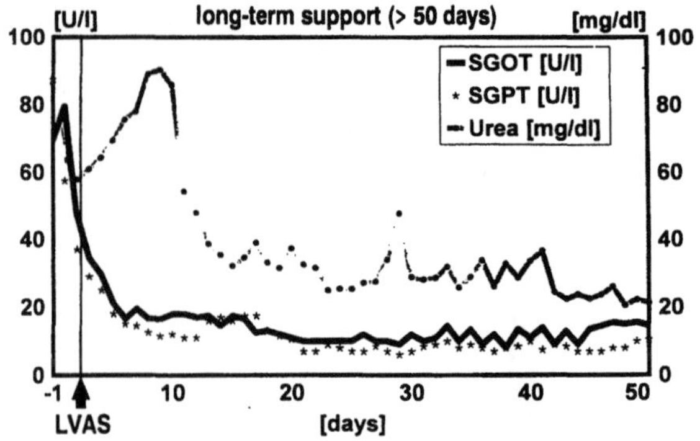


**Fig. 5.** Time course of the hepatic and renal function of the three long-term patients supported by the Novacor left ventricular assist system (LVAS). Parameters normalized on average after 20 days of mechanical circulatory support. SGOT, Serum glutamic-oxaloacetic transaminase; SGPT, serum glutamate pyruvate transaminase

**Table 3.** Complications and outcome of bridge-to-transplant patients supported by the Novacor left ventricular assist system *(LVAS)*

| Patients | Complications | Blood loss (ml) | Days on LVAS | Outcome | Time since HTx (mos) |
|---|---|---|---|---|---|
| 1 | CT day 1, RF | 3190 | 3 | Working | 21 |
| 2 | RF | 1900 | 2 | Died post Tx | – |
| 3 | CT day 2 | 5830 | 5 | Working | 17 |
| 4 | CT day 3 | 2900 | 7 | At home | 14 |
| 5 | CT day 8, CVA day 40 | 6400 | 52 | Working | 8 |
| 6 | None | 5410 | 5 | Working | 7 |
| 7 | CVA day 31, WR, infection | 3910 | 50 | Rehabilitation | 2 |
| 8 | CT days 15 and 22, RF, WR | 6200 | 122 | Transplanted | – |
| Mean | | 4468 | 18 | | |
| ±SD | | 1710 | 23 | | |

*HTx*, Heart transplantation; *CT*, cardiac tamponade; *RF*, renal failure; *CVA*, cerebrovascular accident; *WR*, wound revision

patients a rethoracotomy was performed twice for cardiac tamponade. One patient underwent a revision of the subcutaneous area of the abdominal pocket because of a hematoma.

Two long-term patients had a cerebrovascular accident (thromboembolism) during left ventricular circulatory support (Table 3) which occurred on the 40th (serious impairment of visual function) and on the 31st day (hemiparesis) of support. As reasons for the occurrence of these thromboembolic events we suggest that in one patient the platelet function became normal while he was neither on ASA nor on dipyridamole medication. Additionally, there was a period of low pump output (<3.5 l/min) due to hypovolemia. In the second patient the thromboembolic event occurred when the cardiac rhythm converted spontaneously from atrial fibrillation to sinus rhythm.

The suggested source for thromboembolism was found in the two long-term patients after explantation of the Novacor LVAS. Varying degrees of deposition of thrombotic material were found on the convex and concave sides of the inflow

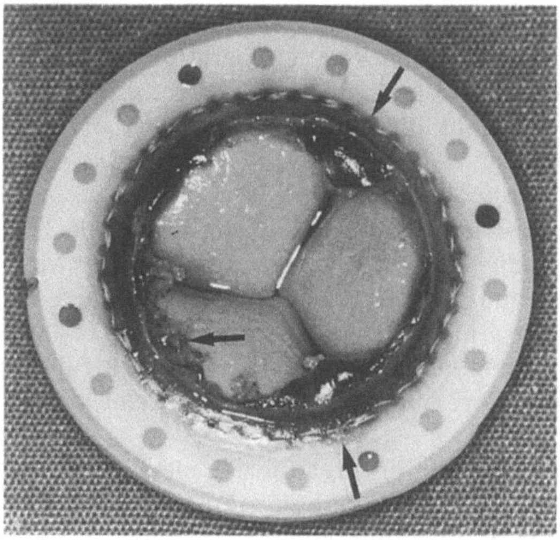

**Fig. 6.** An explanted inflow bovine pericardial valve prosthesis 52 days after Novacor implantation. Concave side reveals areas of thrombus formation (*arrows*)

pericardial valve prostheses (Fig. 6). The neurological lesions which resulted from the thromboembolic events resolved completely in one patient; in the other patient only a minor neurological deficit remained.

### Outcome

The first five patients were supported for a short term (<7 days) and the following three patients for a long-term or chronic period (≥50 days). One patient had been on the support device for 122 days. Orthotopic heart transplantation was performed in eight patients. Cardiopulmonary bypass was established by cannulation of the femoral vessels and the chest was carefully reopened. One patient died 2 days after transplantation due to unspecific donor heart failure. The remaining seven patients are alive and well 4–24 months after heart transplantation. Four patients returned to work, one patient was already retired before the operation, and one patient is currently in rehabilitation.

## Comments

This series of patients who underwent bridge-to-cardiac transplantation with the Novacor left ventricular assist system shows that mechanical circulatory support can be done with low mortality and leads to a significant hemodynamic improvement and physical rehabilitation. Hemodynamic data show that parameters of left heart function can be improved significantly within 24 h of left ventricular circulatory support. In the majority of patients pump operation was performed in the "fill-rate-trigger mode" immediately after Novacor implantation, providing a pump output ranging between 4.5 and 8.0 l/min. As a result, impaired renal function improved rapidly within hours or within the first 2 postoperative days. Only in two patients was continuous hemofiltration necessary in the early postoperative phase. Despite severe impairment, the right heart function improved significantly during left ventricular support only. The implantation of a right ventricular assist device was not indicated. In a clinical study Kormos et al. [9] demonstrated an improvement of the right heart function in most of their patients after implantation of the Novacor system.

At our center the Novacor LVAS has proved to be a highly reliable system to assist the failing heart. Technical faults were not detected during operation. The long-term patients were trained to handle their own "power supply"; they were able to change and recharge batteries and prepare for out-of-hospital walks on their own. Noise of the pump was not a major problem for the patients. The development of the wearable system was a major step forward, providing more mobility for long-term patients and therefore improved quality of life during the waiting period.

However, thromboembolism remains the major threat during mechanical circulatory support. Since we have used a triple-drug therapy consisting of heparin (intravenously or subcutaneously), ASA, and dipyridamole no more thromboembolic complications have occurred in our long-term patients. Obviously, the housing of the inflow prosthetic valve is susceptible to such a phenomenon. Even in patients without clinical evidence of thromboembolism the inflow valve frequently showed some degree of deposition of thrombotic material (Fig. 6). Wagner et al. [10] investigated explanted bioprostheses from 23 Novacor patients. They found that valve thrombus deposition located on the inflow valve of the Novacor system and low pump output were related to the occurrence of thromboembolic events. Therefore, multiple factors have to be taken into account in order to prevent thromboembolic complications.

In summary, the Novacor LVAS provides a safe and sufficient method of mechanical circulatory support in bridge-to-transplant patients. In order to reduce thromboembolic complications, changes in the design of the pump inflow appear to be necessary.

*Acknowledgements.* The authors gratefully thank Mr. Steger and Mrs. von Yorck from the Deparment of Photograhy and Graphics at Grosshadern Hospital.

## References

1. Ramasamy N, Portner PM (1993) Results with bridge to transplant and chronic support. In: Ott RA, Gutfinger DE, Gazzaniga AB (eds) Cardiac surgery. Mechanical cardiac assist. Hanley and Belfus, Philadelphia, pp 363–377
2. Hetzer R, Hennig E, Schiessler A, Friedel N, Warnecke H, Adt M (1992) Mechanical circulatory support and heart transplantation. J Heart Lung Transplant 11:175–181
3. Kormos RL, Murali S, Dew MA, Armitage JM, Hardesty RL, Borovetz HS, Griffith BP (1994) Chronic mechanical circulatory support: rehabilitation, low morbidity, and superior survival. Ann Thorac Surg 57:51–58
4. McCarthy PM, Portner PM, Tobler GH, Starnes VA, Ramasamy N, Oyer PE (1991) Clinical experience with the Novacor ventricular assist system. J Thorac Cardiovasc Surg 102:578–587
5. Oyer PE, Stinson EB, Portner PM, Ream AK, Shumway NE (1980) Development of a totally implantable electrically actuated left ventricular assist system. Am J Surg 140:17–24

6. Buckberg GD (1987) Strategies and logic of cardioplegic delivery to prevent, avoid, and reverse ischemic and reperfusion damage. J Thorac Cardiovasc Surg 88:726–741
7. Kratzer M, Born GV (1985) Simulation of primary hemostasis in vitro. Hemostasis 15:357–362
8. Szukalski EA, Reedy JE, Pennington DG, Swartz MT, McBride LR, Miller LW (1990) Oral anticoagulation in patients with ventricular assist devices. ASAIO Trans 36:M700–M703
9. Kormos RL, Gasior T, Antaki J, Armitage JM, Miyamoto Y, Borovetz HS, Hardesty RL, Griffith BP (1989) Evaluation of right ventricular function during clinical left ventricular assistance. ASAIO Trans 35:547–550
10. Wagner WR, Johnson PC, Kormos RL, Griffith BP (1993) Evaluation of bioprosthetic valve-associated thrombus in ventricular assist device patients. Circulation 88 (pt 1):2023–2029

# Clinical Results of the HeartMate Implantable Blood Pump

V. Poirier and K. Dasse

## Introduction

Cardiac transplantation has become a widely accepted therapy for patients with end-stage heart disease. The demand for donor organs, however, far exceeds the supply. Consequently, a significant percentage of transplant candidates die while waiting for a donor heart. Temporary mechanical circulatory support for patients waiting for donor organs was introduced by Cooley and co-workers in 1969. Subsequent research has led to the development of ventricular assist devices for use as a bridge to transplantation. The results with these devices have been highly encouraging for the support of postcardiotomy, postinfarction, and end-stage cardiomyopathy patients, with support now extending beyond 16 months.

Among the currently available left ventricular assist devices (LVADs), two are specifically designed for long-term mechanical circulatory support. Thermo Cardiosystems (TCI, Woburn, MA, USA) and Novacor (Oakland, CA, USA) have developed implantable, pusher-plate type LVADs that are undergoing clinical evaluation under Food and Drug Administration (FDA)-approved investigational device exemptions. Both devices have been successfully employed as a long-term bridge to transplant with the TCI device, the HeartMate blood pump, having supported a patient for 503 days. The purpose of this report is to summarize the results obtained with the TCI HeartMate air- and electrically driven LVAD, which have been under evaluation since August 1985.

To extend the use of LVADs to the clinical community, sufficient data must be gathered and presented to the FDA to prove, scientifically, that the device is safe and effective. To be considered safe, the device must be reliable and must not jeopardize the ability to transplant the patient; that is, the device should not be associated with severe adverse effects, such as infection, bleeding, hemolysis, end-organ dysfunction, or thromboembolic complications. To be considered effective, the device must improve the hemodynamic status of the patient, enhance the likelihood of survival, and, ideally, promote a higher quality of life than would be otherwise possible without the device.

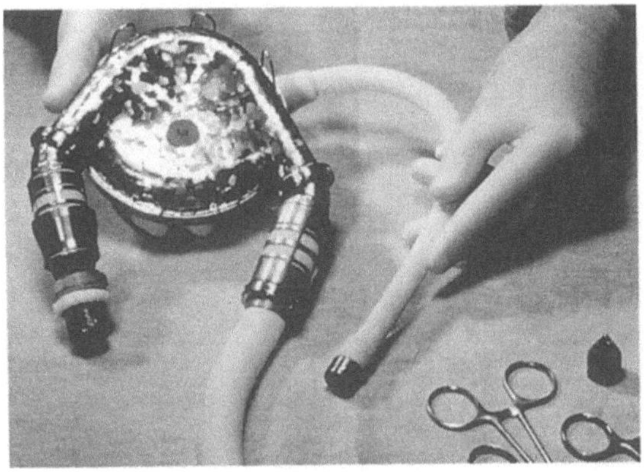

**Fig. 1.** The HeartMate blood pump. Stroke volume 83 ml, up to 11 pm. porcine xenograft valves

# Materials and Methods

## Description of the Device

Patients with acute LV failure have different requirements than those who will require long-term support. We have chosen to concentrate our efforts on supporting patients with chronic LV failure and, as such, have designed systems for long-term use. The requirements for these systems are that they must be implantable to reduce the threat of infection, portable, durable, and simple to operate and must reduce the likelihood of thromboemoblic complications.

Considering all of these factors, TCI's concept was to develop an implantable blood pump that could be driven by either air or electrical energy. It is imperative that systems be as flexible as possible and that they present the safest choice to the patient. Electric systems are by far the most portable systems. An electric system that can also be operated with an air driver is a major advantage and provides an excellent backup system in the event of an electrical or mechanical failure of the system.

Both the air-operated and electric versions of the system utilize exactly the same blood pump as shown in Fig. 1. The air-operated HeartMate LVAD consists of a pusher-plate blood pump driven by a portable external console via a percutaneous driveline. The pump consists of a titanium alloy housing measuring 11.2 cm in diameter and 4.0 cm in thickness. Inside, a flexible polyurethane diaphragm is bonded to a rigid pusher plate. The diaphragm divides the pump housing into two halves: a blood chamber and an air chamber, as shown in Fig. 2. Programmed pulses of air are delivered from the console to the air chamber behind the pusher-plate diaphragm. As the air accumulates, the diaphragm is displaced, propelling the blood through the outflow graft into the arterial circulation. Porcine xenograft valves (25 mm) are placed in the inlet and outlet conduits to ensure unidirectional blood flow.

Two types of air drivers are used to activate this blood pump: a portable console which is fully instrumented and shown in Fig. 3, and a noninstrumented

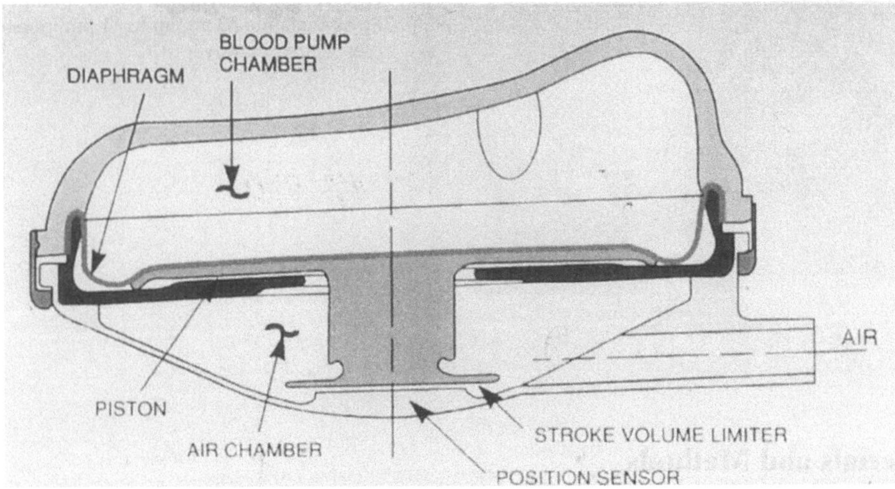


**Fig. 2.** Cross-ectional view of the HeartMate implantable pneumatic blood pump for long-term use

miniature version shown in Fig. 4. Both consoles are battery operated, with the miniaturized version providing up to 7 h of use from one set of batteries.

Both consoles are designed for long-term use and for portability. The consoles provide programmed pneumatic pulses up to a maximum rate of 140 bpm. Two control modes are available: fixed rate and auto rate. The fixed rate is selectable from a minimum of 20 bpm to a maximum of 140 bpm, while the auto rate continuously varies, depending on blood flow into the pump. In the auto mode, the pump will eject when it is 90% full. Rates will automatically adjust to meet this criterion.

The electrically operated version of the HeartMate LVAD utilizes the same blood pump as the air-operated version. As shown in Fig. 5, the electromechanical driver consists of an electronically commutated low-speed torque motor that drives the pusher plate through a pair of nested helical cams. The torque motor itself consists of a stationary copper wave-wound stator, a rotating magnet assembly, and an electronic commutator. The electronic commutator uses solid-state Hall-effect devices to sense rotor position and, through electronic logic, switches the power transistors that control power distribution to the windings. This starts from any position when power is applied. No start-up sequence is required.

The motor operates at physiologic speeds, with one motor revolution corresponding to one pump ejection cycle. As the magnet assembly of the torque motor rotates, two diametrically opposed ball-bearing cam followers bear against nested helical face cams. These face cams are fixed to the pusher plate and serve to convert the rotary motion of the pump to the linear motion of the pusher plate.

The LVAD reacts to each ejection cycle as an individual event. When the commutator receives a start signal, it rotates one revolution and stops. The motor then sits in the standby configuration until another start signal is received. There

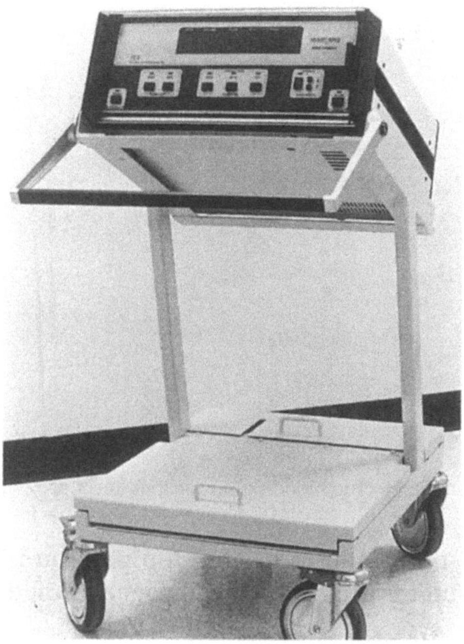

**Fig. 3.** Hospital-based pneumatic console for the HeartMate blood pump

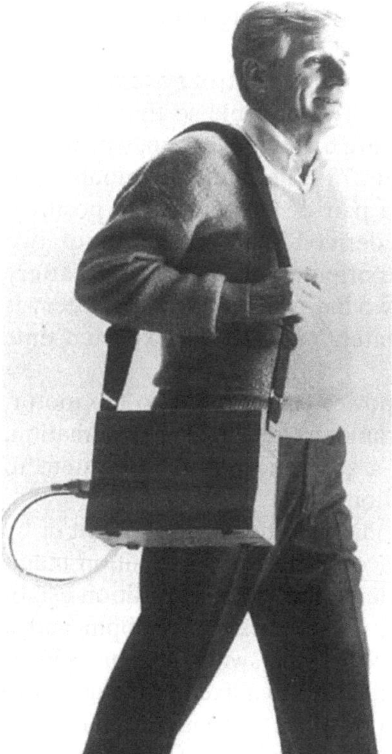

**Fig. 4.** Portable, battery-operated pneumatic console for the HeartMate blood pump

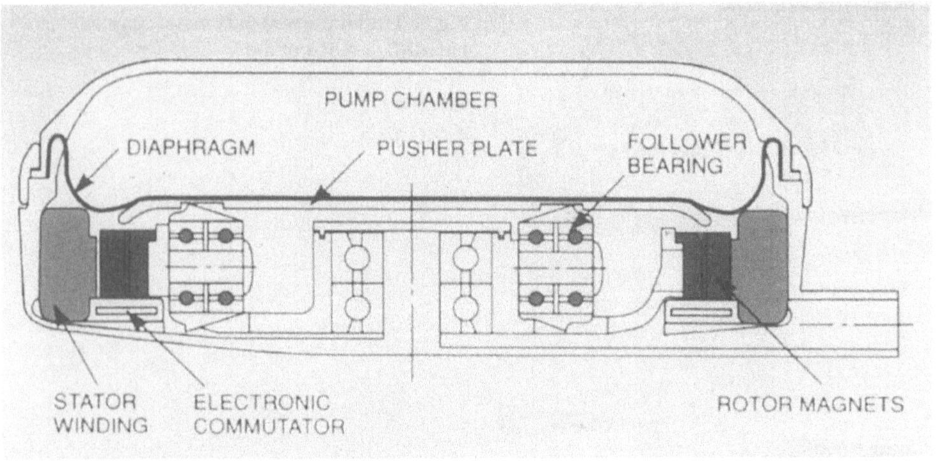


**Fig. 5.** Cross-ectional view of the HeartMate implantable electric blood pump for long-term use

is no need to predict future events based on past history. The stop position is determined by a Hall Sensor on the commutator ring and a small magnet buried in the titanium hub of the rotor.

The weight of the combined pump, torque motor, and energy converter is 908 g, and the displacement is 460 cc. The conduits weigh an additional 161 g, and the displacement is 174 cc. This includes all protective housing, cables, tubes, and connectors.

The vented electric system is operated by a portable control system which is worn by the patient. It is designed to be as small as possible so that it can be conveniently clipped onto a belt. Its dimensions are $6.2 \times 7.6 \times 1.9$ cm, with a total weight with attached cables and connnectors of 275 g. Permanently mounted to the housings are two leads which connect to a pair of batteries via a positive-acting, push-type sealed connector. Power is derived from either one or two batteries to provide redundancy. The preferred orientation to maximize battery life is to use the system coupled in parallel to two batteries. When one battery is used, battery life will be reduced to approximately one half the expected time that two batteries would provide.

The control system is designed to provide power conditioning to the motor, rate control, documentation of operating parameters, diagnostic information, and basal level default capability, as well as a sophisticated alarm system to provide the patient with a warning of malfunction.

Motor rate control is optional and can be modified either by the patient or by the attending physician. The control system incorporates a two-position membrane switch that can be controlled by the patient. The primary position establishes a predetermined fixed rate that can be varied between 50 bpm and a maximum of 120 bpm in increments of 1 bpm. When the switch is depressed by the patient, the control function will be changed either to a fixed rate augmentation by a step difference between 1 and 20 bpm or to an “auto mode.” The auto mode automatically varies the rate as a function of the volume of blood entering

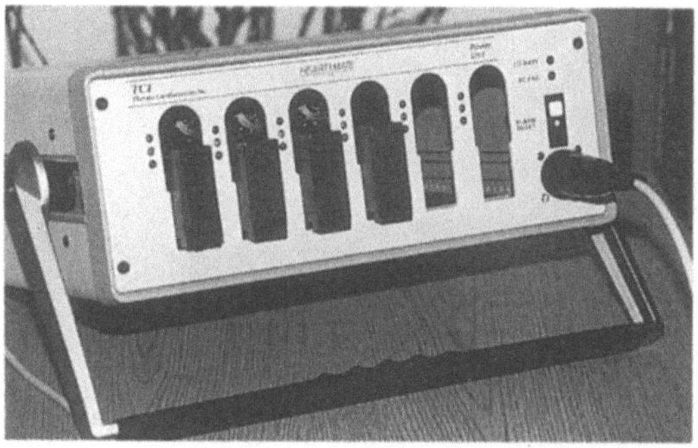

**Fig. 6.** Power-base unit consisting of a 12-V power supply for nighttime use and a six-position battery charger

the pump chamber to maintain the pump stroke volume at 75 ml per beat. The rate of change can be adjusted between 1 and 5 bpm.

The control system digitizes the analog signal of motor current and voltage. These wave forms are used to calculate stroke volume as well as to determine motor operating voltage. In addition, the wave forms can be accessed through our software systems for display on a personal computer or for permanent storage on disk. System performance can then be documented on a real-time basis to establish wear trends over time.

This system utilizes two commercially available gel-type lead acid batteries. These standard six-cell packs are inexpensive and are 18 × 6 × 2 cm and weigh 636 g.

A power unit, shown in Fig. 6, provides the patient with an isolated 12-V power source to energize the electric system during periods when the batteries are not appropriate. In addition, this unit recharges up to six batteries at a time to provide the patient with freshly charged batteries. A digital display can also be attached to this power unit to continuously display stroke volume, rate, and flow.

## Blood-contacting Surfaces and Recommended Anticoagulation

The HeartMate LVAD employs textured biomaterials to interface with the blood. Sintered-titanium microspheres are used on the pump housing and conduits, and integrally textured polyurethane is utilized on the flexing pusher-plate diaphragm, as shown in Fig. 7. The rationale for using textured surfaces is to encourage the formation of a thin, well-adhered, pseudointimal lining on the inside of the pump. The resultant biologic lining serves as the primary interface with the patient's blood. A typical lining that has developed after 233 days in a human being is shown in Fig. 8.

The need for anticoagulation with this device has been greatly reduced by the use of porcine bioprosthetic valves in combination with the textured surfaces. In the majority of patients, an antiplatelet regimen consisting of 80 mg aspirin once a day and 75 mg dipyridamole three times daily has been used beyond the intraoperative period. Heparin and/or coumadin have been utilized only during implantation and in patients with mechanical valves in the native heart.

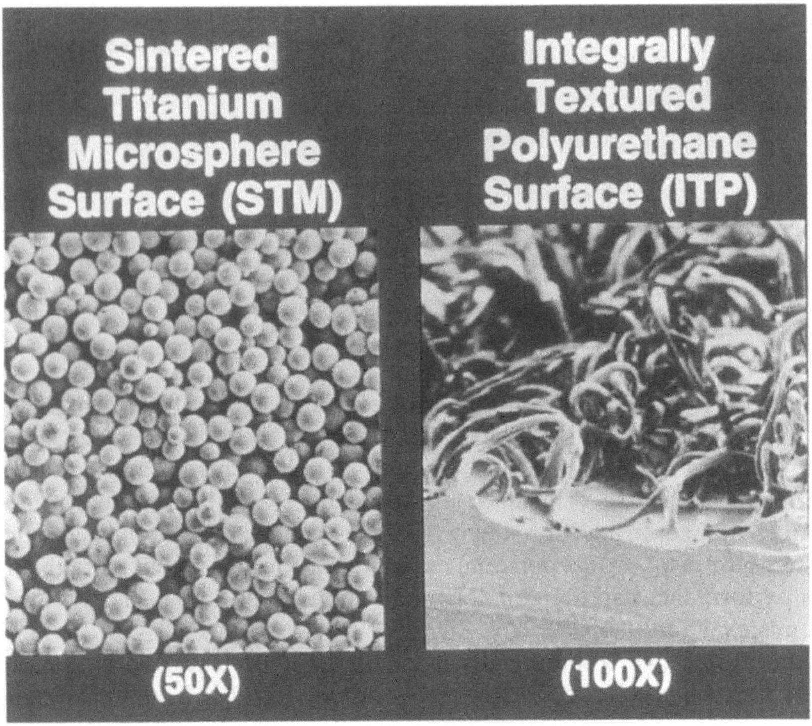


**Fig. 7.** Textured surfaces of the HeartMate blood pump

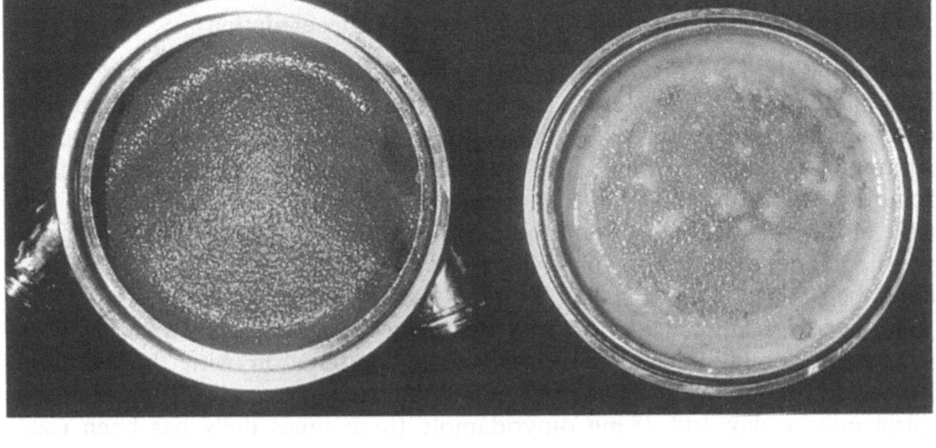

**Fig. 8.** Biologic lining produced by the textured surfaces of the HeartMate blood pump after 233 days in man

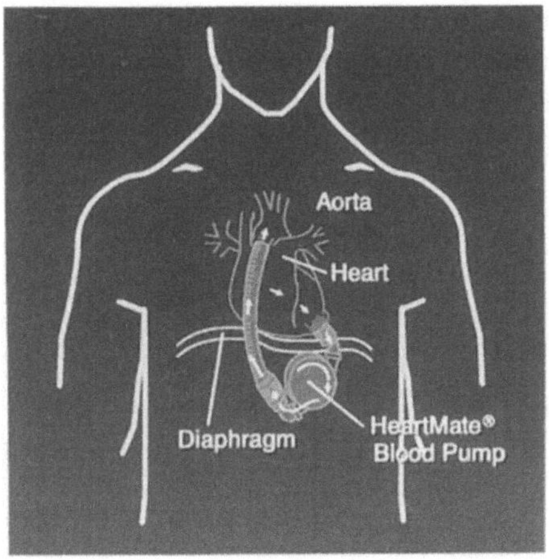


**Fig. 9.** Anatomic positioning of the implantable, long-term HeartMate blood pump

## Device Implantation

Device implantation is accomplished through a median sternotomy, with the incision extending just above the umbilicus, and cardiopulmonary bypass is instituted using standard techniques. The left ventricular apex is cored, and the opening is reinforced with a sewing ring. The pump is then placed in the left abdominal cavity below the diaphragm. An incision is made in the diaphragm, through which the inlet conduit is passed and then secured to the apical opening. The outflow graft (preclotted Dacron) is passed over the diaphragm and anastomosed end-to-side to the ascending aorta. Finally, the pneumatic or electric driveline is tunneled through a stab incision in the left lateral abdominal wall, above the iliac crest. After the pump has been implanted, the patient is gradually weaned from bypass, and the median sternotomy is closed. Figure 9 illustrates the implant position.

## Criteria for Inclusion

Both the air-driven and the electric version of the HeartMate blood pump are being evaluated in patients under two separate Investigational Device Exemptions (I.D.E.). The study protocol is identical for both systems and is restricted to patients that have been approved for cardiac transplantation. These patients have experienced nonreversible damage to the myocardium and require additional circulatory support to sustain life. Patients in acute LV failure thought to be reversible were not included in this study.

The majority of candidates entered into the study suffered from end-stage cardiac failure. Additional patients who had experienced a recent myocardial infarction (MI) were also included, providing they were approved transplant candidates and were over the acute stage of the insult, i.e., that more than 7 days had passed since the onset of the MI.

The decision to implant the device was made if (a) the patient met one of the following categories of acceptance criteria, and (b) the patient was not subject to the exclusion criteria.

*Category I*
(a) Approved transplant candidate
(b) On inotropes
(c) On a ballon pump (if possible)
(d) LAP or PCWP $\geqslant$ 20 mmHg with:
  1. Systolic BP 80 mmHg or less, *or*
  2. Cardiac index 2.0 l/min/m$^2$ or less

*Category II*
(a) Approved transplant candidate
(b) On inotropes; on IABP, if possible
(c) Cardiac arrest
(d) Systolic BP = 60 mmHg or less

## Results

A controlled clinical investigation has been in progress since August 1985 to study the safety and effectiveness of the air-operated HeartMate LVAD. The device has been evaluated for the temporary support of patients in severe left ventricular failure as a bridge to transplantation. One hundred thirty-three patients were enrolled in the study: 92 LVAD patients and 41 untreated control patients. A safety analysis was performed on all patients.

Eighty-eight patients met the study patient selection criteria and were included in an analysis to determine device effectiveness: 57 LVAD and 31 untreated control patients. The average duration from the time of enrollment into the study to either death or transplantation was 12 days for the control patients and 67 days for the LVAD-treated patients. The demographics of the patient population is shown in Table 1, while the summary of results is shown in Tables 2 and 3.

The results of the study in terms of effectiveness and safety are as follows:

- The device was found to provide adequate hemodynamic support for periods of up to 324 days.
- Sixty-eight percent of the LVAD patients underwent transplantation, compared with 39% of the control patients.
- Sixty-three percent of the LVAD patients survived 60 days or longer, compared with 32% of the untreated control group.
- The device was hemodynamically effective. The average pump index (flow/body surface area) for all LVAD treated patients was 48% greater than the baseline cardiac index.
- Minimal damage was done to the cellular elements of the blood. The average plasma-free hemoglobin value for all patients was less than 10 mg/dl.
- Renal and hepatic function improved for LVAD survivors as a result of left

**Table 1.** Patient characteristics

| Parameter | LVAD patients $n = 57$ (%) | Control patients $n = 31$ (%) |
|---|---|---|
| Average age | 46 | 47 |
| Age range | 14–64 | 21–67 |
| Male | 49 (86) | 24 (77) |
| Sex | | |
| Female | 8 (14) | 7 (23) |
| Indications | | |
| Idiopathic cardiomyopathy | 28 (49) | 12 (39) |
| Ischemic cardiomyopathy | 24 (42) | 18 (58) |
| Subacute myocardial Infarction | 5 (9) | 1 (3) |

**Table 2.** Summary of results in the LVAD group

| | |
|---|---|
| Number of LVAD-treated patients | 57 |
| Number of patients who died prior to transplantation | 18 (31) |
| Number of patients who received a transplant | 39 (68) |
| Number of patients who died before 60 days post transplantation | 3 (8) |
| Number of patients alive ≥60 days post transplantation | 36 (92) |
| Percent survival of LVAD-treated patients | 63 |

**Table 3.** Summary of results in the control group

| | |
|---|---|
| Number of control patients | 31 |
| Number of patients who died prior to transplantation | 19 (61) |
| Number of patients who received a transplant | 12 (39) |
| Number of patients who died before 60 days post transplantation | 2 (17) |
| Number of patients alive ≥ 60 days post transplantation | 10 (83) |
| Percent survival of control patients | 32 |

ventricular assistance, based on marked reductions in total bilirubin, SGOT, SGPT, creatinine, and blood urea nitrogen levels.
- There were only two device-related thromboembolic complications with patients being principally anticoagulated with only aspirin and persantine.
- Eighteen percent of all LVAD patients had percutaneous driveline infections; 94% of these patients underwent transplantation and survived.

To date there have been no significant differences between patients utilizing the air-operated version or the electrically operagted system. As shown in Table 4, results are quite similar with both systems.

**Table 4.** Comparison of hemodynamics using pneumatic or electric pump

| | Pneumatic | Electric |
|---|---|---|
| Total number of patients | 123 | 8 |
| Cumulative duration of support (years) | 23 | 3.5 |
| Longest support to date (days) | 343 | 503 |
| Pump Index (l/min/m²) | 2.7 | 2.7 |
| Average pump flow (l/min) | 4.8 | 5.8 |
| Maximum pump flow (l/min) | 10.1 | 9.6 |
| Mean arterial pressure (mmHg) | 90 | 97 |
| Hematocrit (%) | 33 | 37 |
| Hemoglobin (g/dl) | 11 | 12 |
| Plasma-free hemoglobin (mg/dl) | 8 | 8 |
| Platelet count (×10³/ml) | 256 | 228 |

## Discussion

Clinical results of the HeartMate blood pump are very encouraging. After 27 patient years of experience, we are now confident that the device can produce the blood flow required for extended periods of time with adequate pressures and minimal blood damage. Utilizing this device in the bridge-to-transplant category is merely the first step in the development of this technology. Our goal is to use the HeartMate blood pump as an alternative to transplant, not only as an alternative to medical treatment. We are now proceeding in that direction with recent approval from the FDA to discharge patients to their home environment. We now have approval to implant the HeartMate blood pump, allow the patient to recover fully, and release the patient from the hospital to his or her home where they can wait comfortably for a donor heart.

Patients released to their home environment can have a high quality of life with full freedom for an active and productive existence. Heart-assist technology must lead to this end if it is to be useful to society. The initial steps in meeting this goal have been accomplished after 25 years of development. The development of this technology must continue to provide an alternative to the thousands of people every year who die needlessly while waiting for a scarce donor heart.

# The Abiomed BVS 5000 for Treatment of Postcardiotomy Cardiogenic Shock

P.A.M. Everts, J.P.A.M. Schönberger, and C.H. Peels

## Introduction

Improvements in myocardial protection techniques during open heart surgery have reduced the incidence of perioperative ventricular failure and myocardial infarction [1, 2]. Despite these advances, postcardiotomy ventricular failure is observed in nearly 4% of all patients undergoing cardiopulmonary bypass (CPB) procedures [3, 4]. Conventional inotropic therapy and/or application of the intra-aortic ballon pump (IABP) are indicated in these patients [5, 6]. However, myocardial function does not improve in all these patients, despite these measures. Therefore, for approximately 0.7% of all patients undergoing open heart surgery, more effective circulatory support devices are needed [7]. These temporary mechanical circulatory support devices maintain the systemic and/or pulmonary circulation and unload the left ventricle, creating a condition of myocardial rest in patients with potentially reversible myocardial failure while the myocardium recovers. This report describes our experience in 15 patients with postcardiotomy ventricular failure who were treated with the Abiomed BVS 5000 pulsatile sac-type pump (Abiomed Cardiovascular, Inc., Danvers, MA, USA) [8, 9].

## Patients and Methods

The Abiomed BVS 5000 pulsatile assist device was implanted in 11 male and four female patients ranging in age from 38 to 69 years (mean age 51 years) who were suffering from postcardiotomy cardiogenic shock, not treatable with such conventional therapeutic techniques as volume loading, inotropic support with calcium chloride, dopamine, dobutamine, epinephrine, enoximone, and counterpulsation with an intra-aortic ballon pump (IABP). Cardiogenic shock was defined as a cardiac index less than 1.8 l/min/m$^2$ body surface area, with a peak systolic blood pressure less than 90 mm Hg and a pulmonary artery diastolic pressure and/or right atrial pressure higher than 20 mm Hg.

In all patients the cannulas for the blood pumps were placed during CPB. When left heart support was started, CPB was terminated. Then the right heart support device was started and complete biventricular support with the biventricular assist device (BIVAD) was initiated.

## Device Description

The Abiomed BVS 5000 system consists of an automated electromechanical console, disposable sac-type pulsatile blood pumps, and transthoracic cannulas (Fig. 1). The drive console is a microprocessor-controlled pneumatic drive system. The completely closed loop control system eliminates the need for operator adjustment of flow, pressures, vacuum, timing, and electrocardiogram trimming, which simplifies treatment with this device. The only controls that need to be taken care of are the on/off switch, weaning controls for lowering the level of ventricular support, and the level of gravity drainage. The console continuously displays pump flow and rate. The pumps are most frequently run in the so-called fill-to-empty mode with a maximum stroke volume of 82 ml, whereas the weaning mode is used only when the heart shows signs of recovery. The console drives and adjusts the left and/or right blood pump independent of each other to accomplish pulmonary and systemic circulation.

The disposable heterotopic vertical blood pumps are externally placed on the patient. The pump is designed much like the natural heart. It contains a filling chamber (artificial atrium), which acts as a compliant reservoir, and a pumping chamber (artificial ventricle). The artificial ventricle is situated between two trileaflet valves. The inflow valve resides between the artificial atrium and artificial ventricle. The outlet valve isolates the artificial ventricle from the patient's circulation (Fig. 2). Both pump chambers consist of an elastomeric bladder and are like the valves made from smooth-surfaced polyurethane Angioflex (Abiomed Cardiovascular, Inc. Danvers, MA, USA).

At the top of the blood pump where the artificial atrium is positioned the blood flows into the pump, and thereafter blood is returned to the patient from

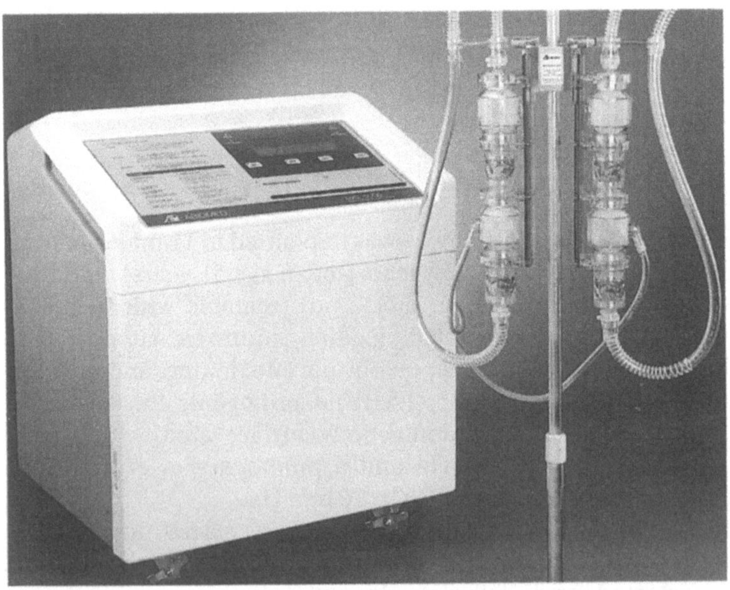

**Fig. 1.** Abiomed console and blood pumps. (Courtesy of ABIOMED Inc.)

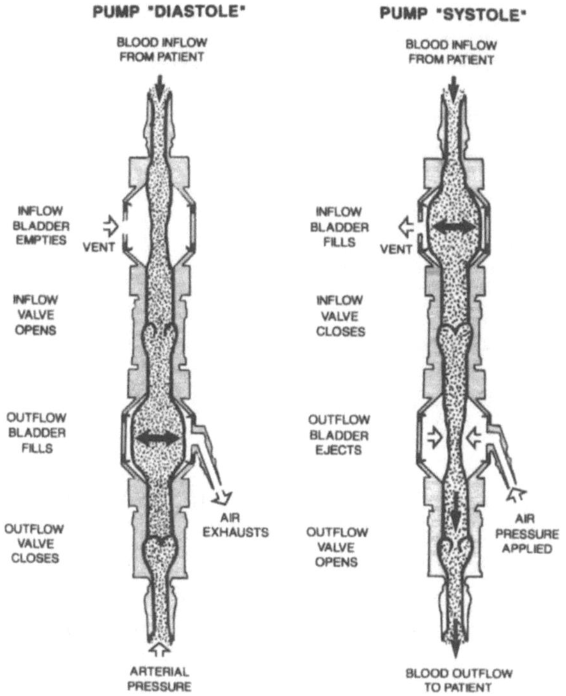


**Fig. 2.** Abiomed BVS 5000 blood pump and circulation pattern within the pump during systole and diastole. (Courtesy of ABIOMED Inc.)

the bottom of the pump. Due to the dual-chambered configuration of the device, the artificial atrium is filled during pump systole by gravity alone, while the inflow valve is closed. This continuous filling by gravity obviates the need for a vacuum. The passive fill design of the BVS blood pump is unique to the Abiomed system, because most pneumatic ventricular assist devices fill the pump by applying vacuum (e.g., Thoratec assist device). The artificial ventricle is collapsed and emptied by a positive pressure pulse from the console, thus ejecting blood into the patient's systemic and\or pulmonary circulation. Beat rates and systolic\diastolic intervals are determined automatically by sensing gas flow to and from the blood pumps. All information for running and controlling the system is obtained through the air line, which is the only connection between the drive console and blood pump.

## Cannulas

The blood pumps and tubing are primed and accurately de-aired with 20% human albumin in Ringers solution. The blood pump is connected to the patient's heart via 0.5-inch class-VI Tygon medical-grade tubing (Norton Plastics, Akron, OH) connected to inflow and outflow cannulas. The cannulas are made from wire-reinforced medical-grade polyvinylchloride, and the exterior surface incorporates a Dacron velour sleeve at the skin interface (Fig. 3). The atrial cannulas incorporate a right-angled 46-F lighthouse tip.

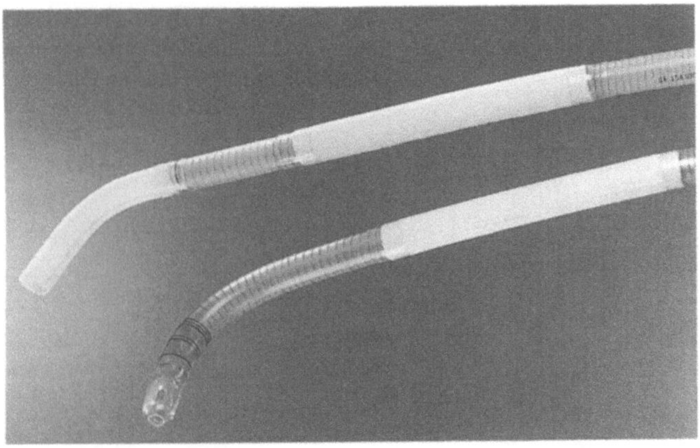

**Fig. 3.** Atrial and arterial BVS cannulas. (Courtesy of ABIOMED Inc.)

The left atrial cannula was situated in the left atrium posterior to the interatrial groove in 12 patients. In three patients, the cannula was placed directly in the left atrium through the left atrial appendage. The right atrium was cannulated in ten patients through the right atrial appendage and in five patients through the right atrial free wall. The pursestring sutures of the atrial cannulas were incorporated with a strip of pericardial tissue to prevent bleeding from the suture holes. The return cannulas consisted of 14-F zero-porosity Dacron grafts connected to the ascending aorta and the pulmonary artery with an end-to-side anastomosis. The cannulas were tunneled through the skin below the costal margin. In ten patients the sternum was closed without compromising the output of the blood pumps. In the remaining patients, the sternum was closed after decannulation.

## Anticoagulation

All patients were anticoagulated with bovine lung heparin during CPB. When the patient could be weaned from CPB with the BIVAD, heparin was neutralized by protamine sulfate at a dose 1.0–1.3 times the total dosage of heparin, to achieve the baseline level of the activated clotting time (ACT) as measured after induction of anesthesia.

For the first 24 h after the initiation of BIVAD therapy, anticoagulation was withheld as long as the pump output was more than 4.0 l/min. The first goal during this period was to control bleeding. If the ACT was prolonged (>150 s) then a bolus of 25 mg protamine sulfate was given until hemostasis was achieved. In general, a continuous infusion of heparin was started 24 h postoperatively, keeping the ACT between 180 and 200 s, as monitored with the Hemochron system (International Technidyne Corp., Edison, NJ).

## Hemodynamic Monitoring and Transesophageal Echocardiographic Studies

Patients were monitored with continuous electrocardiographic tracings, a radial artery line, and a pulmonary artery catheter. Standard thermodilution techniques were used to determine cardiac output and vascular resistances prior to and after the removal of the device. During the period of complete biventricular support no cardiac output determinations were made. The artificial cardiac output was displayed at the console.

During BIVAD support, the systemic vascular resistance (SVR) was calculated from the pump output [10]. The SVR was maintained in the range of 600–1000 dynes-s/cm$^5$ using continuous intravenous infusions of either sodium nitroprusside or phenylephrine. The pulmonary vascular resistance was kept between 100 and 300 dynes-s/cm$^5$ with a continuous infusion of nitroglycerin via the pulmonary artery catheter, directly into the pulmonary artery. During BIVAD support a low-dose infusion of dopamine (2 µg/kg/min) was administered to improve renal function.

Prior to BIVAD implantation and after removal of the device, the left ventricular stroke work index (LVSWI) was calculated to assess the contractility status before and after biventricular support. This formula reflects the amount of work that the left ventricle generates per beat [10].

Perioperative transesophageal echocardiography (TEE) is widely used in cardiac surgery to evaluate reconstructive surgery [11], or to clarify problems related to weaning patients from CPB. Prior to BIVAD implantation, TEE was used to guide the selection of suitable patients for circulatory support treatment. TEE can provide useful information regarding underlying cardiac diseases responsible for the inability to wean from CPB, such as left ventricular hypovolemia in patients with extreme left ventricular hypertrophy or severe valve regurgitation. When severe pump failure was established as the cause of intractable weaning problems, and when dysfunction of a substantial part of the left ventricle was considered to be reversible, then a patient was considered to be a candidate for BIVAD treatment. Postoperatively, during circulatory support, TEE was used to monitor ventricular recovery and function. Furthermore, we wanted to establish a period of time after which no restoration of ventricular function could be expected.

## Laboratory Analysis

Extensive hematological and metabolic parameters were determined prior to, during, and after BIVAD support. At 4-h intervals patients were monitored for plasma-free hemoglobin, fibrinogen levels, hematocrit, platelet number, and fibrin split products. Major organ function was evaluated by examining blood urea nitrogen (BUN), creatinine, total bilirubin, lactic dehydrogenase (LDH), serum glutamic-oxaloacetic transaminase (SGOT), and arterial and venous blood gas values.

## Fluid Management

Fluid regimen consisted of a combination of Ringer's lactate, 5% glucose, and 0.9% saline. The total amount of daily administered fluids was 1 ml/kg/h. The urine output was maintained at more than 1 ml/kg body wt./h, if necessary diuretics like 20% mannitol or furosemide were used.

Volume loading with fresh-frozen plasma, platelet concentrate, packed cells, 20% mannitol, and 20% human albumin was performed according to intravascular filling and kidney function of the individual patient. Furthermore, to provide optimal BIVAD function the pulmonary artery capillary wedge pressure was maintained between 5 and 10 mm Hg, central venous pressure between 5 and 10 mm Hg.

Postoperative bleeding was graded as follows: acceptable-chest tube draining <100 ml/h during the first 6 h; moderate-chest tube draining 100–150 ml/h after the fourth postoperative hour; severe-chest tube draining >150 ml/h after the fourth postoperative hour.

## Weaning

Normally, patients were not able to generate any cardiac output during the first 48 h of biventricular support. Pump on/off data were not obtained before 4 days of myocardial rest. During this period the circulation was completely supported with the BIVAD, as shown in Fig. 4.

Weaning was attempted when changes in arterial and pulmonary artery pressure tracings were seen, and when decreased right and left atrial filling pressures were observed. For evaluation of restoration of cardiac function we allowed filling of the ventricles by decreasing the pump gravity level and reducing pump flow rate for an average period of 5 min, without inotropic support. With TEE the left ventricle was then properly imaged and the reaction to this volume load was carefully monitored and compared with the pre-BIVAD ventricular condition. Recovery of cardiac function was also demonstrated by the patients' arterial pressure waveform tracings, showing broad waveforms from the blood pump ejections and narrow waveforms indicating left ventricular ejection (Fig. 5). Definite weaning was accomplished by decreasing the left and right pump rate/output simultaneously by 0.5 l/min at intervals of 1 h. A minimal flow rate of 1.0 l/min was maintained for 1 h to ascertain that the cardiac function did not deteriorate. Thereafter, the patient was transported to the operating room for decannulation.

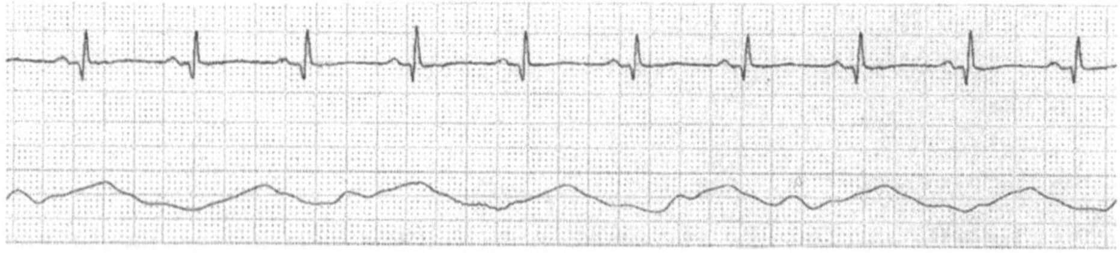

**Fig. 4.** ECG and arterial trace of patient 7 after 24 h of BIVAD support, with flows of >4.0 l/min (arterial blood pressure = 105/55 mm Hg)

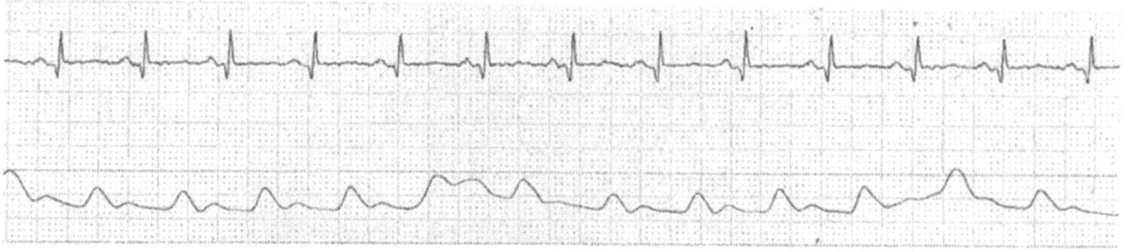

**Fig. 5.** ECG, and arterial pressure trace of patient 7 after 129 h of BIVAD support. Weaning flows have been reduced to 1.8 l/min (arterial blood pressure = 118/59 mm Hg)

In most patients during the weaning period, the hemodynamic status was carefully monitored with TEE to ensure that cardiac function did not deteriorate. However if during weaning the filling pressures rose, or the cardiac rhythm changed drastically with impaired cardiac function, weaning was terminated and the patient was again fully supported for another 24 h. Thereafter new weaning attempts were made.

To prevent thrombus formation during the weaning process, heparin infusion rates were increased and the ACT was kept between 300 and 350 s. With the flow rate set at 1.0 l/min, the ACT was kept above 400 s.

After the patients were weaned, the cannulas and blood pumps were rinsed in saline solution and both macroscopically and microscopically examined.

## Results

From June 1988 until September 1992, 3899 patients underwent cardiac surgery in our hospital. Fifteen of them (0.4%) required treatment with the Abiomed BVS 5000 for postcardiotomy cardiogenic shock. The patient characteristics are listed in Table 1. The patients underwent cardiac operations with standard CPB procedures: roller or centrifugal pump, membrane oxygenator, moderate hypothermia 25–30° C, crystalloid or blood cardioplegia solution. The prime consisted of Ringer's, urea-linked gelatins, and 20% mannitol. To the prime solution of the last nine patients, 2 million Kallikrein Inactivator Units of aprotinin (Trasylol Bayer AG, Leverkusen, Germany) were added [12].

The assist device was implanted in 12 patients who could not be weaned from CPB. The remaining three patients were initially successfully weaned from CPB. However, their cardiac condition deteriorated in the intensive care unit (ICU). They were transported to the operating room for reinstitution of CPB and ultimately the BIVAD was inserted.

Aortic cross-clamp times, total CPB times, and the interval between the first attempt to wean from CPB until insertion of the BIVAD are listed in Table 2. Prior to BIVAD implantation an IABP was temporarily inserted in 12 patients

**Table 1.** Patient characteristics

| Patient number | Age (years) | Sex | Operation | Priority of surgery | Pre-CPB infarction | Pre-CPB CI (l/m/m$^2$) | Pre-CPB PCWP (mm Hg) |
|---|---|---|---|---|---|---|---|
| 1 | 41 | F | CABG 3 | Urgent | Yes; 2 months | 1.7 | 17 |
| 2 | 38 | M | CABG 2 | Emergency | Yes; 1 h | NA | CPR |
| 3 | 54 | M | CABG 3 | Urgent | Yes; 5 months | 3.0 | 8 |
| 4 | 66 | M | CABG 5 | Urgent | Yes; 1 month | 2.3 | 7 |
| 5 | 52 | F | CABG 6 | Semi-urgent | Yes; 2 months | 2.1 | 10 |
| 6 | 42 | M | CABG 3 redo | Urgent | Yes; 9 months | 2.4 | 8 |
| 7 | 48 | M | CABG 4 | Urgent | Yes; 5 months | 3.0 | 11 |
| 8 | 63 | F | CABG 3 | Urgent | No | 2.3 | 8 |
| 9 | 67 | F | VSR repair | Emergency | Yes; 5 days | 1.5 | 22 |
| 10 | 53 | M | CABG 3 redo | Urgent | No | 2.4 | 9 |
| 11 | 42 | M | CABG 4 | Emergency | Yes; 1 h | NA | CPR |
| 12 | 69 | M | CABG 3 | Emergency | Yes; 2 h | 2.1 | 24 |
| 13 | 39 | M | CABG 5 | Semi-urgent | No | 2.4 | 10 |
| 14 | 46 | M | CABG 4 | Emergency | Yes; 2 h | NA | CPR |
| 15 | 57 | M | CABG 2 redo | Urgent | Yes; 4 years | 2.0 | 21 |

*CABG*, Coronary artery bypass grafting; *VSR*, ventricular septal rupture; *NA*, not available; *CPR*, cardiopulmonary resuscitation; *CI*, cardiac index; *PCWP*, pulmonary capillary wedge pressure

**Table 2.** Pre- and postoperative data

| | Mean | Range |
|---|---|---|
| Cross-clamp time | 66 min | 27–106 |
| Total CPB time | 321 min | 220–517 |
| CPB to BIVAD time[a] | 229 min | 101–498 |
| Duration IABP trial | 86 min | 30–180 |
| Duration BIVAD | 132 h | 95–151 |
| Left pump flow | 2.31 l/min/m$^2$ | 1.97–2.65 |
| Right pump flow | 2.21 l/min/m$^2$ | 1.89–2.54 |

*CPB*, Cardiopulmonary bypass; *BIVAD*, biventricular assist; *IABP*, intra-aortic ballon pump
[a] Time from first attempt to wean from CPB until initiation of BIVAD support.

but was removed after initiation of BIVAD treatment. Patient 6 and patient 11 died in the operating room due to exsanguination. In patient 6 the very thin walled left atrium ruptured and led to uncontrollable bleeding. In patient 11 dislodgement of the left atrial cannula was followed by massive air embolism. Thirteen patients were weaned from CPB with the Abiomed operating in a biventricular mode, and they were stabilized in the ICU. Fifteen minutes after the start of BIVAD support, the peak right and left blood pump flows were respectively 2.01 ± 0.23 l/min/m$^2$ and 2.18 ± 0.26 l/min/m$^2$ for all patients in whom full BIVAD support was initiated.

The indication for Abiomed implantation was guided with TEE in eight patients. Postoperatively, Abiomed treatment was closely followed in six of these eight. One patient died shortly after implantation of the device and in one patient logistic problems prevented postoperative TEE follow-up. In the remaining six patients left ventricular pump failure occurred after cardiac surgery. In five patients myocardial stunning was suspected and in one patient a massive anterior infarction preceded the operation. This patient was treated with the assist device because heart transplantation was optional at the time of the operation. These six patients were studied serially with TEE to evaluate whether successful weaning from the BIVAD could be predicted. Four patients showed contraction of the myocardium (hypokinesia or normokinesia) of more than 50% of the left ventricular circumference in the short-axis view in any TEE examination after 96–144 h of biventricular support. These patients were all successfully weaned from the assist device. Two of the six patients revealed less than 50% contraction of the circumference in all examinations; they could not be weaned and died while on the BIVAD owing to persistent pump failure, 2 and 5 days after implantation of the assist device. Postoperatively, laboratory enzyme analysis and ECGs revealed that 11 of the 13 treated patients had experienced a myocardial infarction during the perioperative period.

During the period of myocardial rest, the LVSWI for all the weaned patients increased from 5.5 g.m/m$^2$ (range 1.6–9.4) before biventricular assistance to 19.1 g.m/m$^2$ (range 15.0–24.6) after the device was removed. The increased

LVSWI suggests that recovery of myocardial function is possible in patients suffering from postcardiotomy cardiogenic shock.

## Complications

Bleeding was the most frequent complication associated with temporary ventricular support (Table 3). We observed that patients who survived Abiomed treatment required fewer blood (product) transfusions than patients who did not survive BIVAD treatment (Fig. 6). Ten patients underwent a rethoracotomy in

**Table 3.** Postoperative complications of BIVAD therapy

| Complication | *n* |
|---|---|
| Bleeding | 10 |
| Infection | 5 |
| Sepsis | 3 |
| Renal failure | 4 |
| Respiratory failure | 2 |
| Hemolysis | 0 |
| Embolic events | 0 |
| Neurological | 0 |
| Thrombus in system | 2 |
| Cannula-related | 1 |
| Device failure | 0 |

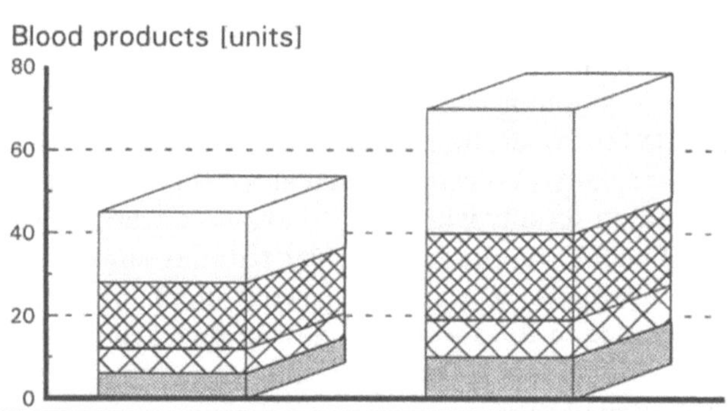


| | Survivors | Non survivors |
|---|---|---|
| Human Albumin | 6 | 10 |
| Platelets | 6 | 9 |
| Fresh Frozen Plasma | 16 | 21 |
| Packed Cells | 17 | 30 |
| | 45 | 70 |

**Fig. 6.** Blood (product) transfusions during Abiomed support. Patients who survived Abiomed treatment required fewer blood (product) transfusions during the course of postoperative biventricular support, although these patients had longer BIVAD support times than the nonsurvivors

**Table 4.** Causes of death among ten patients on Abiomed therapy

| Cause of death | Weaned and died ($n = 4$) | Not weaned ($n = 6$) |
|---|---|---|
| Bleeding | 0 | 2 |
| Cardiogenic shock | 1 | 0 |
| Infarction | 0 | 4 |
| Sepsis | 3 | 0 |
| Multi-organ failure | 0 | 2 |
| Cannula-related | 0 | 1 |

the ICU because of bleeding problems and cardiac tamponade, compromising BIVAD function. In six of these patients, the amount of postoperative bleeding was "moderate", and four patients had severe chest tube drainage. In the early postoperative period, all patients received two or more platelet transfusions. Two patients had acceptable postoperative blood loss, and it was not necessary to perform a rethoracotomy in them. In the last nine patients, we noticed that sternal closure decreased bleeding tendency. Furthermore, in one patient a rethoracotomy was performed to correct a dislodgement of the left atrial cannula.

Hemolysis (plasma hemoglobin levels >30 μmol/l) due to prolonged CPB times occurred in three patients but disappeared during the course of circulatory support, suggesting that hemolysis was unrelated to the application of the BIVAD.

Five patients (45%) developed infections of the urinary tract ($n = 2$), wound ($n = 1$), and upper airway ($n = 2$), originating from *Staphylococcus epidermidis* ($n = 2$), *Streptococcus faecalis, Pseudomonas aeruginosa*, and a *Klebsiella* bacteremia. In three of them sepsis developed, followed by death after the BIVAD was removed.

In four patients dialysis was indicated to treat renal failure (defined as anuria for more than 24 h, with serum creatinine levels >300 mmol/l). Only one patient survived BIVAD therapy in combination with dialysis. In two patients prolonged mechanical ventilatory support (more than 7 days) was necessary to treat respiratory insufficiency after the BIVAD was removed, but this did not lead to death. Four patients died while on the assist device; the causes of death are shown in Table 4. Five patients were discharged from the hospital, with a follow-up of 16–42 months postoperatively. At present they are in NYHA functional classification I or II. Postoperatively, microscopic examination of the blood pumps revealed that two pump systems had visible thrombotic deposits in four blood sacs. Typical places for the adherent thin white hazes were the outlet valves of the artificial ventricles.

## Discussion

The present study of 15 patients in whom a BIVAD was implanted suggests the usefulness, effectiveness, and relative safety of temporary biventricular support with the Abiomed BVS 5000 pulsatile assist system. Our data confirm various clinical studies demonstrating that patients with a postcardiotomy cardiogenic shock can be salvaged by the application of temporary mechanical ventricular support techniques in case of unsuccessful standard resuscitative efforts with the IABP and inotropic support [13–15].

Thirteen patients were stabilized in the ICU. Nine of them were weaned successfully from the BIVAD. Ultimately, five of these patients were discharged from the hospital and are long-term survivors.

The pulsatile blood pumps provided complete support of the systemic and pultmonary circulation with maintenance of satisfactory perfusion of vital organs. With the blood pumps and cannulas the heart was completely decompressed, creating rest for the damaged myocardium and allowing recovery from perioperative myocardial injury.

Several investigators [16–18] reported that right ventricular failure was the most fatal complication after the initiation of only a left ventricular assist device (LVAD). Experimental studies [19, 20] suggest that right ventricular failure can develop during LVAD support, since the interventricular septum contractility is reduced by left ventricular decompression during only LVAD therapy. Early postoperative right ventricular dysfunction also might be related to the effects of complement-mediated polymorphonuclear leukocyte activation [21]. For these reasons we always support our patients with a BIVAD. Dopamine was the only inotropic drug administered, in a low dose ($<3.0\,\mu g/kg/min$), during BIVAD support to maintain renal blood flow. Furthermore, as reported by Sukehiro and Flameng [22], low-dose dopamine might improve blood flow to the intestinal organs during assisted circulation.

Five of our patients who underwent an emergency procedure could not be weaned from the BIVAD because myocardial function did not improve during BIVAD therapy. These results are confirmed by the findings of other investigators [15, 23, 24], who also report that weaning from a ventricular assist device is precluded in patients who have under gone an emergency cardiac operation.

Bleeding continues to be the most common complication during circulatory support. Al-Mondhiry et al. suggested that bleeding is correlated to prolonged CPB times that are caused by surgical repair of the cardiac defect, by resuscitation after surgical repair, and by implantation of the assist device [25]. Furthermore, we assume that hemostatic abnormalities in the postoperative period also might be caused by complement activation during the period of BIVAD support.

Infection is a complication that clearly influences survival of patients with externall placed temporary mechanical circulatory support devices [26]. In three patients infection led to sepsis and ultimately to death, despite successful weaning of the assist device.

As reported in other studies, renal failure indicating dialysis also was an important factor influencing survival of patients on temporary ventricular support [24, 27]. In our series only one patient who was dialysed survived BIVAD therapy.

Current perioperative diagnostic techniques do not allow precise differentiation of patients with potentially reversible myocardial injury like myocardial stunning or perioperative myocardial infarction. In our patients, TEE was a useful technique supporting patient selection prior to BIVAD therapy. In this small group of patients recovery of ventricular function never occurred beyond a period of 6 days of BIVAD support. An improvement in left ventricular function of more than 50% of the left ventricular circumference seems predictive for successful weaning from the Abiomed. Furthermore, guidance with TEE postoperatively can be helpful to optimize patient management and provide prospects of weaning from the assist device [28, 29].

We conclude that postcardiotomy myocardial failure after unsuccessful resuscitation efforts can be successfully treated in carefully selected patients, with potentially reversible myocardial damage, by a temporary mechanical biventricular support device. With the Abiomed BVS 5000 a condition of ventricular unloading was created. Thus myocardial work was decreased and a favorable oxygen demand-to-supply ratio established while the coronary circulation and systemic tissue perfusion were maintained adequately for 6 days. Recovery of ventricular function might be possible after a period of myocardial rest established with the BIVAD. However, an emergency operation followed by BIVAD implantation suggests that improvement in ventricular function and survival will be not successful. Bleeding is a frequent complication, but it alone does not preclude survival.

A considerable amount of information is still needed concerning patient selection, significance of complement activation during assisted circulation, and the importance of intraoperative and postoperative cardiac diagnostics.

## References


1. Barner HB, Kaiser GC, Godd JE et al. (1980) Clinical experience with cold blood as the vehicle for hypothermic potassium cardioplegia. Ann Thorac Surg 24:224–227
2. Buckberg GD (1989) Antegrade/retrograde blood cardioplegia to ensure cardioplegic distribution: operative techniques and objectives. J Cardiac Surg 4:216–238
3. Pae WJ Jr, Gaines WE, Pierce WS, Waldhausen JA (1985) Mechanical circulatory assistance for postoperative cardiogenic shock. Surg Rounds 8:49–63
4. Pennington DG, Samuels LD, Williams G et al. (1985) Experience with the Pierce-Donachy ventricular assist device in postcardiotomy patients with cardiogenic shock. World J Surg 9:37–46
5. Phillips PA, Bregman D (1977) Intraoperative application of intra-aortic balloon counterpulsation determined by clinical monitoring of the endocardial viability ratio. Ann Thorac Surg 23:45–51
6. McEnany MT, Kay HR, Buckley MJ et al. (1978) Clinal experience with intraaortic balloon pump support in 728 patients. Circulation 58[Suppl]:I-124–132
7. Maroko PR, Bernstein SF, Libby P et al. (1972) Effects of intra-aortic balloon counterpulsation on the severity of myocardial ischemic injury following acute coronary occlusion. Circulation 45:1150.
8. Lederman DM (1988) Technical consideration in the development of clinical systems for temporary and permanent cardiac support. In: Akutsu T (ed) Artificial heart, vol 2. Springer, Berlin Heidelberg New York, pp 115–127
9. Guyton RA, Schönberger JPAM, Everts PAM et al. (1993) Postcardiotomy shock: clinical evaluation of the BVS 5000 biventricular support system. Ann Thorac Surg 56:346–356

10. Sprung CL, Rackow EC, Civetta JM (1983) Direct measurements and derived calculations using the pulmonary artery catheter. In: Sprung CL (ed) The pulmonary artery catheter, methodology and clinical application. University Park Press, Baltimore, pp 105–140
11. Stewart WJ, Currie PJ, Salcedo EE et al. (1990) Intraoperative Doppler color flow mapping for decision-making in valve repair for mitral regurgitation. Circulation 81:556–566
12. Schönberger JP, Everts PA, Bavinck JH et al. (1992) Low-dose aprotinin in uni- and bilateral internal mammary artery bypass surgery. Ann Thorac Surg 54:1172–1177
13. Golding LR, Jacobs G, Groves LK, Gill CC, Nosé Y, Loop FD (1982) Clinical results of mechanical support of the failing left ventricle. J Thorac Cardiovasc Surg 83:597–601
14. Pennock JL, Pierce WS, Wisman CB, Bull AP, Waldhausen JA (1983) Survival and complications following ventricular assist pumping for cardiogenic shock. Ann Surg 198:469–478
15. Pierce WS, Rosenberg G, Donachy JH (1987) Postoperative cardiac support with a pulsatile assist pump: techniques and results. J Intern Soc Artif Organs 11:247–251
16. Schoen FJ, Bernhard WF, Khuri SF, Koster JK, VanDevanter SJ, Weintraub RM (1982) Pathologic findings in postcardiotomy patients managed with a temporary left ventricular assist pump. Am J Surg 143:508–513
17. Pennington DG, Codd JE, Merjavy JP et al. (1983) The expanded use of ventricular bypass systems for severe cardiac failure and as a bridge to cardiac transplantation. Heart Transplant 3:38–46
18. Schoen FJ, Palmer DC, Bernhard WF et al. (1986) Clinical temporary ventricular assist, pathologic findings and their implications in a multi-institutional study of 41 patients. J Thorac Cardiovasc Surg 92:1071–1081
19. Farrar DJ, Compton PG, Dajee H, Fonger JD, Hill JD (1984) Right heart function during left heart assist and the effects of volume loading in a canine preparation. Circulation 70:708–716
20. Yada I, Wei CM, Hattori R et al. (1985) Right ventricular function during left heart bypass evaluated by two-dimensional echocardiography. Trans Am Soc Artif Intern Organs 31:17–19
21. Schoen FJ, LaFarge CG, Bernhard WF (1985) Pathology and pathophysiology of temporary cardiac assist. Am Soc Artif Intern Organs J 8:174–181
22. Sukehiro S, Flameng W (1990) Effects of left ventricular assist for cardiogenic shock on cardiac function and organ blood flow distribution. Ann Thorac Surg 50:374–383
23. Pennington DG, McBride LR, Kanter KR, Swartz MT, Miller LW (1988) The effect of acute perioperative myocardial infarction on survival of postcardiotomy patients supported with ventricular assist devices. Circulation 78[Suppl III]:110–115
24. Penninton DG, Kanter KR, McBride LR et al. (1988) Seven years' experience with the Pierce-Donachy ventricular assist device. J Thorac Cardiovasc Surg 96:901–911
25. Al-Mondhiry H, Pierce WS, Richenbacher W, Bull A (1984) Hemostatic abnormalities associated with prolonged ventricular assist pumping: analysis of 24 patients. Am J Cardiol 53:1344–1348
26. Mcbride LR, Ruzevich SA, Pennington DG (1987) Infectious complications associated with ventricular assist device support. ASAIO Trans 33:201–202
27. Parascandola SA, Pae WE, Davis PK, Miller CA, Pierce WS, Waldhausen JA (1988) Determinants of survival in patients with ventricular assist devices. Trans Am Soc Artif Intern Organs 34:222–228
28. Simon P, Owen AN, Moritz A et al. (1991) Transesophageal echocardiographic evaluation in mechanical assisted circulation. Eur J Cardiothorac Surg 9:492–497
29. Kyo S, Matsumura M, Takamoto S, Omoto R (1989) Transesophageal color Doppler echocardiography during mechnical assist circulation. ASAIO Trans 35:722–725

# The Development of Low-cost Temporary and Permanent Circulatory Assist Devices

R.L. WHALEN

## Introduction

There is a growing realization in the United States (US) that the resources available for providing health care are finite. As a direct result of this perceived need for containing health care costs, technological innovation in medicine is increasingly being examined on a cost/benefit basis as well as on the basis of its efficacy. The mere fact that something is technically possible is no longer considered to be sufficient justification for funding continued research or providing patient care with costly treatment modalities. Expressed more directly, the days of preserving life at any cost appear to be over in this country.

The introduction of circulatory assist devices into clinical practice will test the capacity of the health care system to adopt new and potentially costly technology. While long-term circulatory support with cardiac assist devices now appears to be technically feasible [1, 2], this technology will not become generally available unless it can be shown both to be cost-effective and to provide a near normal quality of life to the recipient. As the currently available systems represent technology dating back to the late 1970s, this is doubtful.

Whether we as investigators and clinicians agree with this new emphasis on cost-effectiveness is irrelevant. Either we will adapt to this limitation, or our devices and clinical studies will become footnotes in the medical literature.

Therefore, at Whalen Biomedical Incorporated (WBI) we have placed a growing emphasis on cost-consciousness in the development of new circulatory support systems. A family of devices is evolving for intraoperative, short-term postoperative, and permanent cardiac support. The underlying principles of these systems are design for manufacturing (DFM) and an awareness of the cost implications of the technology.

## Temporary and Intraoperative Circulatory Support

It was a great disappointment to those of us involved in the effort to bring the left ventricular assist device (LVAD) to clinical trials in the 1970s that this technology did not subsequently become widely available. In part, this was a direct result of the increasing regulation of medical devices by government agencies in the US, but it was also a consequence of the design of the available devices themselves.

The temporary LVAD was initially proposed for supporting the circulation of cardiac surgery patients who had undergone apparently successful surgical procedures but were unable to be weaned from cardiopulmonary bypass [3]. It was estimated that there were on the order of 1000–2000 surgical patients with postcardiotomy failure annually in the US who might be temporary LVAD candidates.

The clinical trials of the temporary LVAD were supported by the National Institutes of Health (NIH) over an approximately 7-year period, concluding in 1982. By the end of the study, several groups had reported salvage rates in the range of 30–40% for patients who would otherwise have died [4, 5]. By that measure, the LVADs had been shown to be effective. There were factors other than efficacy, however, that effectively precluded the commercial availability of the systems which had been used in the clinical trials.

Since the primary objective of the NIH-sponsored clinical trials had been to determine the safety and efficacy of temporary left ventricular support, the cost of the devices was never an issue. Thus, the devices which were employed in the trials were configured for maximum safety, and there were few design compromises. For example, the pumps each utilized two commercially available bioprosthetic or mechanical valves, components manufactured for permanent implantation but which were being used for durations ranging from hours to several weeks at most. The valves alone added significantly to the total pump cost, which typically was in the range of $10 000.

The pneumatic drive systems required to operate those pumps were also costly, generally in the range of $60 000–$80 000 per console. A considerable financial investment would thus be required simply to have the capability of employing these systems, and it must be remembered that these were systems usable for only a very small percentage of cardiac surgery patients.

It was not surprising, therefore, that when the NIH-supported clinical trials ended, there was no surge of interest by manufacturers to provide the devices nor any great demand by clinicians to utilize this technology in clinical practice. The average period of circulatory support required for the surviving patients had been only 3–4 days. Thus, while the LVAD systems were shown to be potentially life saving, a $10 000 device cost and the high startup expenses were simply too much for systems to be used for such brief periods of time in small numbers of patients.

Clinical studies with temporary assist devices did continue, however, largely out of academic or promotional interests. At WBI, for example, we sponsored a clinical study in 1985 with one of the devices which had been used in the NIH-supported clinical trials [6]. The decision to proceed with our study was based primarily on marketing considerations by the hospital at which the study was to be conducted. Despite the high cost of the devices, that institution wished to be able to publicize its ability to provide "state of the art" technology in its cardiac surgery services. The potential of the device to offer improved patient care was actually of secondary importance. Thus, it was clear to us that the temporary LVAD was unlikely to become widely used with the devices then available.

We therefore set out to develop a new type of temporary cardiac assist device, designed from the outset for short-term use. The new device was to be low in cost and readily manufacturable. With the support of an NIH grant, the extracorporeal pulsatile assist device (EPAD) was designed and tested. In considering the task of manufacturing a low-cost assist device, we saw no obvious solution to the problem of low-cost valves. Therefore, the EPAD was designed as a valveless pump to be used for providing diastolic augmentation.

Figure 1 is a cross-sectional drawing of the EPAD. The stroke volume of the device is 80 ml, and its total dry weight is approximately 74 g. The composition and method of fabrication of the component parts are indicated. The device is very economically manufactured, the result of a determined effort to apply DFM methodology. For example, the elastomeric pump bladder, the most crucial component in the device, is manufactured by reaction injection molding from silicone rubber. Using this technique, pump bladders may be produced that are both highly reproducible and extremely low in cost. Since the pump is also modular in construction, the most labor-intensive aspects of its manufacture are assembly, testing, and packaging.

The EPAD bladder is designed to collapse with a nonocclusive three-lobe pattern which is highly efficient volumetrically. This may be seen in Fig. 2, an intraoperative photograph of the device being used as a right ventricular assist device (RVAD) in studies conducted at the Massachusetts General Hospital in Boston [7]. In those studies, isolated right ventricular failure was produced by injecting glass beads into the pulmonary artery (PA) of adult sheep, producing pulmonary hypertension and subsequent right ventricular failure. We found that cardiac output augmentation exceeding 50% could be achieved with the device despite its valveless configuration. When the EPAD is used as an RVAD, the outflow valve of the right ventricle in effect functions as a valve for the device to help maintain unidirectional flow.

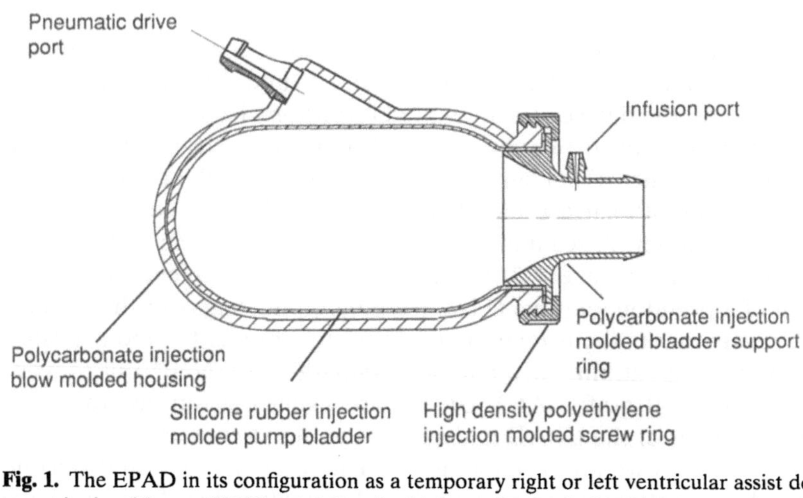


**Fig. 1.** The EPAD in its configuration as a temporary right or left ventricular assist device. Vascular access is via a 16-mm ePTFE arterial graft which attaches to the bladder support ring. All components of the device are manufactured with methods which yield highly reproducible parts at low cost

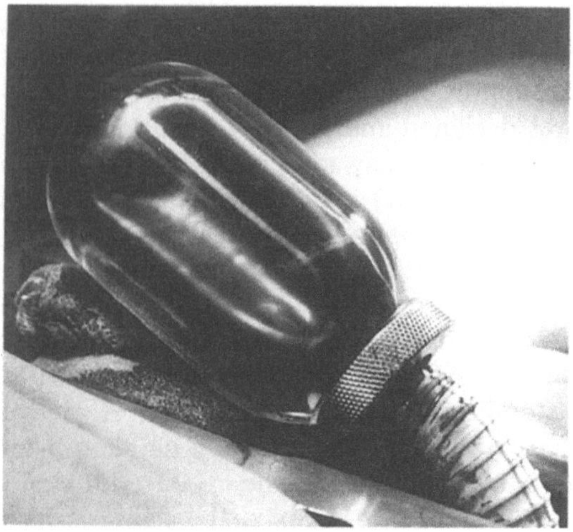

**Fig. 2.** The EPAD during pump systole. The bladder collapses with a three-lobe pattern which is nonocclusive. This design is volumetically efficient, and it promotes good washing of the bladder surface on each beat while avoiding occlusive contact which might produce hemolysis

The EPAD as a valveless device is thus especially suited for right ventricular support because of the anatomy of the pulmonary circulation. It is almost as effective as a valved device for right heart support because diastolic augmentation works best at lower pressures also. This is because the kinetic energy of a moving fluid is a greater fraction of its total energy at PA pressures. Under those conditions, the kinetic energy of the fluid is in the range of 50% of its total energy. The pressure forces acting on the fluid ejected by the EPAD into the pulmonary circulation must overcome the momentum of the fluid to return flow back to the pump; so at PA pressures, there is relatively little retrograde flow and greater augmentation of forward flow. At aortic pressures, in contrast, the kinetic energy is typically only 20% of the total fluid energy, so pressure effects predominate. There is thus considerable retrograde flow back to a valveless pump on each beat in the systemic circulation, lowering the forward flow augmentation provided by the device.

Long-term (to 4 weeks' duration) studies were also conducted using the EPAD as an RVAD or LVAD at the Cleveland Clinic Foundation [8]. To conduct those studies, the device was implanted intrathoracically in 80-kg calves. In order to provide improved blood compatibility in these chronic studies, an integrally textured silicone rubber surface was used on the bladder support ring, such that the only smooth surface blood-contacting part of the device was the elastomeric pump bladder. A scanning electron micrograph of the textured silicone rubber surface is shown in Fig. 3. This type of surface is designed to promote the deposition of a pseudoneointima (PNI) from blood flowing over the surface. The PNI effectively masks the foreign material from continued blood exposure and provides blood compatibility in a manner comparable to the PNI of conventional prosthetic arterial grafts. At WBI, we are using this surface for long-duration in vivo studies of the EPAD and also as the blood-contacting surface in a small-vessel prosthesis we are developing [9]. The integrally textured silicone rubber surface has functioned comparably to other textured surfaces we have investigated which are now being used clinically with good success [10].

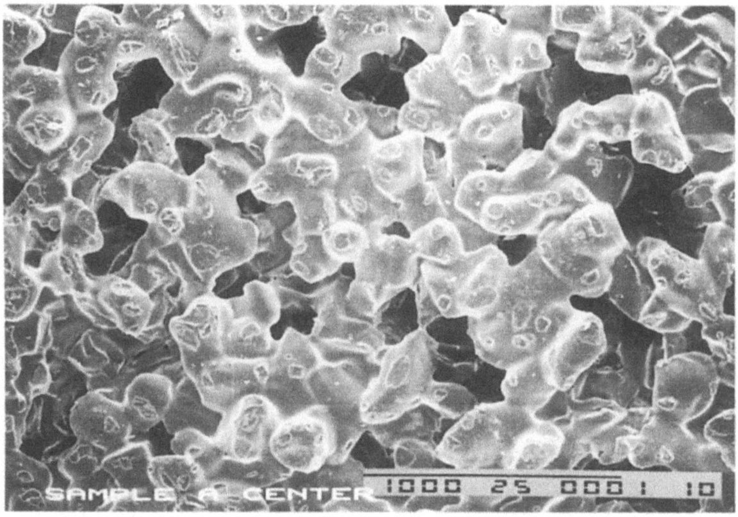


**Fig. 3.** Scanning electron micrograph of the integrally textured silicone rubber surface. This type of surface provides blood compatibility by serving as a matrix to anchor the PNI deposited on the surface by blood flow over the surface

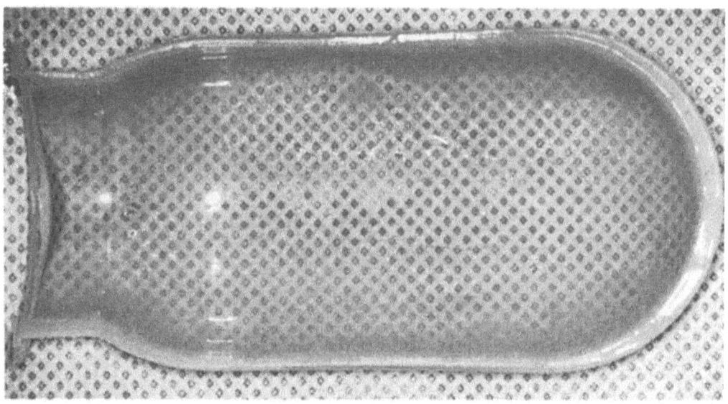

**Fig. 4.** The EPAD pump bladder from Experiment 91022, a 3-week study in which the device was used as an LVAD. There was no macroscopic depositon of thrombus on the smooth surface of the bladder, and no regions of apparent mechanical wear indicative of occlusive contact were seen

One consequence of the nonocclusive collapse pattern of the EPAD bladder is that the device operates with virtually negligible hemolysis, while the bladder surface itself is well washed on each beat to minimize the potential for thrombus deposition. This is illustrated in Fig. 4, a photograph of an EPAD bladder from a 24-day in vivo study in which the device was used as an LVAD. The surface of the bladder shows no macroscopic thrombus deposition or regions of localized wear.

During its development, the hemodynamics within the EPAD were adjusted using in vitro flow visualization testing, and there are no areas of flow separation or damaging shear conditions within the device. Figure 5 illustrates the plasma

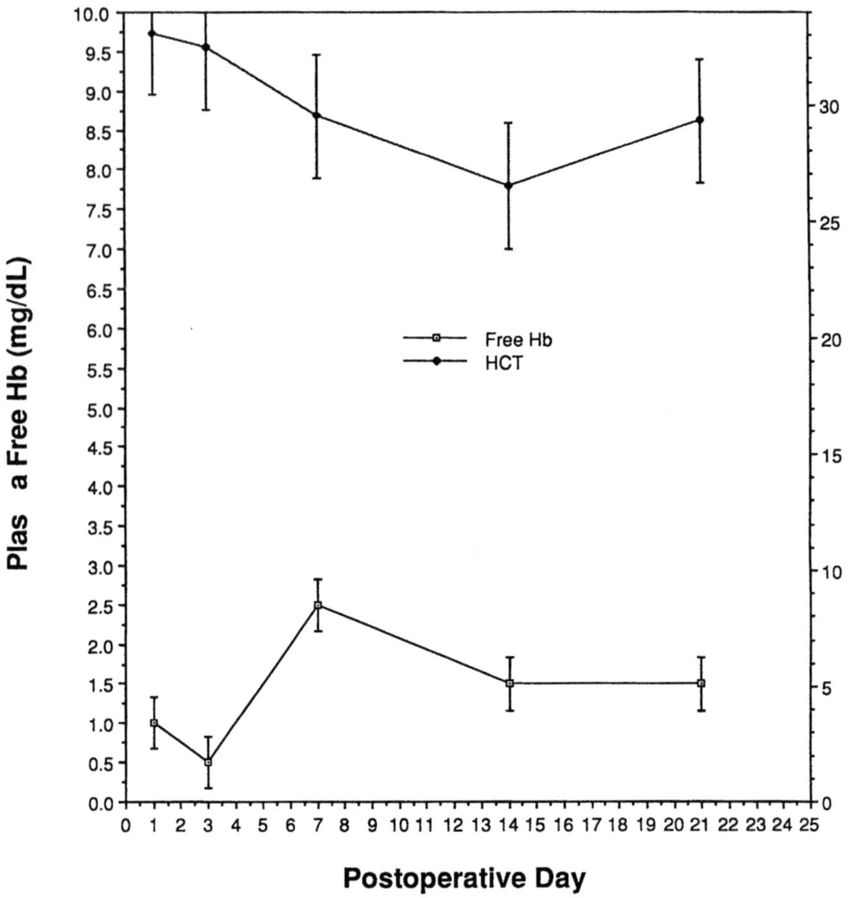


**Fig. 5.** Free plasma hemoglobin levels and hematocrit from the same study as in Fig. 4. The EPAD produced no statistically significant changes in hematocrit or free plasma hemoglobin levels in the long-term animal studies

free hemoglobin and hematocrit from that same animal study. EPAD pumping produced no statistically significant changes in either hematocrit or free plasma hemoglobin in the long-term studies.

When used as an LVAD, the EPAD is able to provide significantly more support than an intra-aortic balloon pump (IAPB) because of its 80-ml stroke volume (SV) and the fact that its output is delivered into the ascending aorta in proximity to the coronary arteries for optimal coronary flow augmentation [11]. One question which has been raised is the utility of a pump SV so much greater than the typical human ventricular SV. The argument has been made that since the ventricular SV establishes the upper limit of the available flow, there is no point to using a diastolic augmentation device with an SV larger than that of the ventricle.

To answer this question, it is necessary to consider the function of the device in terms of pressure effects rather than blood flow. By employing a large stroke volume with the EPAD, the afterload pressure seen by the ventricle during

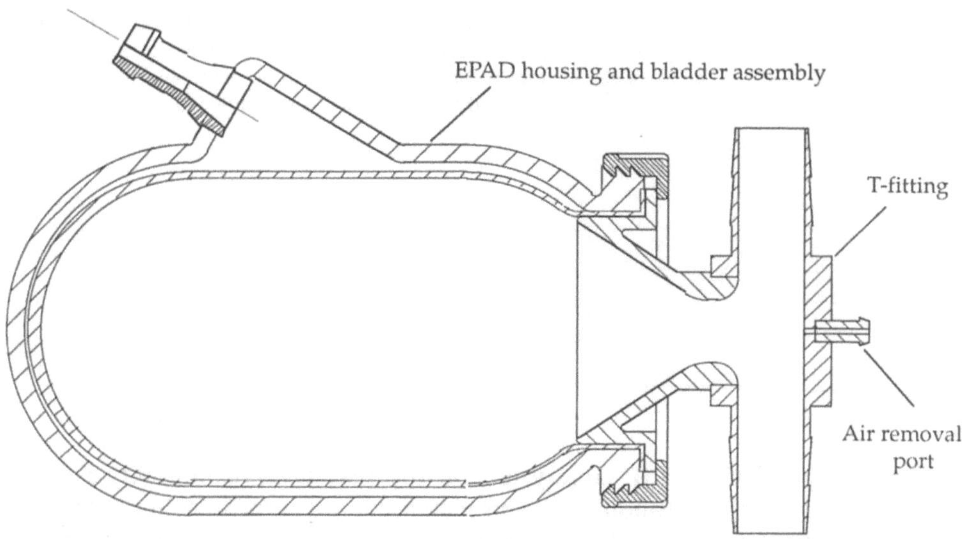


**Fig. 6.** A cross-sectional drawing of the EPAD configured for use in CPB circuits. The device is installed immediately before the aortic cannula in the return line to the patient. In that location, it is highly effective at converting the steady flow output of the bypass circuit to a more physiologic pulsatile flow

ventricular systole is markedly reduced. The chief benefit of the large stroke volume is thus in reducing the pressure work done by the ventricle.

This ability to employ the EPAD to alter the aortic pressure waveform at will actually suggested a use for the device which is likely to be more significant commercially than its application in temporary postoperative circulatory support. By incorporating the EPAD into a cardiopulmonary bypass circuit, the pump provides an ideal way of generating pulsatile cardiopulmonary bypass (CPB). We are now actively pursuing this application for the device in preference to using it for providing postoperative cardiac support, for reasons which we will explain subsequently.

The design of the EPAD configured for CPB is shown in Fig. 6. For use in CPB circuits, the EPAD incorporates a t-inflow fitting, as shown. The t-inflow fitting enables the pump to be installed directly between the aortic cannula and aortic return line from the heart/lung machine. The fitting includes a port which permits air removal from the aortic line at the time of patient cannulation or the measurement of aortic pressures intraoperatively. The t-fitting is molded from polycarbonate resin in three separate pieces, which are ultrasonically welded together to form the complete fitting. The complete disassembled CPB EPAD is pictured in Fig. 7.

Cardiopulmonary bypass, the technique in which oxygenation and circulation of the blood are provided by an external heart/lung machine while the patient's own heart is stopped, is required for open heart surgery. Last year, over 350 000 such procedures were performed in the US alone, mostly for the purpose of coronary artery revascularization. At the present time, however, the complica-

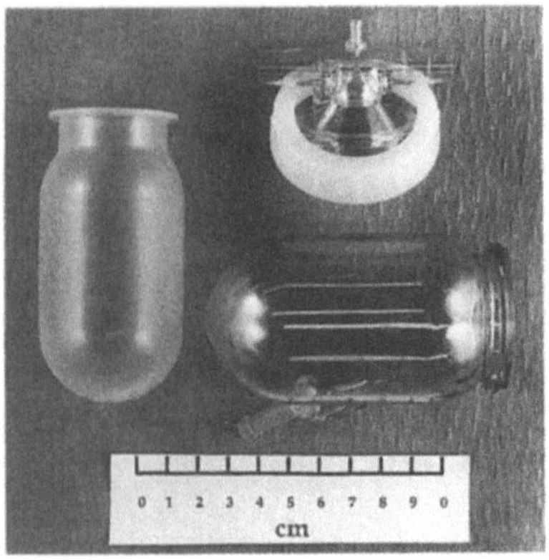


**Fig. 7.** The CPB EPAD disassembled. The device components are all readily manufacturable, an essential feature if the device cost is to be made low enough to fit within the constraints of cost containment

tions associated with CPB surgery are on the rise. Overall mortality is now estimated by the NIH at about 8%. This increase is not surprising, in view of the changing patient population for cardiac surgery. Ten years ago, for example, the average age of patients undergoing coronary revascularization surgery was in the range of 55–60; now it is close to 70. With this shift in the proportion of elderly patients having CPB surgery, the complications associated with CPB and their clinical sequelae have become more prominent. Indeed, in the elderly and very young, overall CPB surgical mortality approaches 15%, according to NIH statistics [12]. It is estimated that one of every 20 adults now requires a cardiac support device following cardiac surgery in the US, usually an IABP.

The clinical experience with patients after cardiac surgery suggests that the acute blood volume distribution resulting from the increased peripheral vascular resistance associated with nonpulsatile blood flow may lead to serious complications, such as fluid accumulation in the lungs and brain [13, 14] and myocardial strain caused by increased afterload [15–17]. While the etiology of these observed effects is certainly multifactorial and also related to complex humoral interactions resulting from exposure of blood to artificial surfaces, one of the possible ways to diminish these perioperative problems is the use of pulsatile CPB. There is evidence that in properly selected patients, pulsatile blood flow improves organ blood flow and perfusion [18, 19] while decreasing fluid retention in the lungs and brain [20–22].

It is generally acknowledged that some of the benefits that are associated with pulsatile flow, specifically improved renal function and a decreased catecholamine stress response to cardiopulmonary bypass, are obtainable with nonpulsatile systems simply by increasing the CPB flow rate to greater than 2.5 l/min/m$^2$, so-called high-flow bypass [23]. We believe it is likely, however, that there are undesirable side effects from high-flow bypass specifically in elderly patients, who as a group are more likely to have diminished vascular compliance and poorer autoregulation of cerebral blood flow secondary to impaired cerebral vasoconstrictor response [24].

Cerebral hyperemia, a possible contributor to increased CPB morbidity in elderly patients, is not a commonly encountered clinical entity. The maintenance of homeostasis is accomplished by intrinsic autoregulatory control mechanisms, and the effects of an externally controlled cardiac output in man have not been extensively studied. The anecdotal experience with the total artificial heart, however, provides some insight. In the first clinical application of the total artificial heart, an attempt was made to improve the patient's renal function by increasing cardiac output from 5–6 l/min to 10 l/min. The result of this externally imposed increase in blood flow was a loss of consciousness by the patient and the occurrence of seizures, an indication that what may be better for the kidney is not necessarily also appropriate for the brain when cardiac output is decoupled from its normal control [25]. It also showed that the normal autoregulation of the cerebral blood flow can be compromised with high flow rates. This experience suggests that cerebral hyperemia is possibly a mechanism of damage with high-flow CPB in elderly patients. Lower flow pulsatile CPB is potentially a way to improve renal function while avoiding the possible risk of cerebral hyperemia in these patients.

The essential argument is that elderly patients are likely to have diminished vascular compliance and impaired cerebral vasoconstrictor response, and this makes them more vulnerable to hyperemia during high-flow CPB. It would be difficult to argue, on the basis of the published literature, that intraoperative cerebral hyperemia is a benign condition. In addition to its potential influence on postoperative complications, there is evidence that the blood/brain barrier is compromised as well [26–28].

The use of pulsatile CPB remains controversial, however, in part because there have been prior but not notably successful attempts to use pulsatile perfusion with CPB systems. The Pulsatile Assist Device (PAD), an in-series pump marketed in the early 1980s by the Datascope Corporation (Pyramus, NJ) was such a device [29]. At that point in time, however, the need for subtle improvements in CPB methodology was perceived to be minimal. Institutions such as the Cleveland Clinic Foundation, for example, were routinely performing coronary revascularization surgery with less than 1% mortality. The Datascope device was thus a commercial failure, primarily because it was introduced at a time when it was not needed routinely. It was also promoted for general use and not just for elderly or high-risk patients, and so we believe it was not addressed to the appropriate patient population.

Because of growing cardiac surgical morbidity and mortality, however, surgeons are now actively looking to improve intraoperative techniques. This interest is evidenced by the fact that approximately 20% of hospitals in the US already have the ability to employ pulsatile CPB in the form of roller pumps using stepped rather than continuous rotation or centrifugal pump systems which employ a variable rotor speed to achieve a time-varying output. The system manufactured by Sarns Inc. (Ann Arbor, MI), which is now the only commercially available pulsatile CPB system in this country, is an example of the latter. The difficulty with both of those approaches is that their effect is dampened by placement of the pulsatile pump at the distal end of the aortic return line, quite far away from the patient. As a result, the resistance and compliance of the comparatively small diameter and physically long return line attenuates the pulsatility obtainable at the patient. Perhaps more importantly, the high shear rates required in these systems, which operate with pump pressures typically in the range of –80 to +700 mm Hg to achieve pulsatile flow in the patient, are more likely to result in hemolysis.

Since the EPAD is positioned at the proximal end of the aortic line, near the patient, it has the advantage of not having to displace the column of fluid in the entire length of the aortic return line on each beat. The losses resulting from aortic return line compliance and resistance are thus eliminated, since the pump ejects only through the aortic cannula on each beat. We believe this makes the EPAD uniquely effective. Our preliminary studies indicate that the EPAD is readily capable of producing a physiologically normal pulsatile flow in the aorta through the aortic cannula without the risk of hemolysis. This is a result of its placement at the patient end of the bypass circuit and also the design of the device itself, which was originally intended for much longer term blood exposure.

To study the efficacy of pulsatile CPB generated by the EPAD, a series of studies using 40- to 45-kg sheep have been conducted. The animals were placed on bypass using a conventional CPB circuit with a roller pump and bubble oxygenator. The EPAD was positioned immediately before an 18-Fr aortic cannula. A typical pulsatile pressure waveform measured in the carotid artery with the device in operation is illustrated in Fig. 8. By adjusting the EPAD SV, pumping rate, and ejection duration, a pulsatile output is easily obtained.

The degree of pulsatility of the output using the EPAD is thus user selectable over a wide range of operating conditions. We do not believe that the actual waveform shape is important, since changes in sympathetic tone and circulating blood volume have a profound influence on the aortic pressure waveform even under normal conditions. Thus, the objective is to obtain not an ideal waveform, but a near-normal pulse pressure. This ability to convert the normally steady flow output of the CPB circuit into pulsatile flow is likely to be useful in clinical situations in which low bypass flow rates are required, such as in the elderly. In the peripheral circulation, the benefits of pulsatile flow are likely to be significant

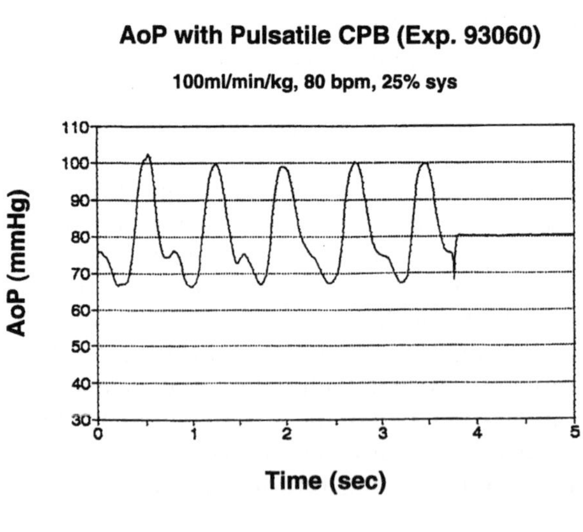


**Fig. 8.** An example of pulsatile flow during CPB as generated by the EPAD. By adjusting the pumping rate, percent systole, and SV, pulsatile CPB is readily obtained without the risk of hemolysis

in those situations, since pulsatile flow can break up fluid boundary layers and thus enhance mass transport occurring by diffusion.

Because the EPAD does not change the net flow rate of the CPB circuit, it was simple to compare the effects of pulsatile versus nonpulsatile CPB using each animal as its own control. As the physiological effects of pulsatile CPB are flow-rate dependent, we chose to examine two distinct flow rates: 60 ml/min/kg, corresponding to a low bypass flow rate, and 100 ml/min/kg, corresponding to a high flow rate. At each flow rate, nonpulsatile flow with the EPAD inactive was followed by pulsatile flow with EPAD in operation. Measurements were made over a 2-h period, with 30 min being allowed for each of the four flow conditions (low rate nonpulsatile, low rate pulsatile, high rate nonpulsatile, and high rate pulsatile) to reach an equilibrium state.

To study organ blood flow, we employed dye-filled microspheres (Ultraspherse, E–Z Trac Inc., Los Angeles, CA). This technique is now being used at the Cleveland Clinic Foundation, where these CPB studies were conducted, to evaluate peripheral blood flow in total artificial heart experiments. The method is elegantly simple.

Hollow, dye-filled polystyrene-divinylbenezene microspheres of $11.9 \pm 1.9\,\mu m$ diameter are injected into the left atrium. The beads are well mixed with the arterial blood when they are ejected by the left ventricle into the systemic circulation. The suspended beads distribute to the target tissue, where they become lodged in the microvasculature. By withdrawing a reference arterial blood sample during infusion, the blood flow in peripheral organs may be determined from the relation:

$$Q_T = \frac{M_T}{\int C_t dt}$$

where: QT = blood flow through the target tissue
MT = number of microspheres in the target tissue
$C_t$ = number of microspheres per milliliter of arterial blood at time $t$

the integration on $C_t$ is obtained experimentally by counting the beads in the simultaneously withdrawn arterial blood sample. By counting the number of spheres in the target tissue, the blood flow to the tissue may then be calculated. This is actually accomplished by digesting the tissue sample and counting the spheres with a hemacytometer using an optical microscope. Samples are routinely taken from the brain, liver, kidneys, pancreas, intestine, and heart. In practice the organs are removed when the animal is killed and frozen for later analysis. Thus, regional organ blood flow may be studied at a later time.

Sequential measurements are possible with this method, since the number of beads employed per measurement is small compared with the number of tissue capillaries. Direct comparisons of this technique with similar measurements using radioactive microspheres has shown a correlation coefficient of $r = 0.98$ [30].

In addition to simplicity, this technique is extremely useful because multiple flow measurements are easily made. The beads are available in eight distinct

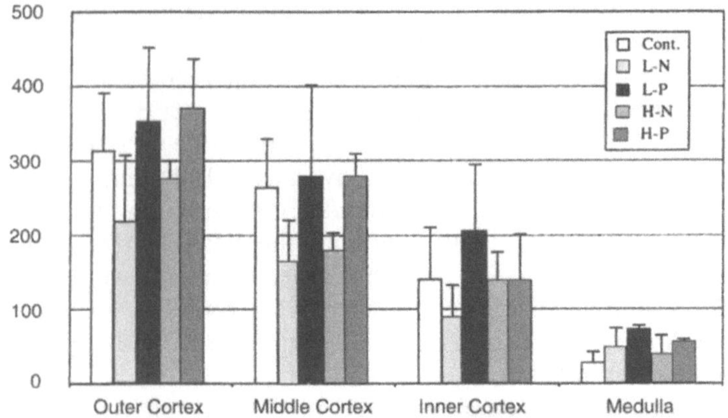


**Fig. 9.** Regional renal blood flow (ml/min per 100 g) measured with low- and high-flow CPB with pulsatile and nonpulsatile flow. With low-flow nonpulsatile CPB, cortical blood flow is reduced from pre-CPB control levels by approximately 30%, while pulsatile flow restores cortical blood flow to pre-CPB values

colors for that purpose. In our experimental studies, we first made a flow measurement immediately before bypass was instituted, then under each of the four CPB flow conditions, and finally after bypass was terminated.

Figure 9 shows the results of these regional blood flow measurements in the kidney from the first three animals. Note that at low CPB flow rates there is a significant drop in cortical perfusion with nonpulsatile flow, but that pulsatile flow using the EPAD restores the flow to control values. At high flow rates the differences between pulsatile versus nonpulsatile flow are negligible. We are continuing these studies and intend to examine in particular the effects of pulsatile flow on the cerebral circulation. It seems clear at this point, however, that at low flow rates, pulsatile flow is beneficial to cortical renal blood flow.

The CPB EPAD is thus a potentially useful device for cardiac surgery in situations where low flow rates are required, such as in the elderly. As this group now constitutes a major fraction of cardiac surgery patients in the US, the device appears to have wide potential applicability.

The key factor to making the CPB EPAD commercially successful in this application is the fact that it can be manufactured with a low-cost device. Even more so that in the case of pumps for postsurgical support, a device which is to be added to CPB circuits must not produce a large incremental cost increase for the procedure. This is a consequence of cost-containment measures already in effect. The reimbursement of hospitals in the US for many surgical procedures has been fixed through a mechanism called diagnosis-related groups (DRGs). Under the DRG system, the institution receives a predetermined fixed amount for a given procedure based on national average costs, regardless of the actual expenses which were incurred. It is therefore difficult for hospitals to begin using new higher cost systems, since this virtually guarantees a financial shortfall until those devices are generally employed. In this way, it is difficult to overstate the potentially limiting effect of cost-containment measures on the introduction of new technology in medical care in this country.

With the EPAD, we believe we have taken the steps necessary to make available a cost-effective device for circulatory support. It is difficult to see how its cost could be further reduced. Its very low cost, however, is the source of a dilemma because of the current regulation of class-III (life-sustaining) devices by the Food and Drug Administration (FDA) in the US. It is estimated that the cost of bringing a class-III device through the FDA regulatory process is on the order of 4–8 million dollars [31]. This explains why we have decided to proceed with the CPB EPAD, rather than use it as an assist device for postcardiotomy patients as originally designed. Given the comparatively small number of postcardiotomy patients annually in whom the device might be used, and considering its low cost, there is simply no way that the money required to bring the device through the FDA approval process could ever be recovered in the life cycle of the product. A device for CPB surgery, particularly if it can be classified as a class-II device (a less regulated category), can be commercially viable because the number of CPB procedures performed each year is so much larger.

The final element in our efforts to develop cost-effective temporary circulatory support devices is a drive system for the EPAD. If circulatory support technology is to be generally useful, we believe it is important to reduce the startup costs associated with using these devices. Therefore, with the assistance of an NIH grant, we have developed a pneumatic drive system addressed to this issue [32]. There were really two cost problems with the old drive systems: the high cost of the hardware itself, as we have previously described, and the functional complexity of the systems, such that highly trained individuals were required to operate them safely. The latter consideration may be as significant a factor as the high hardware cost.

For example, in our clinical trial of the temporary LVAD, it was necessary for us to train cardiac perfusionists to operate the pump console. Because the drive system was so complex, trained perfusionists were the only hospital personnel authorized to operate the system. In the US, cardiac perfusionists (who normally operate the CPB circuit during open heart surgery) are very highly paid technicians. The need to provide 24-h a day coverage with a perfusionist significantly increased the labor costs associated with the clinical trial. Ideally, a drive system for a temporary device should be operable by the available hospital personnel in the critical care unit as a part of their normal duties.

One problem with pneumatically driven systems it that the adjustments of drive pressure and vacuum are interactive with pumping rate and ejection duration settings. Generally it takes considerable experience to operate a conventional pneumatic-drive console with confidence and safety. Therefore, another primary goal in designing a new console was to eliminate the need for pressure adjustments.

This was achieved by using an electromagnetic linear actuator to drive a welded metal bellows to provide a pulsatile pneumatic output. The operation of the linear actuator is controlled using a servo system. The bellows excursion and

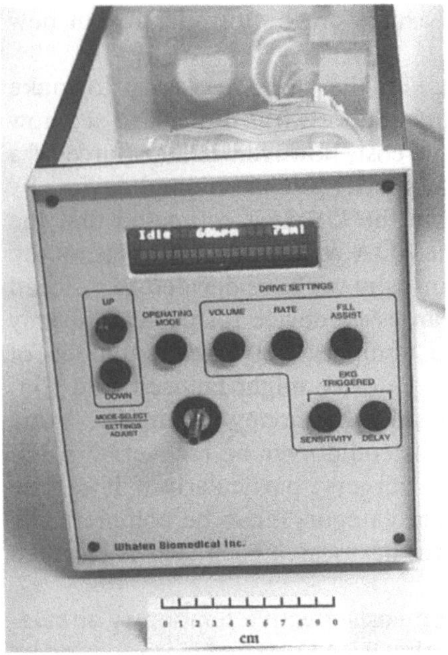


**Fig. 10.** The digitally controlled pneumatic pump drive console. It has only a single moving part, while eliminating those components in conventional drive systems subject to mechanical wear. It also eliminates the need for the operator to make pressure adjustments, permiting it to be safely operated by comparatively untrained hospital personnel

pressure are used as control signals in a feedback loop. The operator merely selects a stroke volume and desired pump-operating mode (fixed rate, counterpulsation, or autonomous variable rate), and the system will then maintain that SV regardless of rate or afterload changes.

Figure 10 is a photograph of the complete drive console. The unit is comparatively small and readily portable. There are no pressure regulators to adjust; instead, the operator specifies operating conditions as read on a fluorescent display. Mechanically, the drive system has only a single moving part, and those components in conventional pneumatic drive consoles subject to wear such as air compressors, pressure regulators, solenoid vales, or sliding seals are all eliminated. The new drive system is thus highly reliable. The control functions are handled by a microprocessor which works as an 8-bit controller, offering more than enough precision for this application. While the new console is simple to use and reliable, it is also low in cost. It can be manufactured such that its final cost will be in the range of $10 000, a fraction of the cost of a typical IABP drive system. This low-cost drive system is the final element in our attempts to produce cost-effective systems for temporary circulatory support.

In summary, by employing low-cost blood pumps and drive systems, and also by designing systems which can be safely operated by less specialized hospital personnel, we are confident that the high costs previously associated with temporary circulatory support systems can be significantly reduced, the principal reason being that our systems have been designed to be truly manufacturable, and they are addressed to the specific clinical requirements of temporary as opposed to permanent circulatory support. These new devices are thus better able to fit within the limited resources which cost containment mandates.

## Permanent Assist Devices

The chief problem with permanent cardiac assist systems is not device cost, but the quality of life provided. While the device cost is not an insignificant factor, what will make his technology acceptable is the degree to which it permits a patient to lead a productive life. Devices which merely maintain life are unlikely to be supported by a health care system which increasingly will make decisions on the basis of cost/benefit analysis.

In its 1991 review of artificial heart research in the US, the Institute of Medicine (IOM) of the National Academy of Sciences determined that "the need for a fully implantable, long-term VAD is substantial" and that "an annual pool of between 35 000 and 50 000 candidates to receive either a VAD or total artificial heart now exists." This report further stated that "if continuing development efforts result in a device whose performance approaches transplantation outcomes (now about a 70% 5-year survival rate), the size of the candidate pool will increase by perhaps another 200 000 per year, as of about the year 2020." The IOM report concluded that: "Taking full advantage of the potential of VADs is thus a vital goal" [33].

We were pleased to testify before the IOM committee during its deliberations, and we share the perspective of the IOM report. During the time we have followed VAD development, significant progress has been made in the area of mechanical circulatory support, but a fully intracorporeal VAD has remained an elusive goal.

In the early 1970s, we participated in studies investigating the use of radioisotope power sources for cardiac assist devices, and in the course of that work actually conducted animal experiments with nuclear-fueled VADs [34]. The appeal of the nuclear-fueled VAD was the power source, a radioisotope (plutonium 238) with a half-life of 87 years. Here was a power source which, at least in theory, would permit a VAD recipient to lead a normal life, unencumbered by the need for external power to operate the implanted blood pump.

The nuclear-fueled devices, however, were totally impractical. They were excessively large, extremely complex, and of poor mechanical reliability. Even if successfully developed, their widespread use would have posed a substantial risk to the general public because of the toxicity of the nuclear fuel itself. For these reasons, nuclear powered VADs, while technically possible, are not a workable option. Thus, in its efforts to develop long term VADs, the National Heart, Lung, and Blood Institute (NHLBI) focused its support on electrically powered devices beginning in the late 1970s. Electrically powered devices, while requiring external power input to operate the pump, were seen as a possible compromise.

Currently, there are two electrically powered VADs developed originally with NHLBI support which are being used clinically for bridging patients to cardiac transplantation. These are: the TCI Heartmate (Thermo Cardiosystems Inc., Woburn, MA) and the Novacor LVAS (Novacor Division, Baxter Healthcare, Oakland, CA). These systems are pulsatile pumps which employ an electric motor to actuate the blood pump, a low-speed torque motor and a solenoid mechanism, respectively. Both devices have been used to support patients for extended periods of time (up to 17 months in one case) with an improved quality of life [1, 2]. Patients are able to wear external battery packs which permit them periods of untethered operation of 6–8 h, depending upon their level of physical activity.

The bridge experience with the TCI and Novacor devices has demonstrated that during mechanical circulatory support, the hemodynamic status of the recipient is stabilized, while peripheral organ function improves such that the results at transplantation are actually improved with increasing periods of support using the VAD [35]. There is now a general perception that these clinical studies of bridging to transplantation have validated the feasibility of mechanical circulatory support with a VAD, notwithstanding the limitations of these existing VADs, which represent hardware designed originally in the early 1980s.

It should also be pointed out that both the TCI and Novacor devices are vented systems with a percutaneous vent and electrical power input line. Their utility as long-term VADs is thus subject to question, since infection is likely to be a limiting problem. To make these devices suitable for long-term use, percutaneous lines would have to be eliminated by the addition of a transcutaneous energy transmission system and a compliance chamber system. The additional hardware burden and complexity raises significant questions regarding the feasibility of these systems.

For this reason, a new generation of VADs are being developed which employ more current technology. Among the more intriguing approaches is the use of nonpulsatile blood pumps [36, 37]. Nonpulsatile pumps eliminate the need for volume compensation, while the pumps themselves are remarkably small and light in weight. There remain some unanswered technical problems for these devices at present. These issues include such questions as the seal design if a rotating drive shaft is used to couple the motor to the blood pump impeller, or the feasibility of magnetically suspended rotors if a directly coupled drive shaft is to be eliminated. There is also the fact that nonpulsatile pumps have a "hard" failure mode. Since there are no valves in these devices, failure of the pump produces a likely fatal left-to-left shunt flow.

Nonpulsatile centrifugal or axial pumps do have the potential to permit the use of much smaller, simplified VADs compared with pulsatile pump systems. While there is still some question regarding the long-term physiologic effects of nonpulsatile blood flow, there is experimental evidence suggesting that these devices will prove to be safe and effective [38]. The chief disadvantage of these devices, however, is that, like all electrically powered pump systems, they require the patient to be connected to external electrical power sources at all times. It is doubtful, in our estimation, that large numbers of patients would find the quality of life provided by such systems to be an acceptable compromise.

Currently, a possible new approach for powering VADs has emerged which, in our estimation, literally renders the electric motor-powered devices obsolete for all but bridging patients to transplantation. Progress in the area of tissue engineering in which skeletal muscle is electrically stimulated to make it fatigue resistant and able to perform cardiac work has now made available a potentially ideal VAD power source. Initially, this research was oriented towards cardiomyoplasty. Cardiomyoplasty is a technique in which skeletal muscle is wrapped around the heart and synchronously stimulated to augment cardiac performance. It is now an accepted procedure in some areas of this country, though many questions remain regarding its long-term efficacy.

The chief problems associated with cardiomyoplasty have been insufficient power output from the muscle and loss of muscle mass, contractile speed, and performance with time [39–41]. Recent investigations have identified a possible methodology, however, that appears to yield results which will permit conditioned skeletal muscle to serve as a VAD power source. With a muscle-powered VAD, the only electrical energy needed to operate the device is the battery power to operate the implanted stimulator, a power level comparable to that of a cardiac pacemaker and supplied by a battery in the stimulator having a life of 5 years or more.

From the perspective of 20 years of work in the area of mechanical circulatory support, we have little doubt that this approach represents a quantum leap in VAD technology. Devices which must be tethered to external sources of electrical power and which provide limited periods of untethered operation using external battery packs are not likely to be an acceptable approach for long-term VADs. When compared with a VAD powered by the patient's own metabolism and which does not require constant attention and vigilance, the electric motor-powered devices may be viewed as a technologic anachronism, comparable in acceptability to the "iron lung" once used for chronic respiratory support. The electrically powered VADs did, however, serve to validate the efficacy of long-term mechanical circulatory support, and they are certainly of use in bridging patients to cardiac transplantation.

The most serious potential competition to the skeletal muscle-powered VAD, in our estimation, will likely come from xenograft transplants. It has been suggested that by using transgenic animal models, it will be possible to genetically engineer animal organs which will be comparable in antigenicity to homologous tissue. This is an active area of research, as evidenced by the fact that there were over 25 abstracts at the most recent annual meeting of the American Heart Association dealing with transgenic models [42]. Even assuming success in that endeavor, however, there are still many problems associated with cardiac transplantation, not the least of which is cost.

Less appreciated generally, but well detailed in the IOM study, is the fact that most of the significant costs associated with cardiac transplantation occur after the surgical procedure and involve the maintenance of immunosuppression and the treatment of opportunistic infections and rejection episodes. In essence, transplantation is expensive technology, and it goes without saying that cost is now a driving factor in determining the applicability of new medical technology. Thus, even if unlimited numbers of donor organs are made available by xenografts, there are real questions as to whether the health care system could deal with the huge expense of maintaining these patients postoperatively.

It is here that the skeletal muscle-powered VAD has advantages compared with transplantation. Ultimately, we expect progress in immunology to make possible transplants with minimal complications, but that possibility does not

**Table 1.** VAD systems and transplantation compared

| System type | Advantages | Limitations |
|---|---|---|
| Electric-powered pulsatile | ? | Requires external power source<br>Requires volume compensation<br>Requires transcutaneous energy transmission system<br>High system cost, complexity |
| Electric nonpulsatile | Mechanically simple<br>Light weight | Requires external power source<br>Requires transcutaneous energy transmission system<br>Hard failure mode |
| Muscle-powered VAD | No external power<br>Extreme simplicity<br>Low weight<br>Low system cost<br>Autologous tissue | Requires second surgery |
| Homologous transplant | Proven approach | Limited donor availability<br>Requires immunosuppression<br>High cost to maintain |
| Xenograft transplant | Unlimited availability | Unproven technology |

appear to be in the immediate future. We have summarized the benefits and limitations of the different approaches to long-term circulatory support and transplantation in Table 1. Of all of the mechanical circulatory support approaches, the skeletal muscle-powered VAD now seems to us to be the most promising.

We are thus focusing our efforts on skeletal muscle-powered VADs using the EPAD as the blood pump. This type of VAD employs only autologous tissue, so the technical problems associated with transplantation and immunosuppression are completely avoided. The relative cost factor is also significant. Currently, the average expense simply to harvest a donor organ in the US is approximately $20 000. While it is unrealistic at this point to project the cost of the muscle-powered VAD accurately, it is difficult to see how the cost of the device, including the stimulator, would exceed $10 000. The skeletal muscle-powered VAD thus has the potential to be an extremely cost-effective solution to the problem of long-term circulatory support. It is an example of where tissue engineering, as opposed to genetic engineering, may be the more useful approach.

The techniques which we are employing to develop a skeletal muscle-powered VAD owe much to the pioneering work of Dr. Norbert W. Guldner (University Hospital, Brussels, Belgium). He has shown that high performance is obtainable from skeletal muscle in a wrapped configuration when it is dynamically conditioned [43]. Typically, when skeletal muscle is conditioned to perform continuous work, losses of 80% in muscle power, 60% in muscle mass, and 75% in contractile velocity are observed. Thus, until quite recently, it was thought that skeletal muscle could not be conditioned to generate sufficient power to drive a VAD in the systemic circulation.

Guldner and his associates have achieved remarkably improved results. They have been able to demonstrate in animal experiments conditioned latissimus dorsi muscle capable of generating pressures greater than 200 mm Hg with preserved contractile velocity and a power output of more than 9 watts [44]. The thickness of the conditioned muscle was increased by a factor of three compared with the contralateral muscle. Putting this into perspective, the maximal performance of the human left ventricle is approximately 3 watts, and it would thus seem that more than enough power is obtainable to power a VAD with muscle conditioned in this way.

The conditioning protocol used to achieve those results is surprisingly simple. It requires a two-stage process. During a period of about 2 weeks, the wrapped muscle contracts around a low resistance load as the rate of contraction is increased from one contraction/min to a rate of 50–60. At that point, the load on the muscle is gradually increased until usable power levels are obtainable. This generally takes 8–12 weeks.

We believe that transapical left ventricular bypass is the preferred pump configuration for a muscle-powered VAD. With transapical bypass, the left ventricle functionally becomes an atrium for the assist device. The pressure created by the ventricle may be used to provide some of the preload on the muscle, an important factor in maintaining muscle performance. It is likely that the failure of conventional myoplasty in some cases arises from insufficient preload. Some investigators thus favor a linear puli rather than a wrapped system to more efficiently use the muscle [43].

To adapt the EPAD for transapical left ventricular bypass, it is necessary to add valves to the device and to redesign the pump inflow. The physical configuration of the modified device is dictated somewhat by its implantation site. Anatomically, the pump will be positioned intrathoracically to rest on the left hemidiaphragm in the costodiaphragmatic recess. The pump inflow will thus be close to the left ventricular apex, and the inflow conduit of the pump will be very short in length. The pump outflow graft will be routed to the ascending aorta anteriorly.

The complete hydraulically driven VAD is shown schematically in Fig. 11. The conditioned latissimus dorsi muscle is wrapped in two layers around the hydraulic drive bladder. Muscle contraction displaces fluid from the hydraulic bladder to produce EPAD ejection. The relative orientations of the EPAD pump housing and the hydraulic drive bladder are easily adjustable, and we have shown them parallel only for the sake of clarity. The modified pump inflow fitting holds the pump valves, which establish unidirectional flow through the device. We have chosen to employ 23-mm St. Jude tilting disk valves (St. Jude Medical Inc., Minneapolis, MN), a valve we have used on other blood pumps.

It is unreasonable to expect that a patient who might be a candidate for a VAD, typically someone in New York Heart Association class-IV failure, should undergo major surgery 8–12 weeks before receiving a functional device, the time required for muscle conditioning. Therefore, the skeletal muscle-powered VAD design must allow the pump to be implanted and driven pneumatically until the muscle is ready. This is accomplished simply by using a detachable

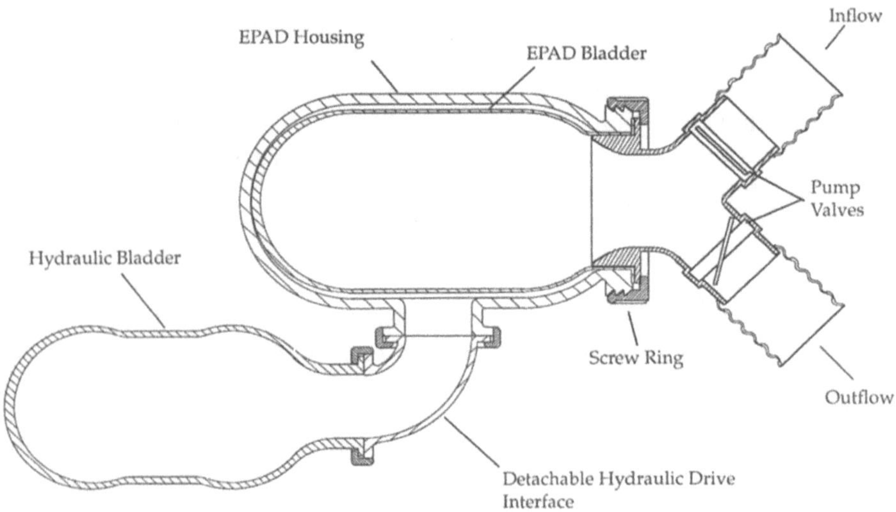


**Fig. 11.** The skeletal muscle-powered VAD. The conditioned latissimus dorsi muscle is wrapped around the hydraulic bladder which drives the EPAD assist pump. While the muscle is being conditioned, a detachable pneumatic-drive fitting is used on the pump in place of the hydraulic-drive interface. It is essential that the hydraulic-drive bladder be closely coupled to the EPAD if the system is to have acceptable total efficiency and not be subject to gravitational/positional effects. The total hardware weight will be under 200 g, and there are only four moving parts including the pump valves

pneumatic-drive fitting on the EPAD housing during the period of muscle conditioning.

The first surgical procedure thus consists of implanting the blood pump and a muscle-conditioning appliance. The muscle-conditioning appliance, consisting of the hydraulic bladder with an attached inflatable side chamber, is also implanted intrathoracically. The latissimus dorsi muscle is wrapped around the hydraulic bladder in a double layer. The exterior of the hydraulic bladder is velour covered to promote attachment of the tissue to its surface. The volume of the side chamber is externally controlled to adjust the load against which the muscle works while the muscle is being conditioned. During this time, the patient's circulation will be supported with the pneumatically driven EPAD.

When the muscle has been adequately conditioned, the pump will be surgically exposed via a left thoracotomy, and the hydraulic drive interface attached to the pump housing. The conditioned skeletal muscle and hydraulic drive bladder of the device are attached, and the pump is then operated as a muscle-powered VAD with no external power input.

As we have previously pointed out, the experience with bridge to transplantation VAD systems has suggested that VAD implantation may be useful to stabilize the condition of a critically ill patient prior to transplantation. Thus, we do not believe the two-stage procedure needed with a muscle-powered VAD will result in increased morbidity and mortality. Indeed, it may actually serve to improve overall results. The procedure to switch the pump from external pneumatic to muscle-powered hydraulic actuation will require a thoracotomy, but not cardiopulmonary bypass or cardiac manipulation.

The great advantages of the muscle-powered VAD system, other than the fact that it does not require external power input, are that the device is extremely simple, low in cost, and thus potentially reliable. There is a strong correlation in our experience with simplicity and dependability. While it does require two surgical procedures, that cost is offset by the low device cost and the likelihood that postoperative follow-up costs will be minimal compared with the alternatives, including xenograft transplants.

Our current efforts to develop a permanently implanted VAD have thus undergone considerable evolution from our initial work with the nuclear-fueled devices, or even from our previous contribution to the first edition of this text in 1979 [46]. At that time, we were pursuing the development of an electrically powered assist device, and there seemed to be few alternatives to that approach. It is characteristic of this field that new ideas are constantly emerging which have the potential to change the direction of one's work.

Because of the growing emphasis on cost/benefit analyses of new medical technology and increasing government regulations of medical devices, however, it is becoming difficult to bring new technology into clinical practice, at least in this country. Unless we are able to adapt to this changing environment for medical device research, future editions of this text will not reflect the conceptual diversity and spirit of innovation which has made this field so interesting.

*Acknowledgments.* We wish to acknowledge the support and assistance of the following individuals, without whom the work we have described could not have been accomplished. At the Cleveland Clinic Foundation: Hiro Harasaki, M.D., Ph.D., J. Utoh, M.D., F. Fukumura, M.D., K. Fukamachi, M.D., and C. Davies, M.S. At the Massachusetts General Hospital: Warren M. Zapol, M.D., W.E. Hurford, M.D., M. Skoskiewicz, M.D., and T.R. Wonders, B.S. At Whalen Biomedical Incorporated: D.L. Jeffery, M.D., F.R. Inhaber, M.D., and M.A. Bowen, B.S.

## References

1. McGee MG, Myers TJ, Abou-Awdi N, Dasse KA, Radovancevic B, Lonquist JL, Duncan JM, Frazier OH (1991) Extended support with a left ventricular assist device as a bridge to transplantation. ASAIO Trans 37(3):M425–426
2. McCarthy PM, Portner PM, Tobler HG, Starnes VA, Ramasamy N, Oyer PE (1991) Clinical experience with the novacor ventricular assist system. Bridge to transplantation and the transition to permanent application. J Thorac Cardiovasc Surg 102:578–587
3. Norman JC, Whalen RL, Daly BDT, Migliore JJ, Huffman FN (1972) An implantable left ventricular assist device (LVAD). Clin Res 20(5):855
4. Bernhard WF, Berger RL, Stetz JP et al. (1979) Temporary left ventricular bypass: factors affecting patient survival. Circulation 60[Suppl]:131–141
5. Pierce WS (1985) Effective clinical application of ventricular bypass. Ann Thorac Surg 36: 2–3
6. Whalen Biomedical Inc (1985) Investigational use of a temporary left ventricular assist device. IDE no G850097-A1
7. Whalen RL, Hurford WE, Skoskiewicz M, Wonders TR, Zapol WM (1987) A new right ventricular assist device: the extracorporeal pulsatile assist device (EPAD). ASAIO Trans 10(3): 222–226

8. Utoh J, Whalen RL, Wilkerson BR, Fukamachi K, Harasaki H (1993) Chronic in vivo function of a new ventricular assist device: the extracorporeal pulsatile assist device (EPAD). Int J Artif Organs 16:91–95
9. Whalen RL, Cardona R, Kantrowitz A (1992) A new all silicone rubber small vessel prosthesis. ASAIO Trans 38(3):M207–212
10. Whalen RL, Murakami T, Ozawa K, Snow J, Nose Y (1979) Powder metal surfaces as a blood interface material. Trans Soc Biomat 3:39
11. Nose' Y, Schamann M, Kantrowitz A (1963) Experimental use of an electronically controlled prosthesis as an auxiliary left ventricle. Trans Am Soc Artif Intem Organs 19:269–274
12. National Heart, Lung, and Blood Institute (1990) Mechanisms of damage caused by cardiopulmonary bypass. (RFA 90-HL-12-H)
13. Dernevik L, Advidsson S, William-Olsson G (1985) Cerebral perfusion in dogs using pulsatile and non-pulsatile extracorporeal circulation. J Cardiovasc Surg 26:32–35
14. Matsumoto T, Wolferth CC, Perlman MH (1971) Effects of pulsatile and nonpulsatile perfusion upon cerebral and conjunctival microcirculation in dogs. Am Surg 37:61–67
15. Landymore RW, Murphy DA, Kinley CE et al. (1979) Does pulsatile flow influence the incidence of postoperative hypertension? Ann Thorac Surg 28:261–268
16. Philbin DM, Levine FH, Kong K et al. (1981) Attenuation of stress response to cardiopulmonary bypass by the addition of pulsatile flow. Circulation 64:808–812
17. Roberts AJ, Niarchos AP, Subramanian VA et al. (1974) Systemic hypertension associated with coronary artery surgery. J Thorac Cardiovasc Surg 74:846–859
18. Boucher JK, Rudy LW, Edmunds LH (1974) Organ blood flow during cardiopulmonary bypass. J Appl Physiol 36:86–90
19. Steed DL, Follette DM, Foglia R, Mahoney JV, Bruckberg GD (1985) Effects of pulsatile and nonpulsatile flow on subendocardial perfusion during cardiopulmonary bypass. Ann Thorac Surg 26:53–58
20. Salerno TA, Charrett EJP, Kieth FM (1980) Hemolysis during pulsatile perfusion: clinical evaluation of a new device. J Thorac Cardiovasc Surg 79:579–581
21. Mori F, Ivey TD, Itoh T, Thomas R, Breazeale DG, Misbach G (1987) Effects of pulsatile reperfusion on postischemic recovery of myocardial function after global hypothermic cardiac arrest. J Thorac Cardiovasc Surg 93:719–727
22. Andersen K, Waaben J, Husum B et al. (1985) Nonpulsatile cardiopulmonary bypass disrupts the flow-metabolism couple in the brain. J Thorac Cardiovasc Surg 90:570–579
23. Frater RWM, Wakayama S, Oka Y, Becker RM, Desai P, Oyama T, Blaufox MD (1980) Pulsatile cardiopulmonary bypass: failure to influence hemodynamics or hormones. Circulation 62[Suppl I]:19–25
24. Faraci FM (1993) Cerebral circulation during aging. In: Phillis JW (ed) The regulation of the cerebral circulation. CRC, Boca Raton, chap 31
25. DeVries WC, Anderson JL, Joyce LD, Anderson FL, Hammond EH, Jarvik RK, Kolf WJ (1984) Clinical use of the total artificial heart. N Engl J Med 310(5):273–278
26. Sadoshima S, Masatoshi F (1993) Hypertension and the autoregulation of cerebral blood flow. In: Phillis JW (ed) The regulation of the cerebral circulation. CRC, Boca Raton, chap 21
27. Maxwell WL, Irvine A, Adams JH, Graham DI, Gennarelli TA (1988) Response of the cerebral microvasculature to brain injury. J Pathol 155:327
28. MacKenzie ET, McCulloch J, O'Keane M, Pickard JD, Harper AM (1976) Cerebral circulation and norepinephrine: relevance of the blood-brain barrier. Am J Physiol 231:483
29. Bregman D (1978) Clinical experience with a new pulsatile assist device (PAD) during open heart surgery. Artif Organs 2:244–248
30. Kowallik P (1991) Measurement of regional myocardial blood flow with multiple colored microspheres. Circulation 83:974–982
31. (1990) MDDI Rep 16(30):16–18
32. Whalen RL, Briskman RN (1988) An electromagnetic pneumatic blood pump driver. ASAIO Trans 34(3):721–725
33. Institute of redicine of the National Academy of Sciences (1991) The artificial heart. A report. National Academy Press, Washington DC, p 191

34. Norman JC, Molokhia FA, Harmison LT, Whalen RL, Huffman FN (1972) An implantable nuclear-fueled circulatory support system I. Systems analysis of conception, design, fabrication, and initial in vivo testing. Ann Surg 176(4):492
35. Dasse KA, Frazier OH, Lesniak JM, Myers T, Burnett CM, Poirier, VL (1992) Clinical responses to ventricular assistance versus transplantation in a series of bridge-to-transplantation patients. ASAIO Trans 38(3):M622–626
36. Antaki JF, Butler KC, Kormos RL, Kawai A, Konishi H, Kerrigan JP, Borovitz HS, Maher TR, Kameneva MV, Griffith BP (1993) In vivo evaluation of the nimbus axial flow ventricular assist system. ASAIO Trans 39(3):M231–236
37. Akamatsua T, Nakazeki T, Itoh H (1992) Magnetically suspended centrifugal blood pump. Artif Organs 16:305–308
38. Golding LR, Murakami G, Harasaki H, Takatani S, Jacobs G, Yada I, Tomita K, Yozu F, Valdes LK, Fujimoto S, Koike S, Nose Y (1982) Chronic nonpulsatile blood flow. ASAIO Trans 28: 81–85
39. Salmons S, Jarvis JC (1992) Cardiac assistance from skeletal muscle: a critical appraisal of the various approaches. Br Heart J 68:333–338
40. Carpentier A, Chachques JC, Grandjean (eds) (1991) Cardiomyoplasty. Futura, Mt Kisko
41. Grandjean PA, Austin L, Chan BS (1991) Dynamic cardiomyoplasty: clinical follow-up results, J Card Surg 6:80–88
42. Circulation supplement (1993) Am Heart Assoc 88(4)(pt 2): I-819
43. Farrar DJ, Hill JD (1992) A new skeletal linear-pull energy convertor as a power source for prosthetic circulatory support devices. J Heart Lung Transplant 11(5):S34150
44. Guldner NW, Tilmans MH, DeHaan H, Ruck K, Bressers H, Messmer BJ (1991) Development and training of skeletal muscle ventricles with low preload. J Card Surg 6[1 Suppl]:175–183
45. Guldner NW, Eichstaedt HC, Klapproth P, Tilmans MHI, Thaudet S, Umbrain V, Ruck K, Wyffels E, Bruyland M, Sigmund M, Messmer BJ, Bardos P (1994) Dynamic training of skeletal muscle ventricles: a method to increase muscular power for cardiac assistance. Circulation (in press)
46. Whalen RL (1979) Toward a blood pump for long-term circulatory support. In: Unger F (ed) Assisted Circulation. Springer, Berlin Heidelberg New York

# Progress Toward a Completely Implantable Left Ventricular Assist Device at the Pennsylvania State University

W.J. WEISS, G. ROSENBERG, A.J. SNYDER, J.H. DONACHY, G. FELDER, J.S. SAPIRSTEIN, W.E. PAE, and W.S. PIERCE

## Introduction

A multidisciplinary effort has been underway at Penn State University's Hershey Medical Center and University Park campus to build a left ventricular assist device (LVAD) which will be suitable for patients requiring long-term circulatory support. Substantial progress has been achieved by the successful testing of a sealed, wireless LVAD system in vitro and in vivo.

Over 70 patients have received the Pierce-Donachy pneumatic ventricular assist device at our institution since 1976, to provide circulatory support as a bridge-to-transplantion or pending myocardial recovery [1–3]. The worsening donor organ shortage and the demonstrated effectiveness of LVAD support in bridge-to-transplant patients for periods of months suggest that 25000–60000 patients per year will benefit from permanent LVAD support [4].

The major emphasis of our recent effort has been the integration of blood pump, motor drive, control electronics, transcutaneous power, and telemetry functions into an implantable system. Five complete LVAD systems have been built and tested in ten Holstein calves, with the longest implant surviving 244 days. These completely sealed systems employ a compliance chamber, transcutaneous energy transmission, and bidirectional telemetry. We have placed additional emphasis on manufacturability and documentation for manufacturing, in preparation for device readiness testing.

## System Description

The ventricular assist system is shown in Fig. 1 as configured for implantation in the calf. The major components are the blood pump and energy converter assembly, the implanted electronics assembly, the implanted energy transmission coil, the compliance chamber, and the external energy transmission coil and electronics [5–8]. Figure 2 shows the system as envisioned in the human recipient.

### Energy Converter

The energy converter uses a roller screw mechanism [9] to convert 4.75 revolutions of rotational motion to a 1.9-cm pusher-plate stroke. The roller screw consists of a central threaded shaft surrounded by seven threaded planetary

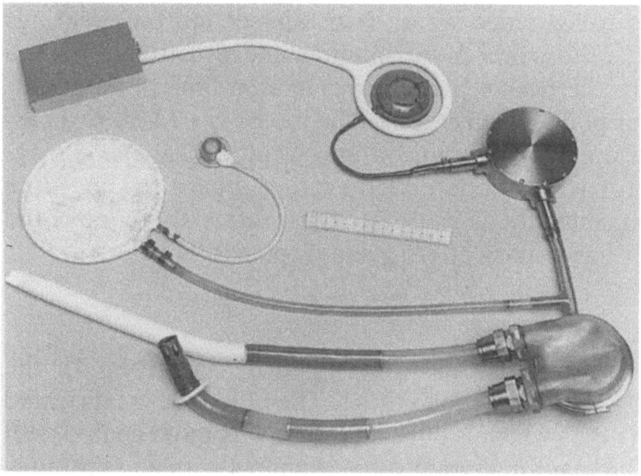

**Fig. 1.** The Penn State implantable LVAD system. (*Counterclockwise from lower right*), the blood pump and roller-screw energy converter with inlet cannula (*lower*) and outlet cannula (*upper*), the implanted electronics canister containing the control electronics and backup batteries, the energy transmission coils, the energy transmission external electronics, and the compliance chamber with attached access port

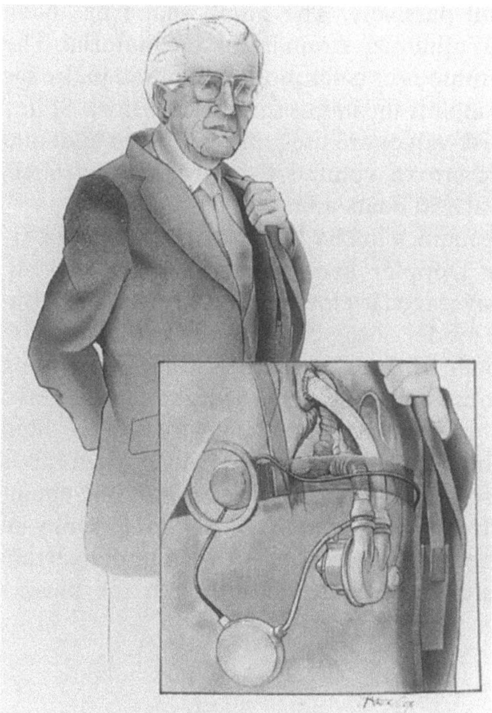

**Fig. 2.** The LVAD system configuration for permanent human implantation. The pump assembly and electronics canister will be implanted within be abdominal wall. The TETS coil will be implanted subcutaneously over the ribs

rollers which roll between the outer nut and the inner shaft. This mechanism distributes axial and radial loads over a large number of rolling point contacts, thereby requiring minimal lubrication and exhibiting low friction and excellent durability. Energy converters have accumulated over 1 year of operation in animals with no measurable roller screw wear. Two thin-section ball bearings hold the roller-screw nut and motor rotor in the titanium energy-converter housing. A guide shaft attached to the pusher plate moves in a bushing in the motor housing to prevent the pusher plate from rotating. The motor is a 14-pole, three-phase brushless DC motor using neodymium-iron-boron rotor magnets. A magnet ring mounted to the rotor is positioned over a circuit board having three Hall-effect sensors. The 3-bit sensor code is used to commutate and control the motor. The energy converter has a mass of 425 g and displaces 95 cc.

**Blood Pump**

The blood pump is fabricated using methods developed by our group for the manufacture of pneumatically actuated blood pumps. The blood sac is fabricated of segmented polyurethane (SPU) which is dip cast over a wax mold coated with silica-free silicone rubber. The resulting blood sac is seamless with an extremely smooth blood-contacting surface. The sac is mounted in a rigid polysulfone pump case by attachment at the inlet and outlet ports. The sac is not attached to the pusher plate, allowing the pump to fill passively. The pump shape has been designed so that the sac sidewalls roll to minimize strain in the sac material. The orientation of the ports encourages continuous circular motion of blood in the sac throughout the pump cycle in order to inhibit thrombus formation. Bjork-Shiley (Sorin, Irving, CA) monostrut Delrin disk valves are used, in size 27 mm inlet and 25 mm outlet. The maximum dynamic stroke volume is approximately 60 cc, yielding a maximum output of 9 l/min at 150 beats/min.

Quantitative studies of the fluid mechanics in the blood sac have been performed using a two-component laser Doppler anemometer (LDA) [10–14]. Measurements of the mean (ensemble-averaged) velocities and Reynolds (turbulent) stresses at over 150 locations in a model of the blood pump chamber using a blood analog solution have been obtained. In addition to the main pumping chamber, the critical near-valve regions, including the regurgitant jets, have recently been mapped. These studies suggest that the shear stresses are high enough to promote good washing of the sac wall, thereby preventing thrombus deposition and growth. The fluid stresses are low enough in the pumping chamber to prevent blood cell damage, but stresses in the valve regurgitant jets may be significant. In addition, cavitation has been found to occur in vitro under certain conditions [15, 16]. We continue to study these effects, although the plasma hemoglobin levels in the animal studies have been low.

**Compliance Chamber**

The compliance chamber, which functions as a reservoir for the gas displaced by the blood sac during pump filling, is a flexible sac implanted in the thorax. The compliance chamber measures 1.1 cm thick and 15 cm in diameter and is made of SPU approximately .020 inches thick and covered with Dacron velour. The size of the compliance chamber is chosen to supply the 60 cc of displacement per pump cycle as well as a buffer volume for loss of gas by diffusion through the chamber walls. Gas is replaced through the subcutaneous infusion port using a standard access-port needle. In animal studies, the chamber is refilled at approximately 4-week intervals with a mixture of sulfur hexafluoride and room air. Research into alternative low-permeability materials has been ongoing [17].

## Control Electronics

The electronics canister houses the electronics for motor control, power supply, battery charging, and telemetry, as well as backup batteries. Electrical power is normally supplied by the transcutaneous energy transmission system (TETS). The backup batteries supply power for up to 30 min (at 5 l/min) whenever the TETS coils are decoupled, for example during bathing, or during accidental coil misalignment. In the current system, the batteries are recharged at a constant current 14-h rate. The recharge time will be reduced to 3–4 h in the next-generation system. The battery pack consists of nine nickel cadmium 600 milliamp-hour size 2/3 $A_f$ cells, which account for approximately 60% of the electronics canister volume. Higher energy density batteries will allow the package size and weight to be reduced in the future. The titanium electronics canister currently measures 3.7 cm thick and 9.7 cm in diameter.

The implanted controller consists of a single-chip microcontroller (Intel 87C196), with added memory, logic, power supply, and safety (watchdog) circuits. The controller shares a single printed circuit board with the motor-power switching, energy transmission, telemetry, and battery charge circuits. The microcontroller is responsible for both control of the blood pump and supervisory tasks such as control of battery charge and reporting its status to external equipment.

Control functions are organized as shown in Fig. 3. Using only the three Hall-effect rotation sensors mounted in the motor, the pump control software effects

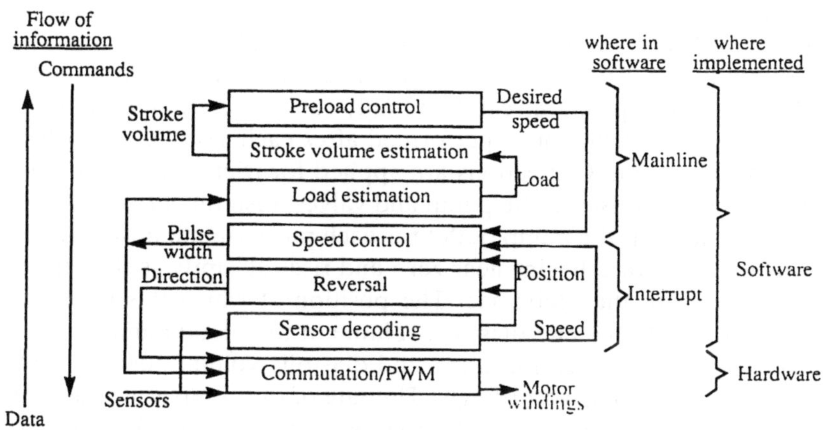


**Fig. 3.** Organization of the control system. Commands that alter operation flow down from higher-level to lower-level tasks. Data needed to make the higher level decisions flow back up. Commutation and pulse width modulation (*PWM*) are performed in hardware. Time-critical tasks are performed at the interrupt level

smooth, repeatable pusher-plate motions, estimates the pump's end-diastolic volume and outlet pressure, and determines the beat rate and systolic duration of the pump [18, 19].

At startup, the controller locates the energy converter's diastolic end point by moving in the diastolic direction until no further Hall sensor changes occur. From that point on, barring loss of power or of sensor integrity, the pusher-plate position is known by tracking the changes in the Hall sensor code, which repeats six times per motor revolution. In the event of a missed or illegal code, the end-point search is repeated and pumping resumes.

Motor speed is controlled by a unique algorithm which takes advantage of the device's multiple repetitions of the same movement. A complete pusher-plate motion is broken into 33 increments of equal distance, corresponding to the 33 complete cycles through the sensor code that occur in a full 19-mm stroke. To complete each incremental motion, the controller applies a pre-planned voltage to the motor. By measuring the time required by the energy converter to complete the incremental motion, the motor's speed can be accurately determined. Any discrepancy between the measured speed and the desired speed for the increment results in a modification of the voltage to be used for the same increment on the next repetition of the complete motion (the next pump cycle). Special mechanisms exist for preventing stalling of the motor due to large, abrupt changes in load, but these come into play infrequently, even when pumping asynchronously with a healthy ventricle, as in our animal experiments. The average speed for systole and diastole are determined by the cardiac output control. The instantaneous speed, for each increment, follows a trajectory chosen to limit peak power consumption and avoid excessive inertial forces at reversal. At the end of each diastolic motion, the pusherplate is held motionless for a diastasis period determined by the cardiac output control, typically 40 to 100 ms. This is provided so that the pusher plate can be retracted faster than the pump naturally fills. The pusher plate is therefore kept from impeding filling while in diastole; diastasis time is provided for pump filling to complete.

For a DC motor like that used in the energy converter, the motor current and thus the torque the motor produces can be readily calculated from the motor's voltage and speed. This calculation is performed after each systole, for each of the 33 increments of motion. Corrections are applied for friction in the mechanism, inertia, and viscous losses in the pump and valves, resulting in an estimate of the pressure produced at the pump outlet for each pusher-plate position. The pressure versus position trace begins near zero and rises abruptly as the pusher plate makes contact with the blood sac. The position at which this inflection occurs correlates well with the end-diastolic volume of the blood pump.

The cardiac output control averages the end-diastolic volume for five beats and adjusts the rate of pumping accordingly. The rate of the pump is increased in small steps until a decrease in the end-diastolic volume is detected (a volume change of 1.8 cc is detectable). The rate is then increased in small steps until no further increase in end-diastolic volume is seen. As this cycle repeats, the pump rate moves up and down slightly while the pump provides a full or nearly full stroke on each beat. Rate adjustments are made first by varying the diastasis time; changes are made to the systolic and diastolic stroke speeds only as necessary to keep the diastasis time within its allowable range. The amount of the diastasis increment corresponds to the amount of time we are willing to wait for a small increase in stroke volume: If the diastasis increment is large, we will wait a long time for a 1.8-cc-larger stroke volume. The pump will fill more completely, but pump flow may drop due to the lower rate.

The average calculated pressure load, from the point of pusher-plate contact to the end of systole, correlates well with the mean outlet pressure of the pump. This value is used for diagnostic purposes: excessive elevation above the normal mean arterial pressure could indicate occlusion of the outlet graft.

## Energy Transmission and Telemetry

The TETS supplies power and transmits data to the implanted electronics. The implanted TETS coil consists of 18 turns of litz wire molded in polyurethane in a mound shape approximately 1.9 cm thick at the center and 7.1 cm in diameter. The external coil consists of five turns of litz wire with a mean diameter of 10 cm molded in silicone rubber into a flexible loop that is held loosely in place over the implanted coil with an elastic band. Both coils are series tuned to 158 kHz with low-loss capacitors. The coil configuration and control mode were adapted from a Thermo CardioSystems design [20] and have been tested in calves by our group with minor modifications since 1987 [21]. The coils have been well tolerated in the calves with the exception of a series of animals, in which the internal tuning capacitor was encapsulated in the center of the implanted coil. These animals exhibited necrosis over the center of the coil due to excessive heat dissipation into the overlying tissue layers. Moving the capacitor into the electronics canister, where the capacity for heat rejection is higher, has eliminated the problem.

The TETS external electronics consist of a power oscillator and control circuit which drives the external coil at a frequency of either 160 kHz or 154 kHz as determined by the ingoing data bit. The internal electronics rectify, filter, and regulate the voltage induced in the implanted coil to maintain a regulated DC voltage of approximately 14 volts. The peak power capability is 64 watts continuous with a peak efficiency of 78%. In normal operation, the TETS supplies a mean power of approximately 9 watts for a flow rate of 5 l/min into a 100 mmHg mean arterial pressure.

Outgoing telemetry consists of frequency shift keying (FSK) modulation of a 32.77 MHz carrier which is transmitted from the implanted electronics canister using the TETS implanted coil as a radiating element. The outgoing data rate can be selected for either 300 or 1200 baud and the maximum transmission distance is approximately 10 m. In normal operation, the implant broadcasts a packet of data obtained from a single pump cycle once every 14 s (at 1200 baud) along with a 16-bit error checking code. The broadcast data include pump rate, estimated stroke volume, estimated outlet pressure, and tables of velocity, estimated load, applied voltage, and supply voltage. Ingoing telemetry, via FSK modulation of the TETS carrier, has a maximum data rate of 300 baud and is used to send commands to the implant, typically only during implantation. When commands are sent, the implant electronics switch to a secure bidirectional mode in which the outgoing telemetry is used to verify the ingoing commands [22].

An external power pack is being developed which will allow the patient a high degree of mobility. The power pack contains two battery packs, each containing 12 nickel cadmium size-D cells rated at 5.3 amp-hours. Each battery pack provides a maximum of 5h of operation at 5l/minute. The power pack contains electronics to monitor each battery and an external power source, if present, and to select the appropriate power source. The patient is alerted by audible and visual alarms, which gradually increase in intensity, when a battery pack is depleted. The power pack also monitors the telemetry broadcasts from the implant, logs data, and verifies proper operation of the implanted system.

## Implant Preparation

Extensive in vivo testing has been performed with the ventricular assist systems. This testing is intended to evaluate the performance of the system, assess the physiological responses and biocompatability, and demonstrate durability and reliabilty.

Prior to implantation, each energy converter undergoes a break-in and qualification test for approximately 1 week on a mock circulatory loop [23]. After connection to the electronics, the complete system is again tested for 1 week, while data are collected for correlating the estimated outlet pressure with measured aortic pressure and checking for normal power consumption and telemetry function. For final assembly, a closed-cell polyethylene foam is applied to the outer surface of the the energy converter over the region of the motor stator to limit heat dissipation in that region. The assembled system is then given a 24-h gas leak test, and the compliance chamber and TETS coil are covered with Dacron velour.

The inlet cannula for calf implantation is a 20-mm SPU tube with wire reinforcing near the proximal tip and along the section which passes through the diaphragm (see Fig. 1). The lighthouse tip is SPU-coated stainless steel for insertion into the ventricular apex with a felt sewing ring for fixation. The outlet cannula consists of a partially wire-wound SPU tube bonded to an 18-mm expanded polytetrafluoroethane (PTFE) graft. After packaging, the ventricular assist device, cannulae, and TETS primary electronics are ethylene-oxide sterilized and allowed to de-gas for 10 days at room temperature.

## Animal Implantation

Ten implantations of the completely implanted ventricular assist device were performed in Holstein calves over a 2-year period beginning in November 1991 (Fig. 4). The animals ranged in weight from 82 to 113kg (97kg mean). None of the systems utilized percutaneous leads. Five complete systems were manufactured and refurbished as necessary for these studies.

a 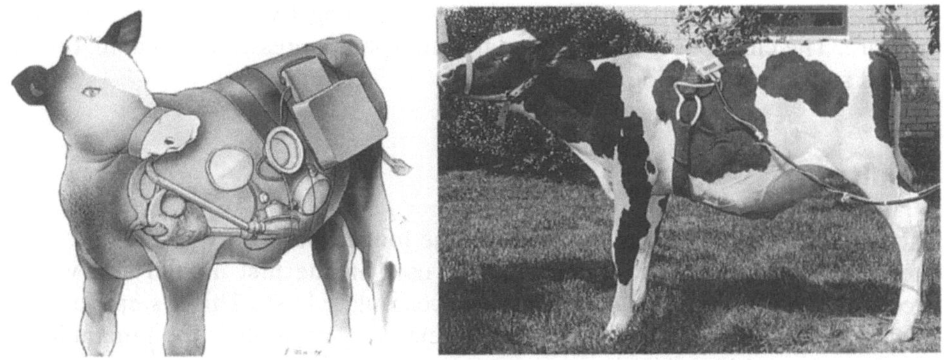 b

**Fig. 4.** **a** Implantation in the Holstein calf. **b** Calf 083 at postoperative day 99. The TETS external coil is held in place with an elastic strap

The cannulae and compliance chamber are positioned in the chest via a left thoracotomy. Cardiopulmonary bypass is not used for ventricular assist device implantation in calves. The outlet cannula is anastomosed to the proximal descending aorta, and the inlet cannula is placed through a cruciate incision in the ventricular apex. The cannulae and compliance chamber conduit connect to the pump through diaphragmatic tunnels.

The pump assembly and electronics canister are placed preperitoneally through a subcostal incision. The implanted TETS coil is tunneled up to the paraspinous area. After de-airing of the pump with heparinized saline, the cannulae are connected and held with titanium collet nuts. The TETS external coil is sutured in place and power is applied. When the pump output has reached 4–5 l/min and normal operation is verified, the compliance chamber is placed over the left hemidiaphragm, connected, and filled with room air. Two chest tubes and an internal mammary arterial line are placed and the incisions are closed.

The animals are able to stand within a few hours postoperatively. Low-molecular-weight dextran (20 cc/h) is begun when the chest tube drainage falls below 50 ml/h. Anticoagulation with warfarin sodium is begun (typically 5 mg/day beginning on day 3) when the chest tube drainage is sufficiently low; we maintain the prothrombin time at 1.5–2 times the preoperative value. Sodium nitroprusside (2–5 μg/kg/min) is given in the immediate postoperative period to keep the mean arterial pressure below 90 mmHg.

After approximately 3 days, all percutaneous lines and tubes are removed. The external TETS coil is held in place with a loose elastic bandage. An audible alarm is triggered when the coil is misaligned. Power supplied to the TETS is measured and recorded. Assist device parameters from the outgoing telemetry are displayed on a computer monitor and recorded hourly. Changes to the implanted control parameters via ingoing telemetry are not normally required.

The compliance chamber is checked every 3–6 weeks. The infusion port is accessed and the pressure is recorded. To determine the baseline volume, gas is then extracted from the chamber until the system monitor shows an increase in estimated outlet pressure and power, indicating a negative compliance chamber pressure. The chamber is then refilled to atmospheric pressure with a mixture of air and sulfur hexafluoride.

## Results

The results are summarized in Table 1. The longest survival was 244 days. The energy converter in this animal was also used in the first animal and was in excellent condition after the 328 days of accumulated use. This system (used in calves 731 and 800) did not have ingoing telemetry capability; the remainder of the systems used both ingoing and outgoing telemetry.

In all cases the animals gained weight normally and remained alert and active. All of the studies were terminated solely due to device failures. The mean plasma hemoglobin value for all animals, after the first 2 postoperative weeks, was 2.81 mg/dl with a standard error of +/–0.78. The minimum plasma hemoglobin our laboratory reports is 2.3 mg/dl. The maximum measured value for the same period was 6.90 mg/dl. The mean hematocrit was 31.0% with a standard error of +/–2.6%. Our calves' preoperative hematocrit values range from 32 to 38%. Routine blood chemistry values were consistently within normal ranges (Fig. 5).

**Table 1.** Implanted LVAD summary data for ten Holstein calves

| Calf no. | Survival (days) | Pump flow (l/min) (mean +/– standard error) | System power (watts) | Findings |
|---|---|---|---|---|
| 731 | 84 | 5.0 +/– .4 | 13.6 +/– 1.4 | Implanted TETS coil failure due to solder migration; no evidence of embolism |
| 760 | 208 | 4.9 +/– .4 | 13.8 +/– 1.6 | Tear in compliance chamber, fluid in motor, shorted Hall sensor; no evidence of embolism |
| 800 | 244 | 5.2 +/– .5 | 16.3 +/– 2.7 | Fractured solder joint on sensor board; infected growth in outlet graft; no evidence of embolism |
| 20 | 130 | 4.6 +/– .4 | 14.2 +/– 1.2 | Electrical short in sensor board, inadequate flux cleaning; outlet graft kinked; no evidence of embolism |
| 41 | 107 | 5.2 +/– .4 | 14.7 +/– 1.5 | Intermittent motor operation, poor solder connections on controller board; infection around electronics canister; no evidence of embolism |
| 9 | 20 | 4.8 +/– .4 | 15.1 +/– 1.4 | Shorted TETS coil, inadequate coating on wires; thrombus in cannulae and blood sac; no evidence of embolism |
| 83 | >167 | 5.6 +/– .4 | 14.9 +/– 1.4 | Ongoing |
| 12 | 25 | 5.8 +/– .3 | 16.6 +/– 1.6 | Motor jammed; mis-dimensioned guide bushing; no evidence of embolism |
| 115 | 27 | 5.0 +/– .5 | 13.2 +/– 1.9 | Motor jammed; thrombus on valves; no evidence of embolism |
| 26 | >20 | 5.4 +/– .5 | 14.6 +/– 1.9 | Ongoing |

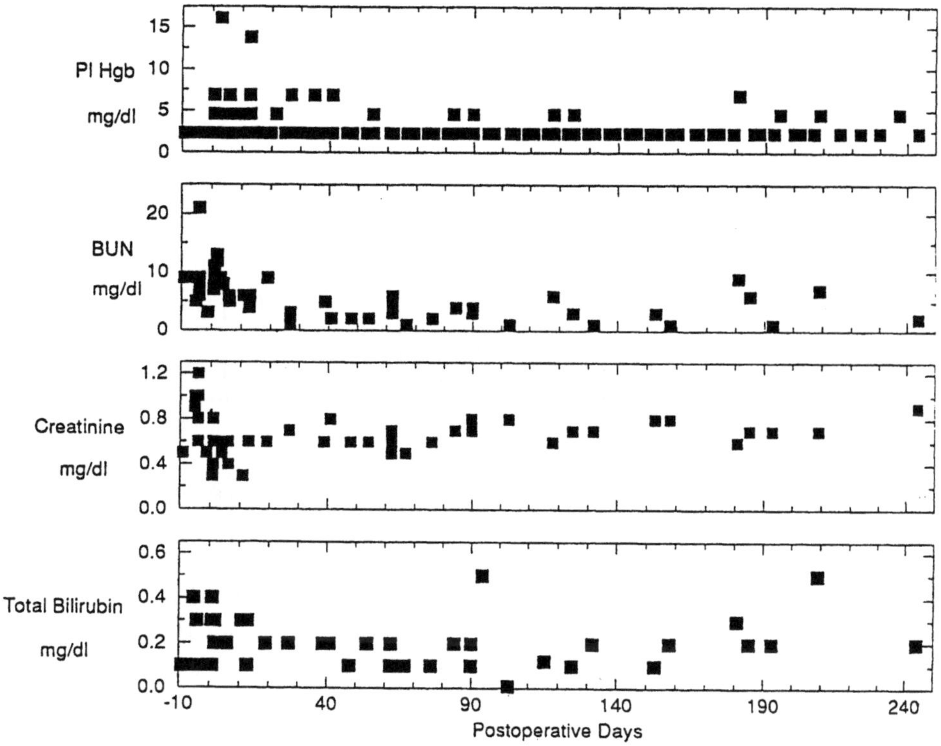


**Fig. 5.** The blood chemistry values, averaged for all animals versus postoperative days

The compliance chamber functioned well in all cases. A thin, pliable, tissue layer was found adherent to the chamber and adjacent lung tissue at explantation, and measurements of compliance chamber pressure during the refilling procedure showed pressure fluctuations of only a few mmHg. Figure 6 shows the gas loss rate from the six longest surviving animals. The compliance chamber used in calf 731 was an experimental design consisting of a polyvinylidene chloride sheet laminated between two sheets of SPU. This composition reduced the diffusion rate but had poor flexibility.

The first four animals developed skin lesions 1–2 cm in diameter over the center of the implanted TETS coil due to heat dissipation from a capacitor encapsulated in the implanted coil. Temperature measurements on the skin surface over the lesions ranged from 37 to 44°C. In the remainder of the animals, the capacitor was located in the electronics canister. The temperature over these coils remained below 35°C and no further problems were encountered. Other than the coil site lesions, there was no gross evidence of thermal injury to tissues surrounding the motor or electronics.

The estimated outlet pressure, shown in Fig. 7 for the five longest survivors, varied significantly among animals and tended to increase over the course of each experiment after the initial postoperative periods. The long length of the outlet graft, the movement of the LVAD, and the compression of the cannulae due to

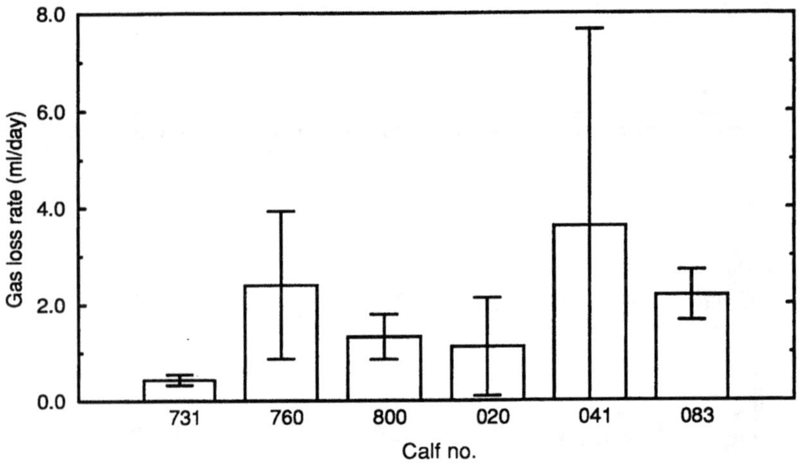


**Fig. 6.** The compliance chamber gas loss rate for the six longest survivors (mean +/–standard error of the mean)

the weight of the animal appeared to contribute to variation in outlet pressure seen by the pump. The LVAD flow rate, which increases with pump filling pressure, increased in some cases and decreased in others over time.

Purulent infections occurred in two animals. Calf 800 developed a hematoma near the pump which subsequently cultured positive for Corynebacterium pyogenes bacteria. At necropsy the outet graft contained a loosely attached pseudoendothelial layer. Calf 41 also developed swelling and pus accumulation around the electronics canister. Systemic sepsis was not evident in either animal.

A number of design changes have resulted from these tests. Two device failures were related to design and manufacturing defects in the Hall sensor assembly which led to failures in the humid implant environment, and one resulted from failure of the assembly when exposed to body fluids directly. As a result, the sensor assembly is being redesigned to allow consistent cleaning and encapsulation. Two failures were caused by shorting of the TETS implanted coil: the capacitor was moved to the electronics canister and the cable design was improved to provide adequate insulation. Two failures were the result of the motor jamming at the end-diastolic position, caused by a combination of inadequte clearance between the rotor and the pusher plate and inadequate electrical braking of the motor. The latter effect was especially evident in animals in which asynchrony between the LVAD and the natural heart (which retains normal function in these healthy calves) caused increased filling pressure during pump diastole not anticipated by the adaptive velocity control. High diastolic speed resulted, causing the motor to overshoot the end-diastolic reversal position and jam. This problem was solved by modifying the control program to use motor velocity during the current stroke while approaching end-diastole to determine the point of application of the motor brake. It was further recognized in the same device build that an improperly dimensioned part resulted in axial play in the rotor mount, yielding a loss of clearance and the potential for jamming and bearing damage.

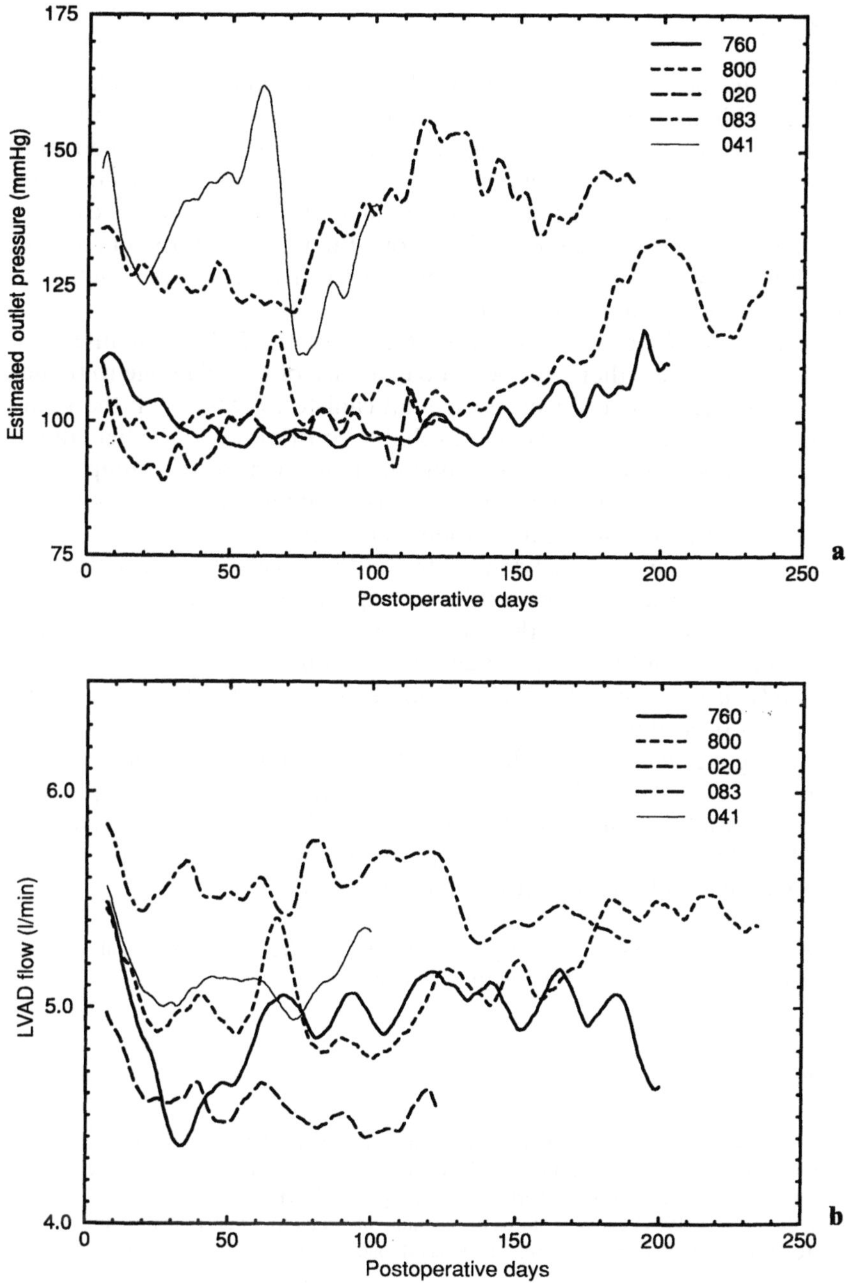


**Fig. 7a,b.** The LVAD estimated outlet pressure (**a**) and LVAD estimated flow (**b**) for the five longest survivors, after two applications of a 15-point running average on data obtained three times per day

## Discussion

Recent progress in the development of the Penn State completely implantable LVAD has been highlighted by the successful integration of blood pump, controller, power delivery system, and telemetry. The system has performed well, and we are gaining a high degree of confidence in the operation of the completely implantable system. Minor design changes are planned. The electronics canister will be redesigned to reduce the size and improve the implantability and assembly. Higher efficiency motor-drive power switches will be used. An improved Hall sensor assembly is being evaluated.

With the exception of the skin lesions associated with the TETS implanted coil capacitor previously noted, there has been no evidence of heat damage to tissues surrounding the energy converter or electronics canister. Pressure on the tissue near the pump due to the animals' weight probably contributed to the hematoma and swelling which occurred in two experiments. Placement of the pump in the preperitoneal position requires long cannulae in the calf model with the potential for kinking as the animal grows and components migrate.

The animal studies have further demonstrated the feasibility of a sealed system utilizing a compliance chamber. While we expect the rate of volume loss to be reduced in the future through the use of lower-permeability materials, the procedure of checking and refilling the chamber can be performed quickly and relatively simply using the subcutaneous infusion port. No infections have resulted from this procedure.

We plan to begin 2-year in vitro durability testing in the near future in order to demonstrate an 80% reliability with 80% confidence for a 2-year life [24, 25]. Chronic animal studies will also be continued [26]. It appears that the implantable LVAD can meet the need for permanent circulatory support while allowing the patient a sufficiently unrestricted life-style.

*Acknowledgment.* This work was supported by grant RO1 HL 13426 from the Public Health Service and by gifts from Mrs. Ruth Lewis and from Arrow International.

## References

1. Quinn RD, Pae WE, Pierce WS (1990) The use of mechanical circulatory assistance as a bridge to heart transplantation: the Penn State experience. In: Hetzer R (ed) Mechanical circulation as a bridge to transplantation. Springer, Berlin Heidelberg New York
2. Pierce WS, Quinn RD (1991) Current status of mechanical circulatory assist devices. In: Weiss J, Bonheim R (eds) Current trends in circulatory assistance, vol 1, no l. Cahners, New York, pp 1–7
3. Pae WE, Miller CA, Matthews Y, Pierce WS (1992) Ventricular assist devices for postcardiotomy cardiogenic shock: a combined registry experience. J Thorac Cardiovasc Surg 104(3):541–553
4. Hogness JR, VanAntwerp MV (eds) (1991) The artificial heart: prototypes, policies, and patients. National Academy Press, Washington DC
5. Weiss WJ, Rosenberg G, Snyder AJ, Donachy J, Reibson J, Kawaguchi O, Sapirstein JS, Pae WE, Pierce WS (1993) A completely implanted left ventricular assist device (LVAD): chronic in vivo testing. ASAIO J 39(3):M427–M432

6. Richenbacher WE, Pae WE, Magovern JA, Rosenberg G, Snyder AJ, Pierce WS (1986) A rollerscrew electric motor ventricular assist device. ASAIO Trans 32:46–38
7. Pierce WS, Snyder AJ, Rosenberg G, Weiss W, Pae WE, and Waldhausen JA (1993) A long-term ventricular assist device. J Thorac Cardiovasc Surg 105(3):520–524
8. Rosenberg G, Snyder A, Weiss W, Cleary T, Pierce WS (1988) A permanent left ventricular assist device, In vivo testing. IEEE Eng Med Biol Soc 65–67
9. Rosenberg G, Snyder A, Weiss W, Landis DL, Geselowitz DB, Pierce WS (1982) A rollerscrew drive for implantable blood pumps. ASAIO Trans 28:1–23
10. Baldwin JT, Deutsch S, Geselowitz DB, Tarbell JM (1990) Estimation of Reynolds stresses within the Penn State ventricular assist device. Trans Am Soc Artif Intern Organs 36:M274–M278
11. Baldwin JT, Tarbell JM, Deutsch S, Geselowitz DB (1990) Reynolds stress measurements within the outet port of the Penn State LVAD. In: Proceedings of the 16th Annual Northeast Bioengineering Conference. pp 17–18 (IEEE Catalogue no 90-CH2834-0)
12. Baldwin JT, Tarbell JM, Deutsch S, Geselowitz DB (1991) Mean velocities and Reynolds stresses within regurgitant jets produced by tilting disk valves. Trans Am Soc Artif Intern Organs 37:M348–M349
13. Baldwin JT, Deutsch S, Petrie HL, Tarbell JM (1993) Determination of prinicipal Reynolds stresses in pulsatile flows after elliptical filtering of discrete velocity Measurements. J Biomech Eng 115:396–403
14. Baldwin JT, Deutsch S, Geselowitz DB, Tarbell JM (1994) LDA Measurements of mean velocity and Reynolds stress fields within an artificial heart ventricle. J Biomech Eng 116:190–200
15. Lamson, TC, Rosenberg G, Geselowitz, DB, Deutsch S, Stinebring DR, Frangos JA, Tarbell JM (1993) Relative blood damage in the three phases of a prosthetic heart valve flow cycle. ASAIO J 39:M626–633
16. Lamson TC, Stinebring DR, Deutsch S, Rosenberg G, Tarbell JM (1991) real-time in vitro observation of cavitation in a prosthetic heart valve. Trans Am Soc Artif Intern Organs 37:M351–353
17. Reid JS, Rosenberg G, Pierce WS (1985) Transmission of water through a biocompatible polyurethane – application to circulatory assist devices. J Biomed Mater Res 19:1181–1202
18. Snyder AJ, Weiss WJ, Nazarian R (1989) Microcomputer control of implantable blood pumps. Proceedings of the 2nd Annual IEEE Symposium on Computer-Based Medical Systems. IEEE, New York, 154–157
19. Snyder AJ, Rosenberg G, Landis D (1985) Indirect estimation of circulatory pressures for control of an electric motor-driven total artificial hear. In: Langrana NA (ed) Advances in bioengineering. The American Society of Mechanical Engineers, New York, pp 87–88
20. Sherman C, Daly B, Dasse K, Clay W, Szycher M, Handrahan J, Schuder J, Lewis M, Worthington M, Hopkins R, Poirier V (1983) Research and development: systems for transmitting energy through intact skin. Final Technical Report N01-HV-0-2903-3, Thermo Electron Corp., Waltham, July 1983.
21. Weiss WJ, Rosenberg G, Snyder AJ, Pae WE, Richenbacher WE, Pierce WS (1989) In vivo performance of a transcutaneous energy transmission system with the Penn State motor-driven ventricular assist device. Trans Am Soc Artif Intern Organs 35:284–288
22. Snyder AJ, Nazarian R, Weiss W (1993) A secure communications and status reporting protocol for implanted devices. In: Kriewall T (ed) Proceedings of the Sixth Annual IEEE Symposium on Computer-Based Medical Systems. IEEE Computer Society, Los Alamitos, pp 253–257
23. Rosenberg G, Phillips WM, Landis DL, Pierce WS (1981) Design and evaluation of the Pennsylvania State Unversity mock circulatory system. ASAIO Trans 4:41–49
24. Dai SH, Wang MO (1992) Reliability analysis in engineering applications. Van Nostrand Reinhold, New York
25. Nelson W (1982) Applied life data analysis. Wiley, New York
26. Ventricular Assist Device (VAD) (1992) Pathology analyses: guidelines for clinical Studies. Society for Biomaterials: Implant Retrieval Symposium – Transactions, Pheasant Run Resort, St Charles, 17–20 Sept 1992, pp 13–20

# Part III
# Nonpulsatile Blood Pumps

# Introduction

F. Unger

Nonpulsatile blood pumps are mechanical devices useful especially in postoperative cardiac failure. Cardiac failure after myocardial infarction is another indication, which should be considered more frequently. Some of the pumps can be used in ECMO or in assisting a part of the circulation during repair of abdomino- or abdominothoracic aneurysms. Different devices are available for clinical use, including impeller, aortic, and spindle-designed devices. Limitations are embolization and hemolysis from the pump.

Since these devices are highly effective and inexpensive, they are the device of choice in direct postoperative cardiac failure.

In this section, Golding reports on his clinical experience using the Biopump. Aboul Hosn explains the Hemopump, which can be inserted directly into the ascending aorta and unloads the left ventricle by means of a cannula through the aortic valves. The device can also be recommended for use in interventional cardiology. Hager reports on progress made in the spindle pump. Finally, Qian reports on the experience using nonpulsatile biventricular impeller pumps in China.

# Centrifugal Pumps – Now and the Future

L.A.R. Golding and W.A. Smith

Since their introduction in the 1970s into the clinical practice of cardiothoracic surgery, many uses have been found for centrifugal pumps (Table 1). It is estimated that these devices have replaced roller pumps in 30% of routine cardiac surgical procedures, especially for procedures that are more prolonged. Their simplicity, reliability, and low cost have also gained for them a major role in the other situations, and it is only in bridging to transplantation that there has been decreasing use as the requirements for longer support (30 days +) and patient mobility have become apparent. Even in some of these patients, however, centrifugal pumps are still briefly deployed to stabilize the patient prior to the decision to utilize a more durable implantable system.

Since 1979, when the program of direct mechanical ventricular support was initiated at our institution, centrifugal blood pumps have had a central role because of their simplicity, low cost, and availability. A few patients have been supported with other devices, e.g., roller pump, Hemopump, and a pneumatically powered pulsatile pump. Initially, the Medtronic Hemadyne centrifugal pump was used [1–5], but when it became unavailable it was replaced by the vortex-shedding Biomedicus Biopump [6–11]. This continues to be the mainstay of our program for short-term support but is infrequently used now for bridging to cardiac transplantation. For the latter indication, we have come to rely on the TCI HeartMate system because of the need for a safe and more durable device that permits patient mobility. The Biopump has also found a role as an integral component of percutaneous emergency bypass systems and in ECMO support.

Our indications for postcardiotomy support have remained constant over the past several years. With only a very few exceptions, left atrial and ascending aortic cannulation sites were used. The cannulae usually were those routinely available for standard cardiopulmonary bypass, but more recently there has been increasing use of heparin-bonded pump heads and tubing. Postoperatively, heparin used to be given by continuous i.v. infusion adjusted to maintain the activated clotting time at about 150 s after postoperative bleeding had been controlled, but we have discontinued this since heparin-coated components became available. In many instances the sternum was not closed initially because of bleeding and edema. In such circumstances closure was delayed for 24 h but in some this was not done until after weaning and device removal and this has not resulted in a higher infection rate. Intra-aortic balloon pumping was continued throughout the support period and for 1–2 days after device removal except where severe atherosclerosis prevented its passage. The maintenance of the

**Table 1.** Clinical uses for centrifugal pumps

| | |
|---|---|
| 1. | Routine cardiopulmonary bypass |
| 2. | Postcardiotomy ventricular support |
| 3. | Percutaneous emergency bypass |
| 4. | ECMO |
| 5. | Bridge to cardiac transplantation |

pump was monitored by a perfusionist in constant attendance during the early years, but this function has been under nursing supervision alone for the past few years with no untoward effects. Nurses are trained to change pump heads in emergency situations, but this has rarely been necessary.

Excluding use in combination with an oxygenator, centrifugal pumps have been used in 108 patients since 1979 – in 91 for failure to wean from bypass or for low cardiac output in the early postoperative period, and for bridging-to-cardiac transplantation as the primary indication in 17 others. Overall there have been 23 survivors (21%), four after bridging to cardiac transplantation.

In the 10-year period from January 1983 through December 1992, 98 patients were supported by ventricular assist with a Biomedicus Biopump – in 81 for postcardiotomy low cardiac output unresponsive to standard measures and in 17 as an attempt to bridge to cardiac transplantation. The 74 male and 24 female patients (3/1 ratio) had a mean age of 51 years (range 1 day to 73 years). Fifteen patients were over 65 years of age, all being postcardiotomy. In four postcardiotomy patients weaning was unsuccessful, but as all other systemic organ functions were good, an attempt to bridge to transplantation was made.

Overall, there were 21 survivors (21.4%) from mechanical ventricular support – 17 after weaning from postcardiotomy support, four after successful cardiac transplantation (Tables 2, 3). There was no significant difference in survival for the two major indications for use (22.1% vs. 19.1%), but based on the poor results of postcardiotomy biventricular support, we believe that such mechanical support should be infrequently used. There was no statistical difference in survival based on sex (male 20% vs. female 25%). The survival rate of 20% (three of 15) for this group differs little from that for patients 65 years of age or less (18/83 = 22%). There were seven patients for whom postcardiotomy support was necessary after transplantation and two survived (29%), both after right ventricular support.

There were 17 patients in whom the primary indication was bridging to transplantation and an additional four in whom weaning was not possible. Transplantation was accomplished in five, and four (19%) were discharged home.

Recently we reported our results for postcardiotomy mechanical support [11]. That analysis showed a high rate of postoperative bleeding, a higher mortality for associated renal failure, but no association of mortality to increasing age. The additional patients since that time have not altered these results. The survival rate of 21.4% is not high but has remained essentially the same in recent years in spite of changing demographics for cardiac surgery patients with higher age,

**Table 2.** Results of centrifugal ventricular support

| Type of support | No. of cases | Survivors n (%) |
|---|---|---|
| Left ventricle | 60 | 15 (25.0) |
| Right ventricle | 20 | 4 (20.0) |
| Biventricular | 18 | 2 (11.0) |
| Total | 98 | 21 (21.4) |

**Table 3.** Results vs. indication for use

| Type of support | Postcardiotomy | | Bridge to transplant | |
|---|---|---|---|---|
| | No. of cases | Survival n (%) | No. of cases | Survival n (%) |
| Left ventricle | 47 | 12 (25.5) | 13 | 3 (23.1) |
| Right ventricle | 17 | 4 (23.5) | 3 | 0 – |
| Biventricular | 13 | 1 (07.7) | 5 | 1 (20.0) |
| Total | 77 | 17 (22.1) | 21 | 4 (19.1) |

more advanced disease, and often at least one previous cardiac operation. We believe that centrifugal pumps are the most cost-effective devices for postcardiotomy mechanical support and that, with the exception of bridging to transplantation, their use should be limited to a maximum of 5 days.

A major effort at this institution has involved studies on the physiological effects of continuous flow [12–21]. We have the largest experience with animals maintained with fibrillating ventricles and nonpulsatile systemic perfusion for 30 days or more and have found that there is an initial transient perturbation of physiology during the initial 7–10 days resulting from a hyperadrenergic response and fluid balance anomalies. Following this phase, however, physiologic function returns to normal and continues so for periods up to the 99-day duration of the longest experiment, provided adequate systemic blood flow and pressure are provided. More recent studies in animals have shown that if fibrillation of the animal's heart is delayed until 7–10 days following surgery, such major transient events are not seen. Thus, it is concluded that these early anomalies were the result of surgery, anesthesia, and immediate depulsation at that time, but adaptation to nonpulsatility occurs. The primary major difference seen in animals maintained with continuous flow is that they may need slightly higher overall volume flow to maintain systemic organ function.

Additional information has also been obtained from patients maintained with continuous-flow blood pumps in attempting to bridge to transplantation [22–24]. We now have experience with some 21 patients, the longest having been supported for a period of 31 days prior to cardiac transplantation. Perhaps most interesting has been the observation that in patients supported with continuous-flow blood pumps, with the passage of time and unloading of the failing left ventricle there is recovery of some ventricular function, and pulsatility returns and is superimposed upon the continuous-flow state.

More prolonged studies in animals and humans, however, have been significantly limited due to the limited durability of continuous-flow blood pumps. In both situations, frequent changes of the device pump head have been necessary and introduced perturbations in physiology. Due to the lack of durability of such devices and the difficulty in patient mobilization, we now reserve its use for postcardiotomy, low cardiac output situations. For bridging to transplantation, more durable implantable, pulsatile assist devices have produced good results [25–27] but also demonstrated that such devices have some limitations in use because of their physical size.

There is an obvious need for a smaller and less costly implantable blood pump which would have a wider range of use in both adults and children, and continuous-flow blood pumps are the greatest hope for such a device. An implantable continuous-flow blood pump providing a nominal 5 l/min blood flow with a size of 5 cm in diameter and 5 cm long would have the potential for significantly reducing cost by virtue of its inherent simplicity. Elimination of flexing diaphragms and cycling valves would remove two of the most critical failure sites of current pumps. Rotodynamic pumps closely follow hydraulic scaling laws, making related devices of higher and lower flows easy to size. The relatively low volume and small surface area, combined with steady flow, make biomaterial and hemocompatibility questions less difficult than in a periodically reversing pump with a large pump chamber that must allow for output, valve regurgitation, and diaphragm-wall clearances. The ports and conduits of pulsatile pumps must also be large enough to accommodate valves which are subject to transient peak flows up to four times higher than the nominal levels.

The major time-limiting technical problem of continuous-flow pumps has been an inevitable deposition at the shaft/seal junction area. There have been several approaches to solving this shaft/seal interface problem, including ferromagnetic fluid seals, perfused seals, and magnetically suspended rotors [28–34]. Another potential solution is to use a blood-lubricated journal bearing to eliminate seals and perfusion fluids, and also the cost and complexity of active magnetic suspensions. We have developed a pump design with a blood-lubricated hydrodynamic bearing which achieves low hemolysis, produces 5 l/min blood flow, and has the potential for long durability.

Hydrodynamic bearing function is described in many texts [35–37]. Hydrodynamic bearings depend on a converging/diverging geometry to create a load-supporting pressure difference around the bearing. With appropriate selection of diameter, length, clearance, rotational speed, temperature, load, and fluid viscosity, the journal will lift off the sleeve and ride on a stable liquid film so that friction is minimal and wear will not occur. If the load is too high or diameter too small, the journal may contact the sleeve and eventually wear out. If the two elements become too close to concentric, the bearing can go into a "whirl" mode with no stable journal position, the resulting vibration leading to destruction of the bearing.

Feasibility studies resulted in a design for a mixed-flow blood pump (CCF Model 2156) with a blood-lubricated journal bearing to eliminate seal problems [38, 39]. The initial design criteria were:

1. Nominal flow of 5 l/min against a 100 mmHg pressure gradient;
2. Electric power input of 10 watts or less
3. No significant damage to blood elements
4. Function for 1 month or more in vivo
5. Biocompatibility
6. Size allowing implantation in any adult or child

This pump was first assembled in May 1990, and the characteristics of the assembled device were: (a) volume 70 ml; (b) weight 170 g; (c) internal priming volume 16 ml; (d) 12 watts power requirement at 5000 RPM to produce 5 l/min and 100 mmHg pressure rise; (e) index of hemolysis approximately 0.1 g Hb/100 l blood pumped. The pump consisted of three main subassemblies; the post-like stator housing which contained the motor windings, an annular rotor containing the motor magnets with "primary" and "secondary" impellers on opposing faces, and a housing, enveloping all components. The motor configuration was inverted from the conventional, the rotating element surrounding the stationary. Blood-lubricated hydrodynamic bearings supported the radial load, while magnet-lamination attraction reacted axial loads.

The major blood flow was from the inlet, through the mixed-flow primary impeller, into the collector, and out the discharge port. Additionally, some blood passed from the impeller discharge through windows in the impeller hub to a secondary flow path. Part of this fluid flowed down through the small-diameter front bearing back to the inlet, providing lubricating and washing flow to this area. Additional flow passed along wider and shallower grooves in the main bearing to a secondary impeller that raised its pressure and sent it along the rotor OD to pump discharge. This secondary pathway for blood provided main bearing lubrication, motor cooling, and wash flow along its path. A significant aspect of this design was to ensure good washing of all blood-contacting surfaces with no crevices, tiny pivots, or other clot-starting features on the center line of the pump, where velocities and centrifugal force gradients to induce flow are inherently very low. Surface velocities and the geometry were configured to generate a surface-separating hydrodynamic film, and only a small amount of blood deliberately recirculated from discharge to inlet. Pump performance data was good, but this prototype had problems with hemolysis and rotor stability. These were resolved and hemolysis improved to 0.1 g Hb/100 l blood pumped, but a brief in vivo study demonstrated significant deposition in the front journal bearing. (Values of 0.02–0.04 g Hb/100 l blood pumped are the hemolysis index values for a Biopump tested in our hemolysis loop as the reference standard.)

Based upon these results, a second prototype (CCF Model 2336) was made with three major design changes: (a) a higher performance alloy for the motor laminations better utilized the neodymium magnets and resulted in a one-third shortening of the motor length; (b) the mixed-flow primary impeller was changed to a radial flow design to eliminate the need for the front bearing, while the larger mean discharge radius reduced the required speed; (c) the original collector-style discharge system was replaced by a more sophisticated volute/diffuser design to more efficiently convert velocity to pressure. Retained were the inverted motor, the grooved, blood-lubricated journal bearing, and the spiral secondary impeller. The stator housing decreased in length due to the motor redesign, shortening the path of blood through the journal bearing. The direction of secondary flow was from a midpoint of the primary impeller, along the bearing, and then into the secondary impeller, on its way over the OD and into the discharge. In vitro testing of this device showed good hydraulic function with 5 l/min flow against 100 mmHg pressure rise at 3000 rpm. The electric power input to produce this performance also dropped to less than 10 watts. Typical performance mapping results for this device are shown in Table 5. The opposing walls of the journal bearing, the rotor ID, and the stator OD were fabricated from titanium alloy (Ti6A14V) with wall thickness of .010 and .018 inches, and any occasional contact of these elements resulted in destruction with device failure. Modification of the stator groove geometry and the offset of the axis of the stator in relation to the motor axis decreased the journal bearing loads and led to improved stability and durability. Other modifications were surface treatment of the opposing members by vapor deposition or by coating with ceramic or silver. The best results were from a nitrided titanium/dry-file epoxy coating pair demonstrating 14 days continuous use, and hemolysis index values improved to 0.07 g Hb/100 l blood pumped. While good results were obtained in vitro, short-term animal implants in vivo showed significant deposition in the grooved journal-bearing area. The spiral blade secondary impeller system was also found to be sensitive to its clearance, relative to the rear shroud.

The significant changes in the present device (CCF Model 2631) are elimination of the grooves in the stator housing and replacement of the spiral impeller blades by simpler straight blades (Fig. 1). The straight blades proved more effective hydraulically and less affected by variation of clearance from the stator flange. Better dynamic balancing of the rotor assembly eliminated vibration and improved durability (Table 4). In vitro studies have now shown 5 l/min blood flow against 100 mmHg pressure rise at 3000 rpm with 7 watts electric power in (Fig. 2). A comparison of the three models is shown in Table 5.

This model also has undergone hydraulic testing in various spatial orientations to show that no significant alteration in performance occurred. Additionally, in mock loop testing the inlet to the device was connected to both mock atrial and

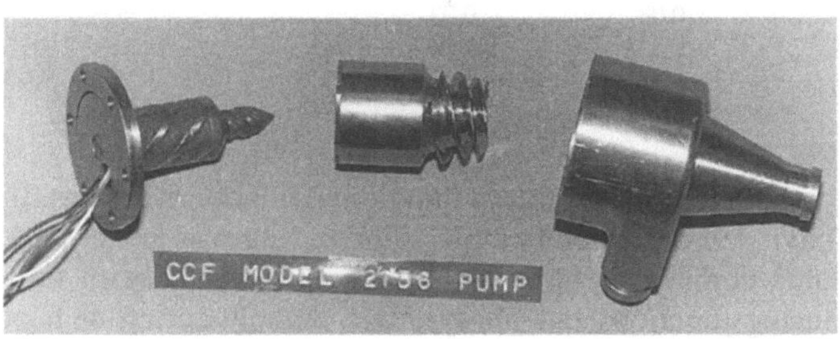


**Fig. 1.** CCF model 2156 pump

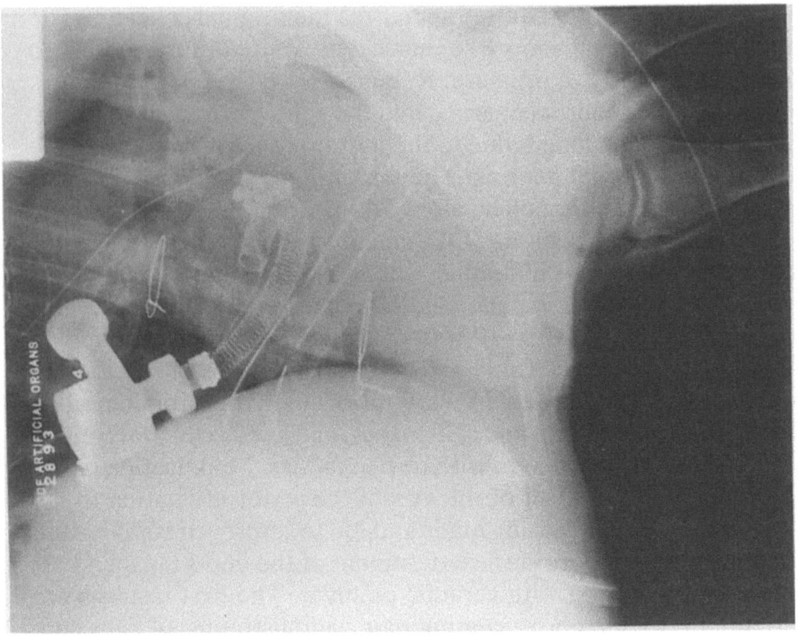


**Fig. 2.** Roentgenogram of implant CCF model 2631

**Table 4.** Performance characteristics of model 2631

| | |
|---|---|
| RPM | 3000 |
| Flow | 5 l/min |
| Pressure rise | 100 mmHg |
| Power | 7.5 watts |
| Δ Temp. windings | 3°C |
| (In blood analog solution of 37°C) | |

**Table 5.** Comparison of three models

| | Model 2156 | Model 2336 | Model 2631 |
|---|---|---|---|
| Volume | 70 ml | 62 ml | 62 ml |
| Weight | 170 g | 216 g | 207 g |
| Priming volume | 16 ml | 13 ml | 12 ml |
| Best HI | 0.1 | 0.08 | 0.03 |
| Power | 12 W | 8.5 W | 7.0 W |

*HI*, Hemolysis index

mock ventricular pressure sources and the pump functioned in both situations. In vitro hemolysis studies have demonstrated hemolysis index values as low as 0.03, and 2-day animal implants confirmed the in vitro hemolysis values with only minor deposition at housing junctions but no systemic emboli during 48 h of function. One pump ran continuously on a mock loop at 3000 RPM, 5 l/min flow against 100 mmHg pressure use for 5 weeks, and intermittent inspection showed no wear at the journal-bearing surfaces.

Variability of hydraulic performance was finally found to be the result of variable magnetic flux of the rotating assembly, as during magnetic assembly the magnets were being variably damaged. This was resolved by demagnetization and led to a significant and constant improvement in performance. Two in vivo studies of 6 and 10 days duration confirmed the low hemolysis levels but did show a problem with deposition on the inflow cannula. This is being redesigned, and simultaneously we are exploring the potential use of plastic and ceramic materials.

Several groups are now working to develop long-term implantable continuous-flow blood pumps. We believe that such devices will be complementary to the existing implantable pulsatile pumps and be a cost-effective option within 10 years.

## References


1. Golding L, Loop F, Peter M, Jacobs G, Gill C, Groves L, Nosé Y (1979) Use of a temporary left ventricular assist system postoperatively. Proceedings of the 2nd Meeting of the International Society for Artificial Organs. Artif Organs 3[Suppl]:394–397
2. Golding LR, Groves LK, Peter M, Jacobs G, Sukalac R, Nosé Y, Loop FD (1980) Initial clinical experience with a new temporary left ventricular assist device. Ann Thorac Surg 29:66–69
3. Golding LR, Loop FD, Sandberg GW, Jacobs G, Lewis RC (1981) Left ventricular assist device support: twenty-one month survival. Cleve Clin Q 48:373–377
4. Golding LAR, Harasaki H, Gill CC, Jacobs G, Loop FD, Nosé Y (1981) Clinical mechanical ventricular support. Proceedings of the 3rd Meeting of the International Society for Artifical Organs. Artif Organs 5[Suppl]:565–567
5. Golding LR, Jacobs G, Groves LK, Gill CC, Nosé Y, Loop FD (1982) Clinical results of mechanical support of the failing left ventricle. J Thorac Cardiovasc Surg 83:597–601
6. Golding LAR (1984) Centrifugal pumps. In: Unger F (ed) Assisted circulation, vol 2. Springer, Berlin Heidelberg New York, p 142
7. Golding LAR, Loop FD, Nosé Y (1985) Clinical and experimental use of the centrifugal pump. In: Attar S (ed) New developments in cardiac assist devices. Praeger Saunders, New York, 92–102
8. Golding LAR, Stewart RW, Loop FD (1989) Centrifugal pumps in clinical practice. In: Unger F (ed) Assisted circulation, vol 3. Springer, Berlin Heidelberg New York, pp 160–166
9. Golding LAR, Oyer PE, Cabrol C (1989) Circulatory support 1988: weaning and bridging. Ann Thorac Surg 47:102–107
10. Golding LAR (1990) Biomedicus centrifugal pump for mechanical cardiac support. In: Sezai Y (ed) Proceedings of Nihon University International Symposium on the Development of Biomation in the 21st Century, May 1990. Saunders, Philadelphia, pp 248–252
11. Golding LAR, Crouch RD, Stewart RW, Novoa R, Lytle BW, McCarthy PM, Taylor PC, Loop FD, Cosgrove DM (1992) Postcardiotomy centrifugal mechanical ventricular support. Ann Thorac Surg 54:1059–1064
12. Golding LR, Jacobs G, Murakami T, Takatani S, Valdes F, Harasaki H, Nosé Y (1980) Chronic nonpulsatile blood flow in an alive, awake animal: 34-day survival. Trans Am Soc Intern Organs 26:251
13. Golding LR, Murakami G, Harasaki H, Takatani S, Jacobs G, Yada I, Tomita K, Yozu R, Valdes F, Fujimoto LK, Koike S, Nosé Y (1982) Chronic nonpulsatile blood flow. Trans Am Soc Artif Intern Organs 28:81–85

14. Golding LAR, Loop FD, Nosé Y (1985) Clinical and experimental use of the centrifugal pump. In: Attar S (ed) New developments in cardiac assist devices. Praeger Saunders, New York, pp 92–102
15. Sugita Y, Golding LR, Jacobs G, Harasaki H, Yozu R, Sato N, Fujimoto LK, Morimoto T, Snow J, Olsen E, Smith W, Murabayashi S, Kambic H, Kiraly R, Nosé Y (1984) Comparison of osmotic and body fluid balance in chronic nonpulsatile biventricular bypass (NPBVB) and total artificial heart (TAH) experiments. Trans Am Soc Artif Intern Organs 30:148–154
16. Takatani S, Golding LR, Jacobs GB, Murakami T, Harasaki H, Ozawa K, Kiraly R, Nosé Y (1979) Comparison of nonpulsatile and pulsatile pumps as left ventricular assist devices. Trans Jpn Soc Artif Intern Organs 9:372
17. Takatani S, Golding L, Harasaki H, Yada I, Koike S, Yozu R, Fujimoto L, Murakami G, Tomita K, Jacobs G, Nosé Y (1983) Nonpulsatile biventricular bypass during ventricular fibrillation. Jpn J Artif Organs 12:254
18. Valdes F, Takatani S, Jacobs GB, Murakami T, Harasaki H, Golding LR, Nosé Y (1980) Comparison of hemodynamic changes in a chronic nonpulsatile biventricular bypass (BVB) and total artificial heart (TAH). Trans Am Soc Artif Intern Organs 26:455
19. Valdes F, Golding LR, Harasaki H, Takatani S, Jacobs G, Nosé Y (1981) Hemodynamic response to exercise during chronic ventricular fibrillation and nonpulsatile biventricular bypass (BVB). Trans Am Soc Artif Intern Organs 27:449–452
20. Yada I, Golding LR, Harasaki H, Jacobs G, Koike S, Yozu R, Sato N, Fujimoto LK, Snow J. Olsen E, Murabayashi S, Venkatesen VS, Kiraly R, Nosé Y (1983) Physiopathological studies of nonpulsatile blood flow in chronic models. Trans Am Soc Artif Intern Organs 29:520
21. Yozu R, Golding LAR, Shimomitsu T, Jacobs G, Watanabe T, Harasaki H, Nosé Y (1985) Exercise response in chronic nonpulsatile and pulsatile TAH animals. Trans Am Soc Artif Intern Organs 31:22–27
22. Golding LAR, Tishko DJ, Stewart RW (1988) Results of mechanical ventricular assist in bridging to cardiac transplantation. Cleve Clin J Med 55:59–62
23. Golding LR, Tishko DJ, Fujimoto LK, Moise J, Nosé Y (1988) Permanent and temporary mechanical ventricular assist. Cleve Clin Found ASAIO Primers 3:31–37
24. Golding LAR, Stewart RW, Sinkewich M, Smith W, Cosgrove DM (1987) Nonpulsatile ventricular assist bridging to transplantation. ASAIO Trans 34:476–479
25. Dasse KA, Frazier OH, Lesniak JM, Myers T, Burnett CM, Poirier VL (1992) Clinical responses to ventricular assistance versus transplantation in a series of bridge-to-transplant patients. ASAIO J 38:M622-626
26. Frazier OH, Rose EA, Macmanus Q, Burton NA, Lefrak EA, Poirier VL, Dasse KA (1992) Multicenter clinical evaluation of the HeartMate 1000 IP left ventricular assist device. Ann Thorac Surg 53:1080–1090
27. Frazier OH (1993) Chronic left ventricular support with a vented electric assist device. Ann Thorac Surg 55:273–275
28. Hamrock BJ (1991) Fundamentals of fluid film lubrication. US Government Printing Office, Washington DC (NASA Reference Publication 1255)
29. Pinkus O, Sternlicht B (1961) Theory of hydrodynamic lubrication. McGraw Hill, New York
30. Shigley JE (1977) Mechanical engineering design, 3rd edn. McGraw Hill, New York, 347–397
31. Jarvik RK (1991) Intraventricular artificial hearts and methods of their surgical implantation and use. (US patent 4,994,078)
32. Moise JC (1988) Magnetically suspended rotor axial flow blood pump. (US patent 4,779,614)
33. Olsen DB, Bramm G, Novak P (1987) Magnetically suspended rotated impeller pump apparatus and method. (US patent 4,688,998)
34. Wampler RK (1986) High-capacity intravascular blood pump utilizing percutaneous access. (US patent 4,625,712)
35. Akamatsu T, Nakazeki T, Hoh H (1992) Centrifugal blood pump with a magnetically suspended impeller. Artif Organs 16:305–308
36. Dorman FD, Bernstein EF, Blackshear PL (1971) Implantable blood pump. (US patent 3,608,088)

37. Isaacson MS, Lioi AP (1992) Hydrodynamically suspended rotor axial flow blood pump. (US patent 5,112,200)
38. Golding LAR, Smith WA, Mitchell D, Wade WF (1990) Continuous blood flow – an alternate approach. Cardiovascular science and technology. Basic and applied II. Oxymoron, Boston, pp 281–283
39. Golding LAR, Smith WA, Wade WF (1991) Sealless pump. (US patent 5,049,4134)

# The Hemopump: Clinical Results and Future Applications

W. Aboul-Hosn and R. Wampler

## Introduction

Cardiovascular disease is the leading cause of death in the United States [1], killing about one million Americans (population 250 million) each year. Seventy million Americans suffer from and nearly two people in five will ultimately die of cardiovascular disease. Acute myocardial infarction kills 500000 Americans each year and of these, 90000 die of cardiogenic shock. Table 1 shows the number of deaths associated with cardiovascular disease and myocardial infarction in the United States.

### Cardiogenic Shock – Background

Cardiogenic shock is a life-threatening condition characterized by severe left ventricular dysfunction, hypoperfusion, and secondary organ failure. Cardiogenic shock may occur secondary to open heart surgery, acute myocardial infarction (AMI), myocarditis, and acute donor graft rejection in heart transplant recipients. Cardiogenic shock complicates the condition of 7.5% of all patients with acute myocardial infarction, making AMI the most common cause of cardiogenic shock [2]. If the heart is unable to provide blood flow sufficient to maintain cellular metabolism, multiorgan failure and death will result.

### Cardiogenic Shock – Treatment

The strategy of the treatment of cardiogenic shock posits that the heart may recover from even severe acute myocardial dysfunction if it is relieved of the requirement to support the circulation and is effectively decompressed. The standard treatment for cardiogenic shock includes pharmacological agents intended to increase heart contractility, reduce myocardial oxygen consumption, and increase tissue perfusion. In severe cases, intra-aortic counterpulsation in combination with pharmacological modalities has been used in an attempt to improve the survival of cardiogenic shock. However, these modalities have been of limited clinical utility in decreasing the high mortality (80–90%) of cardiogenic shock [3–5]. Ventricular assist devices (VADs) provide much greater circulatory support than the IABP and may offer a more effective alternative to the IABP in the treatment of cardiogenic shock. Indeed, LVADs have been shown to affect recovery of noncontractile but viable or "stunned" myocardium in the setting of cardiogenic shock in experimental animals and have demon-

**Table 1.** Number of deaths associated with different types of disease. (From [1])

| Cause of death | New cases per year | Deaths,[a] total | Deaths,[a] male | Deaths,[a] female |
|---|---|---|---|---|
| Cardiovascular disease and stroke | – | 941 815 | 456 113 | 485 782 |
| Acute myocardial infarction | 1 500 000 | 498 021 | 257 524 | 240 497 |
| Cardiogenic shock | 112 500 | 90 000 | – | – |

[a] United States 1989 final mortality

strated limited clinical utility in patients who fail to wean from bypass and as bridges to cardiac transplantation [6–9]. Unfortunately, existing LVADs have not yet evolved to practical devices because current embodiments are large, complicated experimental devices adapted to limited use in surgical patients [10–14]. Consequently, LVADs are rarely used in the treatment of cardiogenic shock secondary to AMI because of the risks of the major surgery needed to implant them. Clearly, if LVADs are to find a place in the treatment of cardiogenic shock, a new technology is needed.

An "ideal" assist device should combine the hemodynamic power of the LVAD with the simplicity and safety of the IABP. Such a device could make it possible to exploit the therapeutic potential of the LVAD in the treatment of cardiogenic shock. The HEMOPUMP embodies many attributes of both the IABP and LVAD.

### Evolution Beyond IABP

The HEMOPUMP [15] represents a significant improvement in LVAD technology because it supports most of the cardiac output, reduces the work load of the heart, and does not require major surgery for implantation. The HEMOPUMP combines the hemodynamic power of the LVAD with the relative simplicity of the IABP. The HEMOPUMP is a catheter-mounted LVAD that can support most of the circulation for up to 7 days and yet be implanted without major surgery.

The HEMOPUMP improves on the IABP because:

1. It does not need to synchronize with the heart rhythm.
2. It does not require some remaining left ventricular contractility to be effective.
3. It has a higher flow capacity.
4. It provides much more effective decompression.

## Hemopump – Design and Performance

A pump is a machine that transfers mechanical energy generated by an external energy source to the fluid flowing through the pump. The HEMOPUMP is based

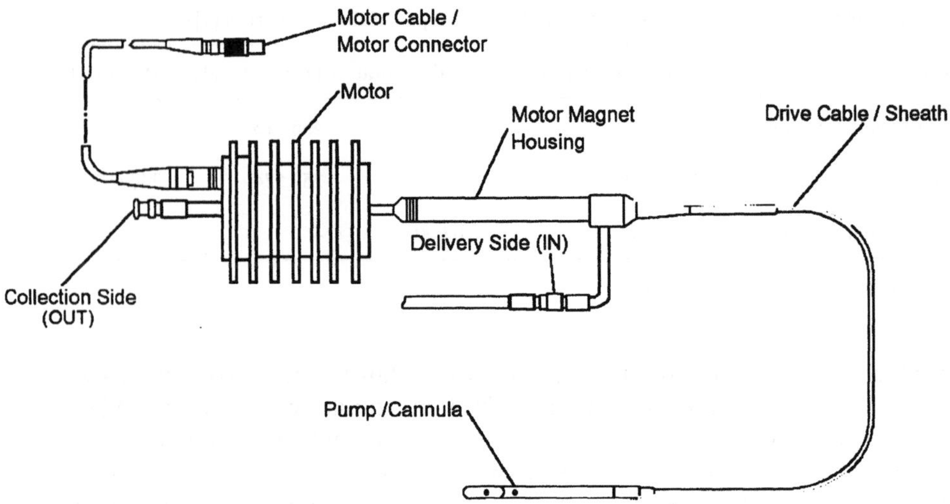


**Fig. 1.** Disposable pump catheter and motor

on the principle of the screw pump developed by the ancient Egyptians and later described by Archimedes in 200 BC. The HEMOPUMP transforms electrical energy into the rotational energy of a high-speed rotor. The rotary energy then accelerates the blood such that it is removed from the low-pressure inlet (left ventricle) to the high-pressure pump outlet (the aorta).

## Design

The HEMOPUMP consists of two main systems: the disposable pump catheter and motor (Fig. 1) and the electrical console (Fig. 2). The main components are described below.

| | |
|---|---|
| *Motor stator* | – Transforms electrical energy into rotational motion. |
| *Magnet housing* | – Transmits rotational motion to the flexible drive cable. |
| *Flexible drive cable* | – Transmits torque from the motor magnet to the hydraulic rotor (impeller). |
| *Pump and cannula* | – Axial flow pump and inflow tube, which conducts blood from the left ventricle to the aorta. |
| *Electrical console* | – Provides power and purge solution to disposable pump. |

The pump's cannula is advanced into the left ventricle via a peripheral vascular access or the ascending aorta. The cannula inlet draws blood from the left ventricle and expels it into the aorta, as shown in Fig. 3. Blood flows against a pressure gradient due to the energy imparted to the blood by the rotor.

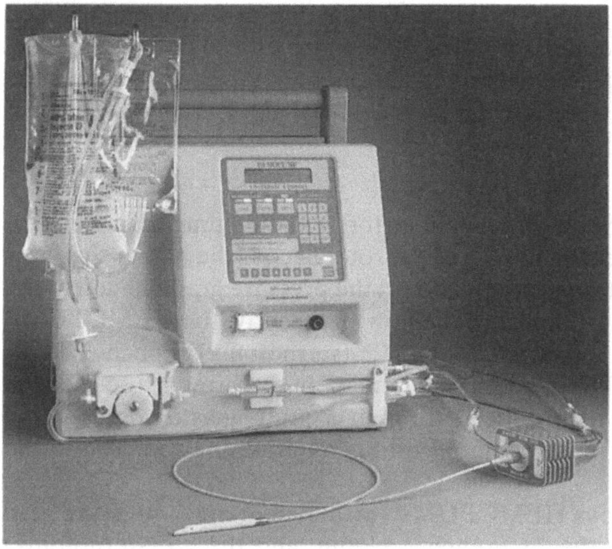

**Fig. 2.** Hemopump electrical console

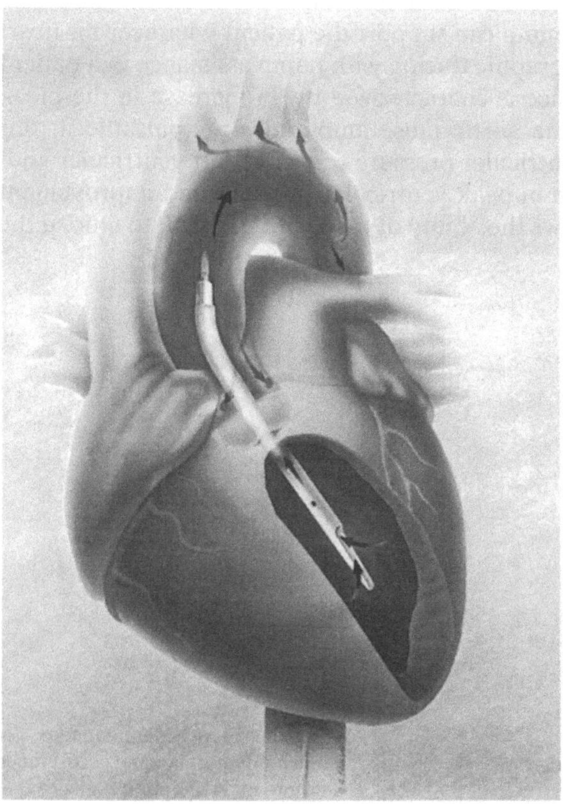

**Fig. 3.** Sternotomy Hemopump in position across the aortic valve

The console is an integrated electronic controller that provides pump speed selection, pump lubrication, and diagnostics. New consoles also provide an electrical signal that can be used to verify correct placement of the cannula across the aortic valve.

**Performance**

The pump's flow is dependent on three main factors: (a) the pump diameter (the larger the diameter, the larger the flow), (b) the rotor speed (the higher the rotor speed, the larger the energy transferred), and (c) the pressure gradient across the pump (the lower the gradient, the higher the flow). Presently, the HEMOPUMP is available in three different sizes; 14, 24, and 26 (sternotomy) French (Fig. 4). The 14-French HEMOPUMP is introduced percutaneously through a specialized introducer, the 24 French is introduced through a graft anastomosed to the femoral artery, and the 26 French is placed through a graft anastomosed to the ascending aorta.

The 14-French percutaneous HEMOPUMP (at 70 mm of mean pressure) can produce a flow of 2.3 l/min, the 24 French 3.5 l/min, and the 26 (sternotomy) French 5.0 l/min. The improved flow of the 26 French over the 24 French is due to the improvement in the 26 French hydraulic efficiency rather than to the size difference.

In contrast to the IABP, the HEMOPUMP does not need to synchronize with a beating heart. Therefore, the pump can support the patient whatever his heart rhythm. Figure 5 shows a physiographic tracing with pump assistance in a patient with cardiogenic shock. Assistance is characterized by an increase in the mean aortic pressure, a decrease in the aortic pulse amplitude (nonpulsatile in this case), and a decrease in peak ventricular pressure wave and left ventricular end-diastolic pressure. The reduction in peak ventricular pressure and improvement in the aortic pressure clearly shows the ability of the HEMOPUMP to unload the left ventricle.

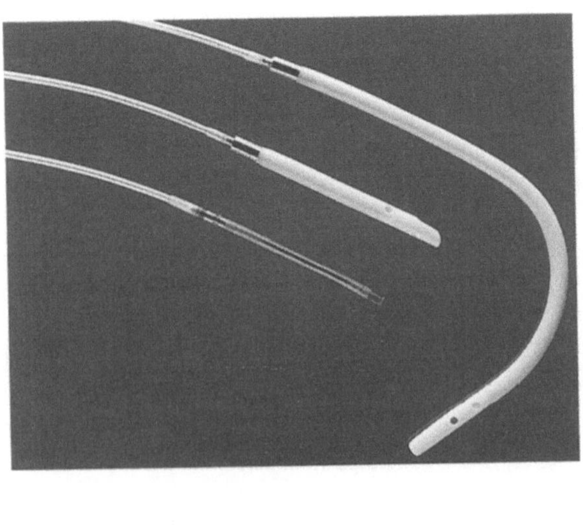

**Fig. 4.** 14-French percutaneous, 24-French femoral, and 26-French sternotomy Hemopump units

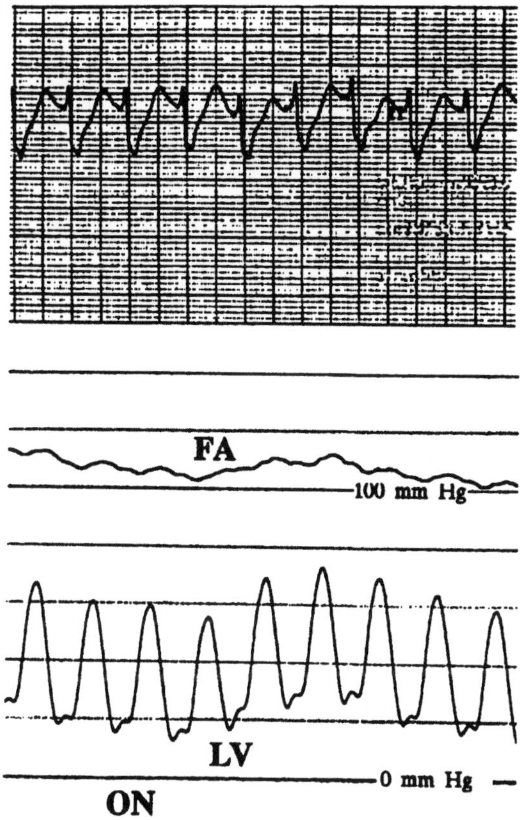


**Fig. 5.** Femoral artery and left ventricular pressure of cardiogenic shock patient assisted with the Hemopump (with permission of Richard W. Smalling, MD., PhD., University of Texas)

## Femoral Hemopump – Phase I

The initial clinical trials [16] focused on the HEMOPUMP in treating cardiogenic shock. Patients were accepted into the trial if shock was secondary to one of the following: acute myocardial infraction (AMI), failure to wean from cardiopulmonary bypass (FTW), low cardiac output (LCO), and other causes (acute donor graft rejection, cardiomyopathy, etc.).

### Phase-I Trials Cardiogenic Shock

*Protocol*

Patients with cardiogenic shock secondary to AMI, FTW, LCO, and other causes were accepted into the trial if they met the following hemodynamic criteria:

1. Pulmonary capillary wedge pressure greater than 18 mmHg
2. Systolic pressure less than 90 mmHg

**Table 2.** Patient summary – successful insertion. (From [17, 18])

| Group | Successful insertion (*n*) | Weaned (*n*) | Survivor (*n*) | Survivor (%) |
|---|---|---|---|---|
| AMI | 34 | 16 | 11 | 32.4 |
| FTW | 35 | 10 | 8 | 22.9 |
| LCO | 17 | 4 | 2 | 11.8 |
| Other | 29 | 16 | 10 | 34.5 |
| Total | 115 | 46 | 31 | 27.0 |

3. Cardiac index less than 2 l/min/m²
4. Patient refractory to drug and volume therapy

The HEMOPUMP was placed through the femoral artery via a 12-mm graft anastomosed end-to-side to the artery. The pump was introduced through the graft and advanced into the left ventricle. Anticoagulation was maintained with intravenous heparin to achieve an activated clotting time (ACT) at 1.5–2 times the baseline.

*Patient Summary*

The mean age was 53.7 years (range 8.6–76 years). All these patients had evidence of "irreversible cardiogenic shock" and were on assisted ventilation. Sixty-eight percent failed to respond to the intra-aortic balloon pump and most had evidence of major organ failure. Table 2 [17] summarizes the diagnosis at the time of entry into the trial. The study included 145 patients. Successful insertion was completed in 79% (115/145) of the patients, 40% (46/115) were successfully weaned from assistance, and 27% (31/115) survived to 30 days.

Patients with AMI who were assisted with the HEMOPUMP had a survival rate of 32.4% (11/34), compared with a survival of 16.7% (2/12) (*p* value NS) for AMI patients in whom the device could not be inserted. Although the failed insertion group was not a prospective control group, these results do suggest that the HEMOPUMP may significantly improve survival in patients with cardiogenic shock secondary to AMI.

*Hemodynamic Response to the HEMOPUMP*

The hemodynamic effects of the HEMOPUMP were verified by measuring the cardiac index (CI), pulmonary capillary wedge pressure (PCWP), and systolic blood pressure. Table 3 [18] shows these values before HEMOPUMP insertion, during HEMOPUMP operation, and 24 h after weaning. The data shown are the results of the first 88 patients.

The average CI before pump insertion for all patients was 1.72 l/min/m², which is consistent with severe cardiogenic shock. The CI increased by 35% for patients weaned from the device. In addition, it improved significantly during the first 24 h of device operation. The average PCWP decreased 57% in patients weaned from

**Table 3.** Patient hemodymanic response. (Source IDE G870192/43 March 13, 1991 JJIS [17])

| | | Pre-insert | During | Post-removal |
|---|---|---|---|---|
| Cardiac index | All patients | 1.72 ± 0.074 | 2.16 ± 0.08 | 2.24 ± 0.08 |
| | *n* | 63 | 71 | 59 |
| | Weaned | 1.87 ± 0.11 | 2.52 ± 0.08 | 2.48 ± 0.08 |
| | *n* | 28 | 36 | 32 |
| | Notweaned | 1.60 ± 0.10 | 1.78 ± 0.11 | 1.96 ± 0.12 |
| | *n* | 35 | 35 | 27 |
| Pulmonary capillary WP | All patients | 25 ± 1.0 | 16 ± 0.5 | 16 ± 0.6 |
| | *n* | 50 | 68 | 60 |
| | Weaned | 23 ± 1.1 | 16 ± 0.7 | 15 ± 0.6 |
| | *n* | 23 | 36 | 33 |
| | Notweaned | 28 ± 1.5 | 17 ± 0.8 | 17 ± 1.2 |
| | *n* | 27 | 32 | 27 |
| Systolic pressure | All patients | 77 ± 2.1 | 74 ± 2.6 | 78 ± 2.6 |
| | *n* | 84 | 81 | 61 |
| | Weaned | 76 ± 2.9 | 89 ± 2.6 | 83 ± 3.2 |
| | *n* | 36 | 36 | 34 |
| | Notweaned | 78 ± 3.0 | 63 ± 3.2 | 71 ± 4.0 |
| | *n* | 48 | 45 | 27 |

support and 38% in all patients. This demonstrates the effectiveness of the device in unloading the heart.

### *Physiologic Response to the HEMOPUMP*

The physiological response to HEMOPUMP assistance was evaluated by measuring the urine output and the fraction of inspired oxygen ($FIO_2$) provided by the ventilator. Table 4 summarizes the urine output and inspired oxygen of the first 88 patients.

**Table 4.** Patient physiological response. (Source IDE G870192/43 March 13, 1991 JJIS Annual Report [17])

| | | Pre-insert | During | Post-removal |
|---|---|---|---|---|
| Urine output | All patients | 116 ± 14.5 | 81 ± 7.4 | 92 ± 11.9 |
| | *n* | 72 | 70 | 60 |
| | Weaned | 109 ± 22.1 | 104 ± 11.4 | 114 ± 17.6 |
| | *n* | 31 | 35 | 33 |
| | Nonweaned | 120 ± 19.4 | 58 ± 8.0 | 65 ± 14.0 |
| | *n* | 41 | 35 | 27 |
| Fraction of inspired $O_2$ | All patients | 0.82 ± 0.027 | 0.70 ± 0.023 | 0.62 ± 0.029 |
| | *n* | 80 | 76 | 57 |
| | Weaned | 0.81 ± 0.038 | 0.61 ± 0.027 | 0.58 ± 0.036 |
| | *n* | 34 | 36 | 31 |
| | Notweaned | 0.83 ± 0.037 | 0.78 ± 0.030 | 0.67 ± 0.047 |
| | *n* | 46 | 40 | 26 |

The urine output was stable in the group successfully weaned, while it decreased by 52% in the group not weaned. The $FIO_2$, which is an indicator of lung edema and gaseous exchange, shows a 25% reduction in weaned patients and no change in those not weaned. The improvement in the $FIO_2$ after 24 h of pump assistance is probably a direct result of left ventricular decompression.

### *Hematological Response to the HEMOPUMP*

Since the HEMOPUMP energizes the blood by transferring velocity from a high-speed rotor, it is logical to expect significant damage to the blood components, especially red blood cells. To evaluate the effect of the HEMOPUMP on cellular elements of the blood, the platelet count, total hemoglobin, and plasma-free hemoglobin were measured. Table 5 shows the platelet count, plasma-free hemoglobin, and total hemoglobin. The data shown are the results of the first 88 patients. A moderate thrombocytopenia was observed, but only a minor elevation in plasma-free hemoglobin was noted.

The resilience of the blood elements to the high velocities in the pump remains a mystery. The exact mechanism that protects blood cells in the harsh environment of the pump is not well understood. Many theories have been advanced to explain why the blood can withstand the shear force of a 27 000 rpm rotor, but none have been proven. One plausible theory suggests the short time (2.5 ms) that the blood is exposed to the pump is not of sufficient duration to result in damage.

**Table 5.** Patient hematological response. (Source IDE G870192/43 March 13, 1991 JJIS Annual Report [17])

| | | Pre-insert | During | Post-removal |
|---|---|---|---|---|
| Platelet count | All patients | 207 ± 11.9 | 122 ± 7.1 | 116 ± 8.1 |
| 1000/mm³ | *n* | 81 | 69 | 59 |
| | Weaned | 210 ± 17.2 | 117 ± 9.5 | 110 ± 8.6 |
| | *n* | 34 | 35 | 34 |
| | Nonweaned | 205 ± 16.5 | 126 ± 10.7 | 125 ± 15.2 |
| | *n* | 47 | 34 | 25 |
| Plasma-free | All patients | 18.5 ± 3.4 | 44.9 ± 6.9 | 35.0 ± 7.9 |
| Hgb mg/dl | *n* | 47 | 65 | 51 |
| | Weaned | 14.1 ± 3.9 | 27.2 ± 3.5 | 30.0 ± 11.9 |
| | *n* | 21 | 33 | 27 |
| | Nonweaned | 22.1 ± 5.2 | 63.2 ± 12.3 | 40.6 ± 10.1 |
| | *n* | 26 | 32 | 24 |
| Hemoglobin | All patients | 11.5 ± 0.24 | 10.4 ± 0.17 | 10.4 ± 0.20 |
| gm/dl | *n* | 87 | 75 | 61 |
| | Weaned | 11.8 ± 0.37 | 11.0 ± 0.19 | 10.8 ± 0.25 |
| | *n* | 37 | 36 | 34 |
| | Nonweaned | 11.3 ± 0.32 | 9.9 ± 0.23 | 9.8 ± 0.29 |
| | *n* | 50 | 39 | 27 |

## Sternotomy Hemopump – Phase II

Although the HEMOPUMP was originally conceived for use in the treatment of cardiogenic shock, we have come to the conclusion that the difficulties of conducting a study of cardiogenic shock that would pass the scrutiny of the FDA may be insurmountable. The phase-II trial for the Sternotomy HEMOPUMP will study its clinical utility for intraoperative non-oxygenator support during aortocoronary bypass (ACB) surgery.

The purpose of this clinical investigation is to show that the HEMOPUMP Cardiac Assist System is equivalent to or better than conventional extracorporeal cardiopulmonary bypass when used to support a subset of patients who would normally be candidates for isolated aortocoronary bypass graft surgery. It is our belief that such a study can demonstrate significant reductions in blood transfusions, complications, recovery time, and cost. Recent experience with surgery on the beating heart and the historical development of ACB surgery supports this hypothesis.

### Aortocoronary Bypass Surgery Without Support

Motivated by the desire to avoid the complications of CPB and the artificial oxygenator, several investigators have reported reduced complications while performing ACB surgery on the beating, unsupported heart. Buffolo et al., Benetti et al., and Pfister et al. investigated the merit of ACB surgery on the unsupported beating heart and concluded that the complications of CPB can be avoided during ACB surgery [19–23].

### Nonoxygenator Aortocoronary Bypass Surgery on the Assisted Beating Heart

Nonoxygenator extracorporeal circulatory support with VADs has been successfully used to support patients during ACB surgery. Use of VADs during ACB surgery avoids the risk of the artificial oxygenator, since the patient's own lungs are functioning, yet allows the surgeon to safely revascularize vessels that were inaccessible in the experiences of Buffolo et al., Benetti et al., and Pfister et al., reported above. Glenville and Ross [24] and Sweeney and Frazier [25] demonstrated that a VAD may be effectively used for intraoperative hemodynamic support and ventricular decompression during ACB surgery. The use of nonoxygenator extracorporeal support during ACB surgery has a number of theoretical advantages.

1. *Ventricular decompression* should decrease myocardial oxygen demand and increase coronary flow to ischemic areas, thereby protecting the myocardium.
2. An *artificial oxygenator* and the associated circuit are not needed, since the patient's own lungs oxygenate the blood.
3. *Aortic cross-clamping and ischemic arrest* are not necessary.
4. The *heparin dosage can be lowered*, with a corresponding potential reduction in blood loss.

Although Glenville and Ross did not exploit all of the theoretical advantages mentioned above, they were the first to successfully use a VAD for circulatory support during ACB surgery. Sweeney and Frazier modified their procedure to exploit more of the theoretical advantages. They reported on 43 patients who presented with either acute or chronic severe left ventricular dysfunction and subsequently underwent VAD-assisted ACB surgery. Six of these patients were in cardiogenic shock. The mean ejection fraction was 22% (range 12–28%). Two of these patients died, for an overall mortality of 4.6%.

Although the results with VAD-supported ACB surgery have been encouraging, currently available VADs are not ideally suited to this application. At this time, VAD-supported ACB surgery adapts a centrifugal pump intended for use in a cardiopulmonary circuit as an extracorporeal VAD. There are several disadvantages to this approach:

1. Use of a large cannula, particularly on the left side of the heart, is cumbersome and complicates the surgical procedure.
2. A hole must be made in the left ventricular apex to achieve good LV decompression.
3. Negative pressures inherent to a centrifugal pump in an extracorporeal blood circuit pose the risk of air embolism.

The Sternotomy HEMOPUMP is an intracorporeal circulatory assist device that, because of its unique design, may avoid the difficulties of extracorporeal VADs [26]. The HEMOPUMP may be particularly well suited to intraoperative support and could be readily adapted to nonoxygenator circulatory support during ACB surgery.

## Phase-II Clinical Trials

The phase-II trial will be a prospective, randomized study. A patient may be entered into the study if he or she meets all of the following criteria:

1. The patient is a candidate for isolated ACB grafting using conventional CPB.
2. One to five grafts are planned.
3. The target vessels intended for bypass are among the following:

   *Left coronary artery*
   a) left anterior descending artery
   b) ramus medianus artery
   c) diagonal artery
   d) obtuse marginal artery 2 cm from the takeoff of the circumflex artery

   *Right coronary artery*
   a) acute marginal artery
   b) posterior descending artery
   c) posterior left ventricular artery

A patient will be excluded from the trial if he or she meets any one of the following criteria:

1. Has a significant blood dyscrasia
2. Has a prosthetic aortic valve or severe aortic stenosis or insufficiency
3. Refuses to accept blood transfusions
4. Has a left ventricular or atrial mural thrombus
5. Has pulmonary hypertension
6. Is a candidate for emergency surgery
7. Has intravascular hemolysis greater than 25 mg%

The clinical utility of nonoxygenator support with the HEMOPUMP and cardiopulmonary bypass will be established by assessing freedom from serious complication and avoidance of heterogeneous blood transfusions. Serious complications will include:

1. Any reoperation due to bleeding
2. Focal neurological deficit following surgery
3. Pulmonary failure, defined as the need for ventilator support 24 h post surgery
4. Low-output state, defined as impaired hemodynamics requiring inotropic drug therapy longer than 24 h post surgery or the use of an IABP
5. Disseminated intravascular coagulopathy (DIC)

Pilot studies based on this protocol began in Europe in the spring of 1993. Approval of an investigation device exemption from the U.S. FDA was granted in 1993. The clinical trial is now in progress in three centers in the USA and one in Europe. To date, 25+ patients have undergone ACB on HEMOPUMP support. One patient could not be completed on HEMOPUMP support and was crossed over to CPB. One to four grafts have been performed. There has been one postoperative death in a patient who crossed over to CPB. Although it is too early to present specific data, the following trends are emerging: (a) postoperative bleeding is significantly reduced in the HEMOPUMP group; (b) the HEMOPUMP-supported patients seem more vigorous in the postoperative period and require less time in the ICU and hospital; (c) fewer patients in the HEMOPUMP group require blood transfusions. Published reports of initial clinical experience are anticipated during 1994.

## Future Use

The technology of a high-efficiency, catheter-mounted, miniature LVAD has already spawned a multitude of applications. The initial trials of the HEMOPUMP were hindered by failed insertions (25%) due to the large diameter of the 24-French femoral device. This fact led to the development of a percutaneous HEMOPUMP, which is a 14-French HEMOPUMP intended for nonsurgical insertion by the interventional cardiologist. The percutaneous HEMOPUMP is undergoing limited clinical trials in Europe for support of high-risk angioplasty. Successful clinical use of the percutaneous HEMOPUMP in high-risk angioplasty patients was first reported by Scholtz et al. [27].

Another potential application of the HEMOPUMP adapts it for use as an extracorporeal blood pump during fetal heart surgery. In the past, fetal surgery which required circulatory support was hindered by the large volume needed to prime to extracorporeal circuit. At the University of California in San Francisco, Hanley et al. have used a modified HEMOPUMP to support the circulation of the ovine fetus during cardiac surgery. Significant reduction in placental dysfunction and dramatic improvement in fetal survival have been observed. This study is still in its initial stages, and published results are anticipated within a year.

Another logical application for the 14-French percutaneous HEMOPUMP is pediatric ventricular support. It was necessary to shorten the inflow cannula to accommodate the anatomical difference between children and adults, but the 14-French device should offer a great advantage over any present technology used for pediatric assistance.

Besides these applications, right ventricular support is possible with the same basic technology, adapted to right heart support. In conclusion, the HEMOPUMP technology could be modified and adapted to many applications requiring the movement of blood.

## Conclusion

The HEMOPUMP is an innovative left ventricular assist device that, for the first time, provides a practical way to exploit the benefits of mechanical circulatory assistance in the treatment of cardiogenic shock and acute myocardial infarction. The initial clinical trials in the treatment of cardiogenic shock and the early experience with supported interventional procedures are very encouraging. New applications for its use continue to emerge as we gain experience and confidence in the safety and effectiveness of the HEMOPUMP. Ongoing clinical experience will define the indications for its use and its clinical utility.

## References

1. American Heart Association (1993) Heart and stroke facts statistics. American Heart Association Press, Dallas, Texas
2. Rutan P, Rountree W, Myers K, Baker L (1989) Initial experience with the hemopump J Crit Care Nursing North Am 1(3):527–534
3. Norman JC, Cooley DA, Igo SR et al. (1977) Prognostic indices for survival during postcardiotomy intra-aortic balloon pumping. J Thorac Cardiovasc Surg 74(5):709–720
4. Parmley W (1983) Cardiac failure. In: Rosen MR, Hoffman BF (eds) Cardiac therapy. Nijhoff, Boston pp 21–44
5. Shoemaker WC, Bland RD, Appel PL (1985) Therapy of critically ill postoperative patients based on outcome prediction and prospective clinical trials. Surg Clin North Am 65:811–833
6. Schoen FJ, Palmer DC, Bernhard WF et al. (1986) Clinical temporary ventricular assist. J Thorac Cardiovasc Surg 92:1071–1081

7. Lass J, Campbell CD, Takanashi Y, Pick R, Replogle RL (1979) Preservation of ischemic myocardium with TALVB using complete left ventricular decompression. Trans Am Soc Artif Intern Organs 25:220–223
8. Takanashi Y, Campbell CD, Laas J, Pick RL, Meus P, Replogle RL (1981) Reduction of myocardial infarct size in swine: a comparative study of intraaortic balloon pumping and transapical left ventricular bypass. 32:475–485
9. Merhige ME, Smalling RW, Cassidy D, Barrett R, Wise G, Short J, Wampler RK (1989) Effect of the Hemopump left ventricular assist device on regional myocardial perfusion and function: reduction of ischemia during coronary occlusion. Circulation 80(5)[Suppl III]:158–166
10. Magovern GJ, Park SB, Maher TD (1985) Use of a centrifugal pump without anticoagulants for postoperative left ventricular assist. World J Surg 9:25–36
11. Bernstein EF, Dorman FD, Blackshear PL, Scott DR (1970) An efficient, compact blood pump for assisted circulation. Surgery 68(1):105–115
12. Golding LR, Jacobs G, Groves LK, Gill CC, Nose' Y, Loop FD (1982) Clinical results of mechanical support of the failing left ventricle. J Thorac Cardiovasc Surg 83:597–601
13. Pae WE, Pierce WS, Pennock JL, Campbell DB, Waldhausen JA (1987) Long-term results of ventricular assist pumping in postcardiotomy cardiogenic shock. J Thorac Cardiovasc Surg 93:431–441
14. Pennington DG, Samuels LD, Williams G et al. (1985) Experience with the Pierce-Donachy ventricular assist device in postcardiotomy patients with cardiogenic shock. World J Surg 9:37–46
15. Wampler RK, Moise JC, Frazier OH, Olsen DB (1988) In vivo evaluation of a peripheral vascular access axial flow blood pump. Trans Am Soc Artif Intern Organs 34(3):450–454
16. Wampler RK, Frazier OH, Lansing AM et al. (1991) Treatment of cardiogenic shock with the Hemopump left ventricular assist device. Ann Thorac Surg 52:506–513
17. Johnson and Johnson Interventional Systems CD-0218 (1993) Final report-pending recovery of the natural heart, May 17 (IDE G870192/43)
18. Nimbus Medical (1990) Pre-market approval application hemopump – temporary cardiac assist system vols 1–4
19. Trapp WG, Bisarya R (1975) Placement of coronary artery bypass graft without pump oxygenator. Ann Thorac Surg 19:1–9
20. Ankeney JL (1975) Coronary vein graft without cardiopulmonary bypass; a surgical motion picture. Ann Thorac Surg 1(19)
21. Buffolo E, Andrade JCS, Branco JNR, Aguiar LF, Ribeiro EE, Jatene AD (1990) Myocardial revascularization without extracorporeal circulation: seven-year experience in 593 cases. Eur J Cardiothorac Surg 4:504–508
22. Benetti FJ, Naselli G, Wood M, Geffner L (1991) Direct myocardial revascularization without extracorporeal circulation. Chest 100(2):313–316
23. Pfister AJ et al. (1992) Coronary artery bypass without cardiopulmonary bypass. Presented at the 28th Annual Meeting of the Society of Thoracic Surgeons, Orlando
24. Glenville B, Ross D (1986) Coronary artery surgery with patient's lungs as oxygenator. Lancet 333:1005–1006
25. Sweeney MS, Frazier OH (1992) Device-supported myocardial revascularization: the benefits of avoiding pump oxygenation and cardiac arrest in operations upon dilapidated hearts. Presented at the 28th Annual Meeting of the Society of Thoracic Surgeons, Orlando
26. Wampler R, Aboul-Hosn W, Cleary M, Saunders M (1993) The Sternotomy HEMOPUMP – a second-generation intraarterial ventricular assist device. ASAIO J 39(3):M218–M223
27. Scholtz K, Figulla H, Schweda F, Smalling R, Hellige G, Kreuzer H, Aboul-Hosn W, Wampler R (1994) Mechanical left ventricular unloading during high-risk coronary angioplasty: first use of a new percutaneous transvalvular left ventricular assist device. Cathet Cardiovasc Diagn 31(61):61–69

# Considerations in the Development of the Mini-Spindle Pump

J. HAGER and F. BRANDSTAETTER

## Introduction

In the recent past, several attempts have been made to develop rotary or nonpulsatile implantable blood pumps for assisted circulation [1–6]. We, too, are engaged in constructing such a device with a design basically identical to that of our 16th prototype of the known spindle pump (Fig. 1).

## Considerations Regarding the Development of the Mini-Spindle Pump

### Theoretical Considerations

The premise which formed the basis for the development of the device(s) – taking into account the experiences with the "large" spindle pump [7, 8] – was to transport about 4 l of water per min in mock circulation with a pressure difference of 90 torr between inflow and outflow port at a speed between 12 000 and 15 000 rpm.

### In Vitro Tests

Primarily, each prototype developed was to be tested in the circulation model; later, if the results met our expectations, its influence on blood corpuscles was to be examined in an oxygenator (Maxima hollow fiber oxygenator from Medtronic). The oxygenator was filled with 1.3 l of human blood and 0.5 l Ringer's lactate, resulting in a hematocrit level of about 30 vol%. This form of investigation was chosen in order to avoid animal experiments (which are frowned upon in Austria).

## Material and Methods

### First Prototype of the Mini-Spindle Pump

*Description of device*

To fill the above-mentioned demands, the first prototype consisted of a U-shaped block-formed Plexiglas housing (9.5 × 3 × 3 cm), a spindle rotor made of Teflon

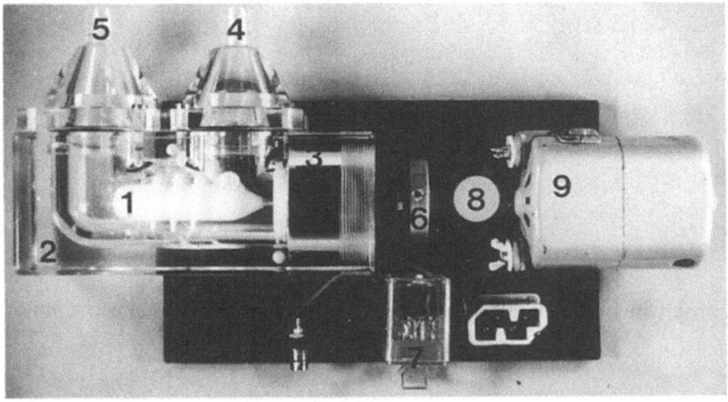


**Fig. 1.** Full view of the 16th prototype of the "large" spindle pump. *1*, Spindle rotor; *2*, Plexiglas housing; *3*, carrier unit for sealing and ball bearings; *4*, inflow port; *5*, outflow port; *6*, aluminium disc; *7*, induction coil for speed measurment; *8*, plastic coupler; *9*, electric motor

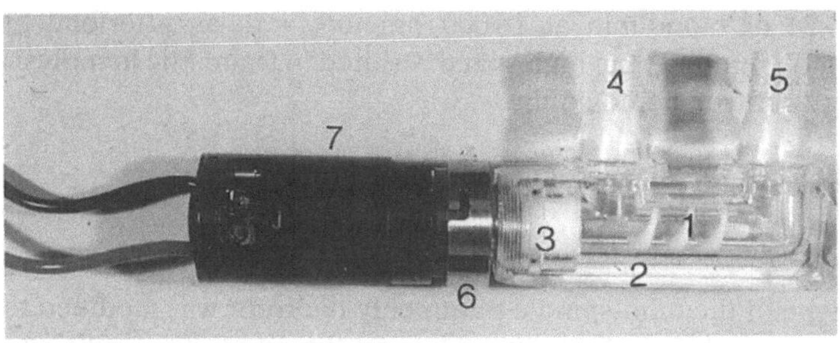


**Fig. 2.** Full view of the first prototype of the mini-spindle pump. *1*, Rotor; *2*, housing; *3*, carrier unit for sealing and ball bearings; *4*, inflow port; *5*, outflow port; *6*, coupler; *7*, drive unit (electric motor without cooling system)

with three windings (outer diameter 1.8 cm; inner diameter 0.62 cm; length 4.5 cm; pitch 1 cm) and an electric motor with a cooling system.

The spindle rotor was mounted on a steel axis (diameter 0.4 cm) and inserted into the first cylindrical chamber (length 6.7 cm; lumen 2 cm) in the block's longitudinal area, i.e., the blood chamber of the pump. Attached to this cylinder is another one (length 2.5 cm; lumen 2.6 cm) for the sealing and the ball bearings.

On one side of the housing, cylindrical holes (inner diameter 2.5 cm) are drilled for the inflow and the outflow connector (length 3.8 cm; lumen 50 French). The rotor is moved by an electric motor, which is connected by a coupler to the end of the driving axis, and combined with a cooling system (Fig. 2).

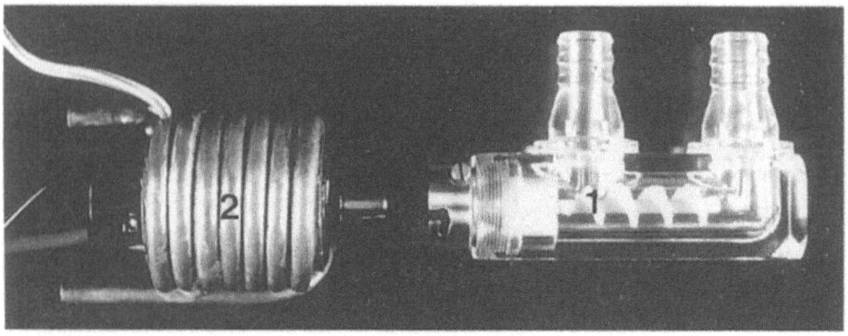


**Fig. 3.** View of the third prototype of the mini-spindle pump (*1*, streamlined rotor; *2*, electric motor and cooling system)

### *In Vitro Results*

In mock circulation the device circulated 7.8 l of water/min at 18 000 rpm with an afterload of 90 mm Hg. Combined with a Maxima oxygenator, the mini-spindle pump transported 4.2 l of blood/min at 18 000 rpm too, with an afterload of 105 mm Hg. After 7 h of pumping, the high speed resulted in traumatic hemolysis of more than 250 mg% of free hemoglobin.

## Technical Specifications of the Second and the Third Prototype

### *Description of the Devices*

In the second prototype of the mini-spindle pump only the rotor was modified to minimize the blood trauma in the inflow area: The first thread of the spindle was rounded up; i.e., the rotor had only 2 1/2 threads. This modification failed to reduce the hemolysis problem.

Therefore, a new prototype – the third in our series – had to be constructed. As a first step the spindle rotor was redesigned; i.e., a streamlined spindle with four threads (Fig. 3) was chosen. In a second step a complete novelty was realized – the flow direction was reversed.

### *In Vitro Results with the Third Prototype*

In mock circulation the third prototype transported 8.9 l of water/min at 15 000 rpm with a pressure difference of 110 torr between inflow and outflow port. In the oxygenator experiment the pump circulated 4.3 l of blood/min at 12 000 rpm with an afterload of 90 mm Hg.

Although traumatic hemolysis was reduced, the results were not satisfying: Up to 9000 rpm, the device circulated about 2.5 l of blood/min; the rate of free hemoglobin was slightly elevated. However, over 9000 rpm a sudden rapid increase of free hemoglobin in the serum was noted; this meant after 8 h of pumping the free hemoglobin value was 180 mg% and therefore still too high.

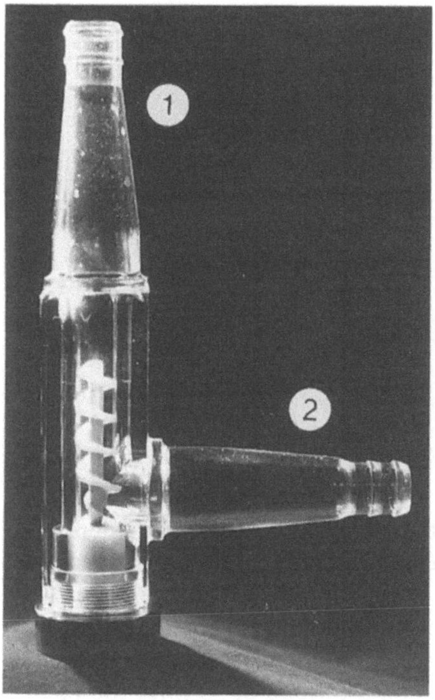


**Fig. 4.** View of the fourth prototype (without the electric motor and the cooling system) with the new inflow (*1*) and outflow tract (*2*)

### Fourth Prototype of the Mini-Spindle Pump

*Description of Device*

Because of the problem with hemolysis, the U-shape of the housing was abandoned and the inflow tract laid axially to the spindle rotor. The housing itself, as well as the spindle rotor, retained the same form as in the third prototype, but in addition, inflow and outflow tract were reconstructed in a large trumpet-shaped form with a length of 7.5 cm (Fig. 4).

*In Vitro Results*

In mock circulation the fourth prototype circulated 9.2 l of water/min at 15 000 rpm with an afterload of 118 torr. In combination with a Maxima oxygenator, this prototype transported 4.5 l of blood/min at 12 000 rpm with a pressure difference of 90 torr between inflow and outflow tract (Fig. 5). After a pumping duration of 7 h the level of free hemoglobin was 220 mg%.

## Discussion

With all four prototypes the hemolysis rate was always tolerable in the oxygenator experiments at revolutions up to 9000 rpm. At this speed the pumps

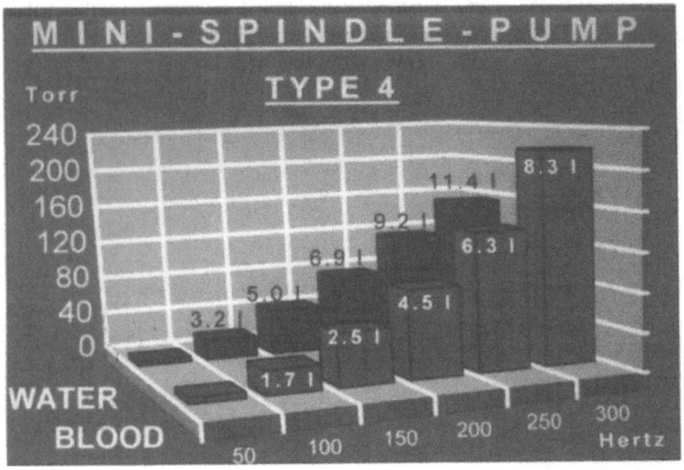


**Fig. 5.** Functional diagram of the fourth prototype. *water*, Function in mock circulation; *blood*, function in the oxygenator

transport only about 2–2.5 l of blood/min. If the number of revolutions increases and the transported volume Spindle Pump increases too, the hemolysis rate increases, and dramatically so.

To find out if the oxygenator might be responsible for this problem, an in vitro test with the 16th prototype of the "large" spindle pump was performed. After 8 h of pumping (4 l of blood/min at 5000 rpm with an afterload of 90 torr) the result of this experiment was almost as expected: The blood trauma was the same as seen with the four prototypes of the mini-spindle pump; i.e., the level of free hemoglobin was 190 mg%.

The oxygenator experiments therefore were not feasible. To verify the function of the fourth prototype of the mini-spindle pump an animal experiment was set up. Under normal cardiac conditions the device was capable of emptying 60–70% of the left ventricle (at a speed of 9000 rpm, about 6 l of blood/min was transported; the afterload was about 75 torr). After a pumping duration of 8 h the hemolysis rate was 90 mg% of free hemoglobin. This result is encouraging and will enable us to continue with further developments of this new device.

## References

1. Schistek R, Genelin A, Hager J, Nagl S, Nessler N, Stoss F, Gschnitzer F, Unger F (1982) Total implantable axial nonpulsatile blood pump for left ventricular assist and total artificial heart replacement. Trans Am Soc Artif Intern Organs 28:589–593
2. Qian KX, Wang YP, Zhao MJ (1987) Toward an implantable impeller total heart. Trans Am Soc Artif Intern Organs 33:704–707
3. Wampler RK, Moise JC, Frazier OH, Olsen DB (1988) In-vivo evaluation of a peripheral vascular access axial flow blood pump. Trans Am Soc Artif Intern Organs 34:450–454
4. Monties JR, Mesana T, Havlik P, Trinkl J, Demunck JL, Candelon B (1990) Another way of pumping blood with a rotary but non-centrifugal pump for an artificial heart. Trans Am Soc Artif Intern Organs 36:M258–M260
5. Schima H, Trubel W, Mueller MR, Papantonis D, Salat A, Schlusche C, Prodinger A, Spitaler F, Krausler S, Losert U, Thoma H, Wolner E (1991) Development of a centrifugal blood pump with

minimal hemolysis. In: Schima H, Thoma H, Wieselthaler G, Wolner E (eds) Proceedings of the International Workshop on Rotary Blood Pumps, Vienna 1991, pp 141–147
6. Westphal D, Reul H, Rau G (1991) Development and in vitro test results of the Helmholtz centrifugal pump. In: Schima H, Thoma H, Wieselthaler G, Wolner E (eds) Proceedings of the International Workshop on Rotary Blood Pumps, Vienna 1991, pp 132–136
7. Hager J, Brandstaetter F, Koller I, Unger F (1989) The spindle pump. Development of a nonpulsatile blood pump for assisted circulation. Trans Am Soc Artif Intern Organs 35:471–474
8. Hager J, Brandstaetter F, Dietze O, Koller I, Unger F (1990) The spindle pump – a nonpulsatile blood pump for assisted circulation. J Biomater Appl 4:225–330

# New Progress with Impeller Pumps in Taiwan*

K.X. Qian

## Introduction

The impeller blood pump program began in the middle of the 1980s in Shanghai and was put on hold a few years later. It has been reactivated in Taipei since 1992 under the support of the National Council of Sciences, with a 5-year plan including animal experiments and human trials of left ventricular and biventricular assist for the failing heart. Both acute and survival experiments with pigs or calves and control experiments with locally made diaphragm pumps or clinically used rollers have been carried out recently. The results demonstrated that the pulsatile impeller blood pumps cause less hemolysis and thrombosis than other blood pumps, can support the failing or healthy heart to maintain the circulation, and can help heart function to recover effectively.

## Left Ventricular Assist Impeller Pump

### Acute Experiments with Pigs

The pump has been described previously [1–3]. It is a motor-driven pulsatile centrifugal pump. The pulsatility of the blood pressure and volume is achieved by changing the rotating speed of the impeller, introducing a square waveform voltage into the motor coil. The impeller vane and shroud are designed according to stream lines in the pump, to reduce the hemolysis and thrombosis caused by the pump.

Five pigs weighing 30–50 kg were used for the acute experiments of left ventricular assistance. The pump delivered the blood from the left atrium to the aorta; the flow rate was detected by a transonic flow meter (Fig. 1) and was adjusted to approximately 40–50% of the total flow by changing the motor voltage. The pump ejected the flow with a fixed frequency of 60/min, independent of the ECG of the natural heart. The systole remained at about 40%. The experiment lasted 6 h in each case. Hematological data such as red blood cell (RBC), white blood cell (WBC), and platelet (PLT) counts, hemoglobin (HGB), hematocrit (HCT), free hemoglobin (FHB), and lactate dehydrogenase (LDH)

* Project Supported by National Council of Sciences, ROC.

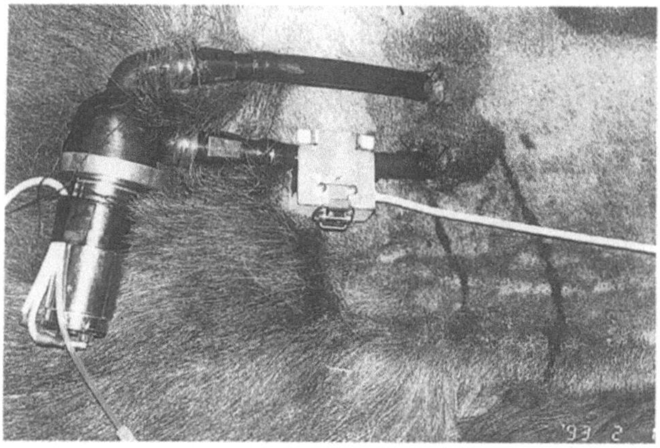


**Fig. 1.** The left ventricular assistance experiment with pigs using a pulsatile impeller pump

were measured preoperatively, at the beginning of the pumping, and every hour during the experiments. In Table 1 the mean values and the standard deviations of hematological parameters are listed. The RBC, HGB, and HCT remained basically unchanged; only from the 5th to the 6th hours did they drop slightly, perhaps because of the dilution of the blood due to intravenous infusion with saline. The FHB remained constant, indicating that the pulsatile impeller pump destroys no erythrocytes. The PLT number decreased and LDH was obviously increased, but within the normal range. This means that platelet damage occurred but was not serious during the bypass experiments.

At heart failure, the aortic flow is provided mainly by the pump and thus the aortic pressure form is determined mainly by the pump pulse (Fig. 2, top). Only a few hours later, the heart has recovered; the aortic pressure then has a complicated form, overlapped by the blood flow from the natural and artificial heart (Fig. 2, bottom). This fact demonstrates that the pulsatile impeller pump can support the failing heart to maintain the circulation, while the heart recovers its function effectively.

The acute experiments of left ventricular assist with the pulsatile impeller pump have proven that pulsatile perfusion with the impeller-type centrifugal pump is feasible and that the pulsatile impeller pump promises to have chronic applications in survival experiments.

## Survival Experiments with Calves

Based on the acute experiments with pigs, the pulsatile impeller pump was evaluated continuously in chronic survival experiments with four calves. The surgical procedure and the postoperative care were the same as in the acute experiments. The pump served again as the left ventricular assist device, delivering blood from the left atrium to the aorta. The bypass flow was adjusted to 40–50% of total flow. The systole ratio was fixed at 40% and the frequency at 60/min. The blood samples for hematological measurement were taken preoperatively, at the beginning of the pumping, 6 h and then every 24 h postoperatively. The

**Table 1.** Hematological variations in pigs ($n$ = 5) during acute experiments of left ventricular assistance with the pulsatile impeller pump

| | RBC ($10^6$/μl) | WBC ($10^3$/μl) | PLT ($10^3$/μl) | HGB (g/dl) | HCT (%) | Fr.Hb. (mg/dl) | LDH (U/l) |
|---|---|---|---|---|---|---|---|
| Preoperative | 6.85 ± 0.62 | 12.90 ± 0.40 | 515.0 ± 164.0 | 11.40 ± 0.71 | 36.00 ± 1.27 | 3.72 ± 1.06 | 1043.7 ± 398.6 |
| Pump on | 6.67 ± 0.86 | 10.00 ± 4.37 | 423.3 ± 133.2 | 9.90 ± 3.33 | 32.40 ± 8.92 | 4.84 ± 3.65 | 1526.0 ± 903.3 |
| 1 h | 6.41 ± 1.12 | 10.40 ± 2.00 | 390.3 ± 137.0 | 9.80 ± 3.78 | 31.30 ± 9.93 | 4.46 ± 4.09 | 1720.0 ± 1145.6 |
| 2 h | 6.80 ± 1.55 | 12.80 ± 3.98 | 384.3 ± 107.2 | 10.23 ± 4.37 | 33.27 ± 12.40 | 5.03 ± 4.72 | 1781.7 ± 1107.5 |
| 3 h | 6.60 ± 1.60 | 12.40 ± 4.32 | 353.7 ± 85.6 | 10.10 ± 4.47 | 32.50 ± 12.50 | 5.49 ± 4.85 | 1806.0 ± 1039.5 |
| 4 h | 6.35 ± 1.99 | 10.70 ± 5.14 | 300.0 ± 82.4 | 9.77 ± 4.68 | 31.47 ± 13.75 | 5.78 ± 5.79 | 2008.7 ± 794.3 |
| 5 h | 5.22 ± 2.76 | 8.37 ± 7.18 | 225.0 ± 53.9 | 8.17 ± 4.97 | 26.50 ± 15.25 | 4.98 ± 4.81 | 1602.3 ± 698.0 |
| 6 h | 5.12 ± 2.97 | 8.03 ± 6.95 | 216.7 ± 57.73 | 8.03 ± 5.18 | 26.10 ± 16.06 | 4.68 ± 4.64 | 1594.0 ± 836.8 |

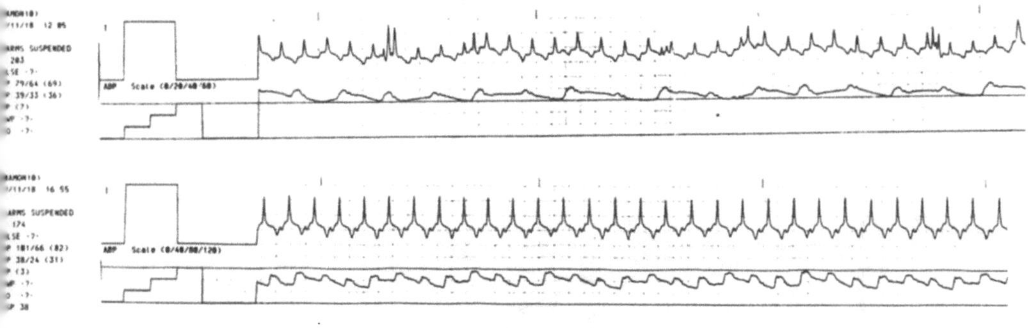

**Fig. 2.** Left ventricular assistance with pulsatile impeller pump can support the failing heart to maintain the circulation (*top*) and can help the heart function (*bottom*) to recover effectively

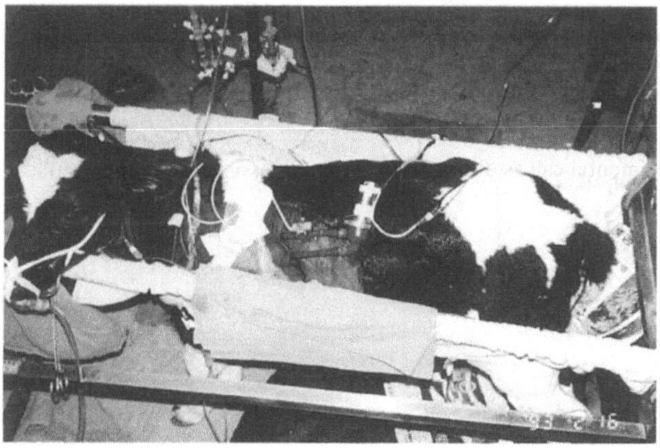

**Fig. 3.** The experimental calves were in good condition during left ventricular assistance with the pulsatile impeller pump

experimental calves awoke shortly after the operation, stood up a few hours later, and were in good condition during most of the experimental period (Fig. 3). Two calves survived 5 days and another two 7 and 11 days, respectively. The termination of the experiments was due to pulmonary failure (two cases), bleeding (one case), and infection (one case); in no case was termination related to the pump itself. Figures 4–10 describe the hematological variations of experimental calves during the survival experiments. The RBC, HCT, HGB, and PLT decreased in the first 4 days and went up thereafter. The FHB decreased in most cases, indicating no erythrocyte damage. The LDH increased but was with in the normal range.

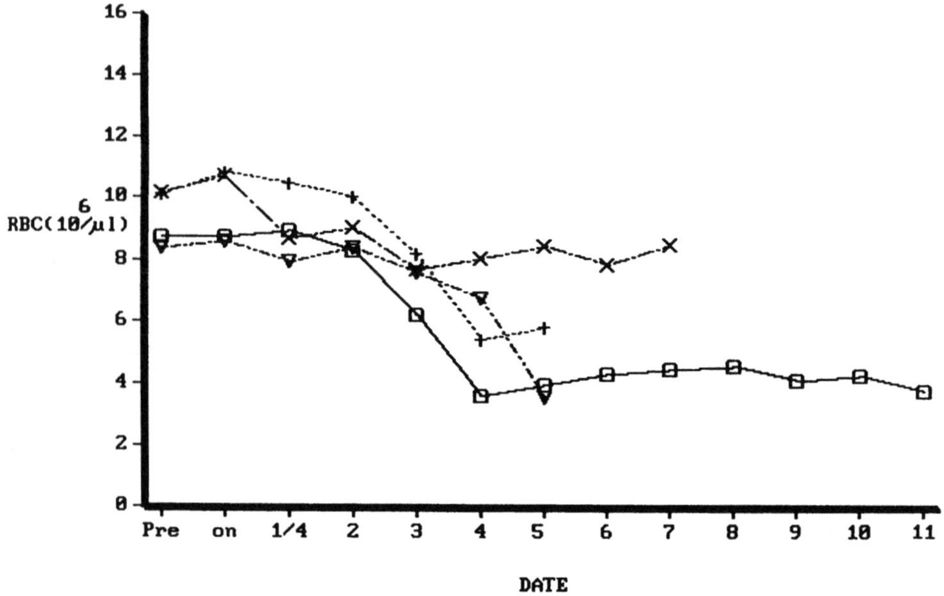


**Fig. 4.** RBC count variations in experimental calves during left ventricular assistance with pulsatile impeller pump

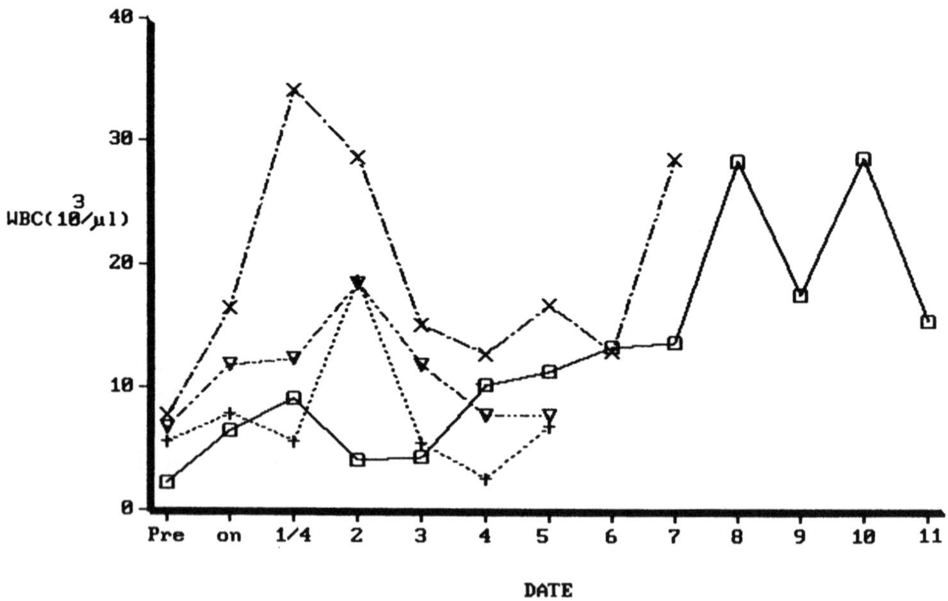


**Fig. 5.** WBC count variations in experimental calves during left ventricular assistance with pulsatile impeller pump

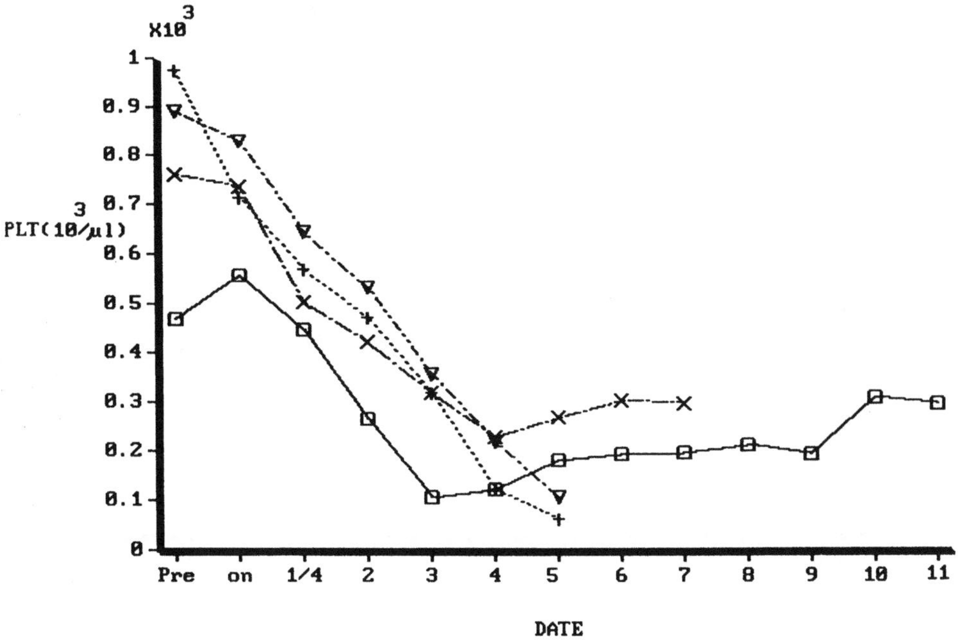


**Fig. 6.** PLT count variations in experimental calves during left ventricular assistance with pulsatile impeller pump

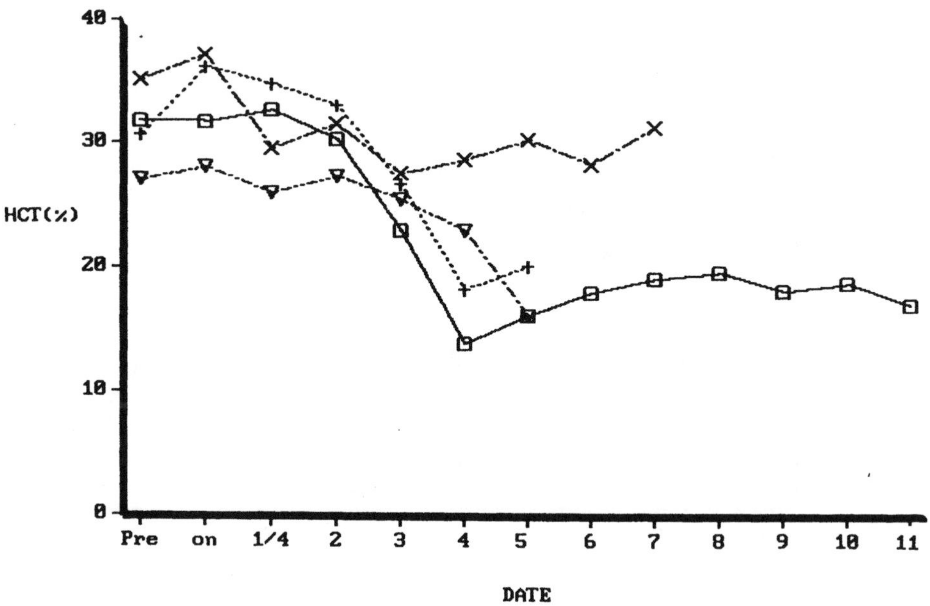


**Fig. 7.** Hematocrit variations of experimental calves during left ventricular assistance with pulsatile impeller pump

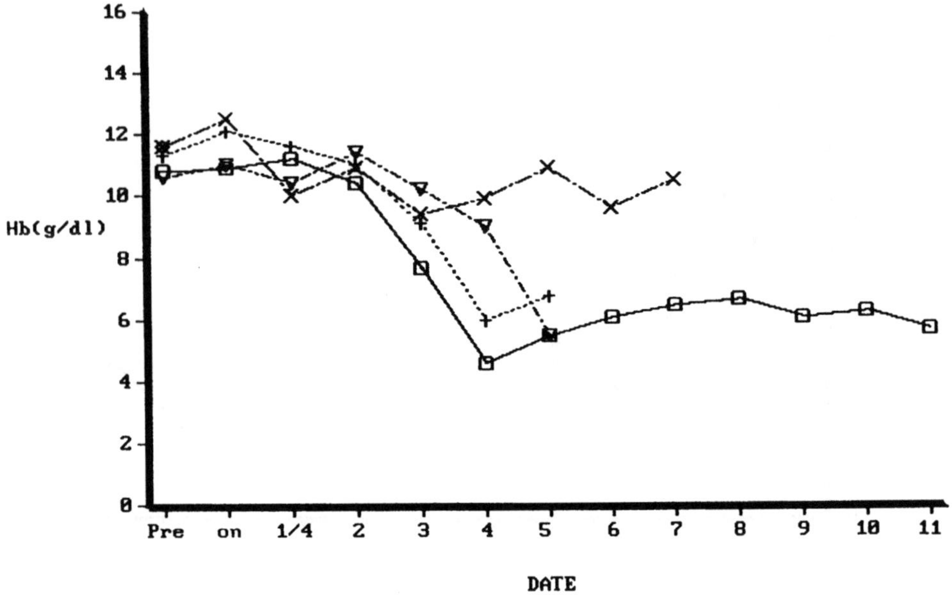


**Fig. 8.** Hemoglobin variations of experimental calves during left ventricular assistance with pulsatile impeller pump

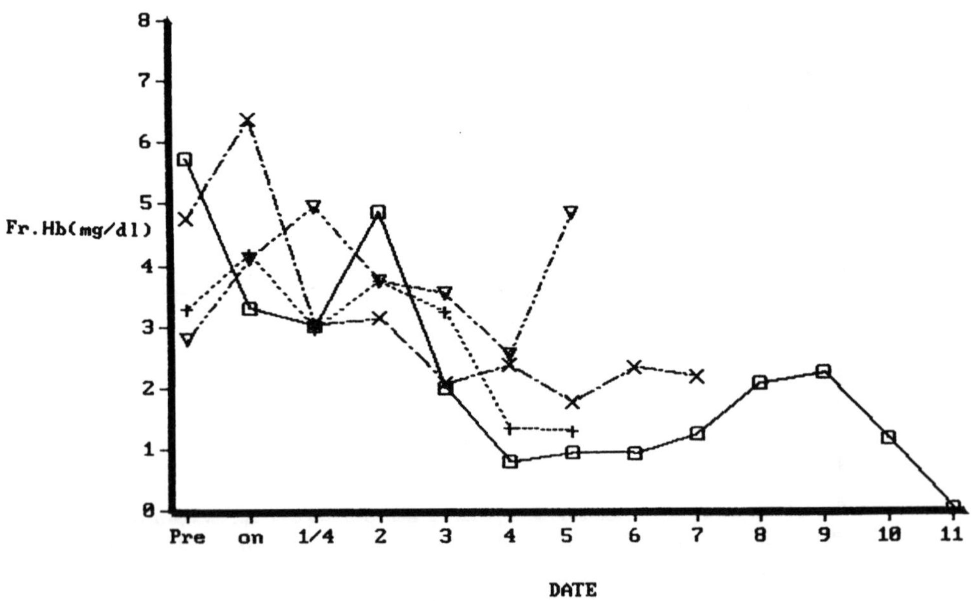


**Fig. 9.** Free hemoglobin variations in experimental calves during left ventricular assistance with pulsatile impeller pump

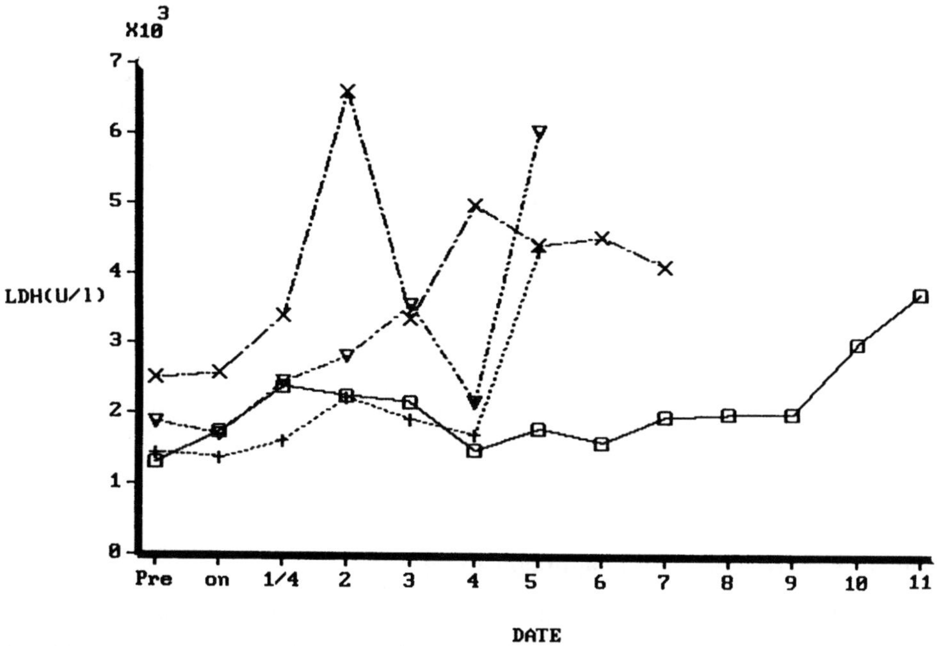


**Fig. 10.** Lactate dehydrogenase variations in experimental calves during left ventricular assistance with pulsatile impeller pump

**Table 2.** Hematological variations in experiments with calves during left ventricular assistance with a locally made diaphragm pump

| | RBC ($10^6/\mu l$) | WBC ($10^3/\mu l$) | PLT ($10^3/\mu l$) | HGB (g/dl) | HCT (%) | FHB (mg/dl) | LDH (U/l) |
|---|---|---|---|---|---|---|---|
| Pre-op | | | | | | | |
| case 1 | 8.36 | 6.7 | 891 | 10.6 | 27.1 | 2.78 | 1 877 |
| case 2 | 8.75 | 10.8 | 730 | 11.5 | 30.7 | 3.75 | 1 960 |
| Pump on | | | | | | | |
| case 1 | 8.59 | 11.9 | 828 | 11.0 | 28.0 | 4.11 | 1 711 |
| case 2 | 11.97 | 24.1 | 707 | 12.9 | 38.1 | 11.70 | 2 380 |
| 6 h | | | | | | | |
| case 1 | 7.93 | 12.3 | 645 | 10.4 | 25.9 | 4.93 | 2 483 |
| case 2 | 12.15 | 11.9 | 244 | 13.2 | 38.5 | 6.09 | 2 130 |
| 2nd day | | | | | | | |
| case 1 | 8.39 | 18.5 | 533 | 11.4 | 27.3 | 3.73 | 2 815 |
| case 2 | 9.97 | 12.6 | 115 | 10.7 | 31.7 | 6.23 | 9 100 |
| 3rd day | | | | | | | |
| case 1 | 7.56 | 11.8 | 354 | 10.2 | 25.4 | 3.53 | 3 565 |
| case 2 (death) | 2.91 | 3.8 | 33 | 3.2 | 10.5 | 21.93 | 14 920 |
| 4th day | | | | | | | |
| case 1 | 6.73 | 7.7 | 219 | 9.0 | 22.9 | 2.55 | 2 167 |
| 5th day | | | | | | | |
| case 1 (death) | 3.55 | 7.7 | 105 | 16.1 | 5.5 | 4.84 | 6 020 |

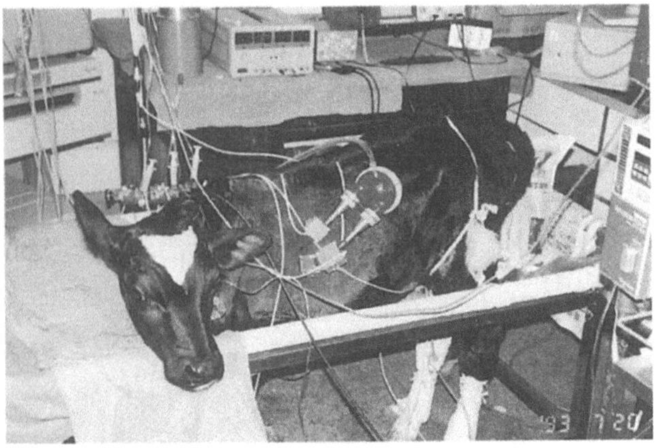


**Fig. 11.** Control experiments with calves using locally made left ventricular assist diaphragm pump

### Control Experiments with Diaphragm Pump

As a control, the same experiments were done with calves (two cases) using a diaphragm pump system (Fig. 11) made by the author [4, 5]. The hematological data demonstrated no obvious difference from those in the experiments with the pulsatile impeller pump (Table 2).

At autopsy after the experiments, however, it was observed that thrombus formation in the diaphragm pump and its connecting tubes was more visible than in the impeller pump and its cannulae, although the activated coagulation time (ACT) in diaphragm pump experiments was controlled to 2.0~3.0 times the normal value, while that in impeller pump experiments was controlled to 1.5~2.0 times the normal value.

## Biventricular Assist Impeller Pump

### Acute Experiments with Pigs

The biventricular assist impeller pump, i.e., the impeller total heart, was developed several years ago [1, 6, 7]; it has only recently been tested in vivo. As the first step, acute biventricular assist in pigs was attempted (Fig. 12). In this device, two impeller pumps are located on both sides of, and are driven by, a single DC motor with a double output shaft (Fig. 13). As the motor changes its rotating speed periodically by introducing a square waveform voltage into the motor, both pumps eject the blood flow simultaneously. To meet with the requirement that the left and right pumps deliver the same blood flow volume while working against different blood pressures, the left and right impellers have the same vane form but different dimensions (Fig. 14). The flow equilibrium of both pumps is achieved automatically without need for any control, because of the self-modulation property of the impeller pump. That is, the output of the impeller pump increases when the afterload decreases, and vice versa.

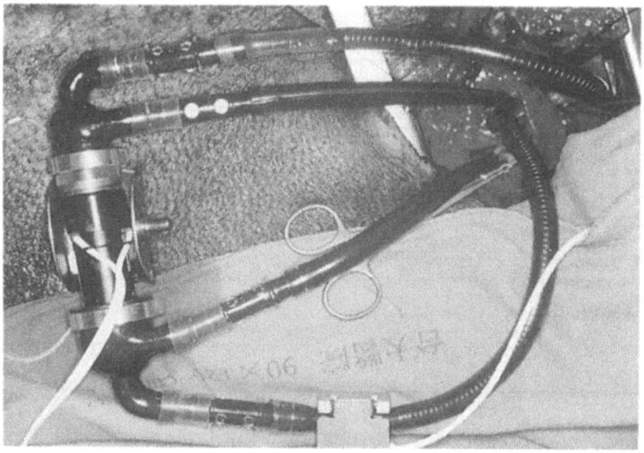

**Fig. 12.** Acute experiments of biventricular assistance with pigs using impeller total heart

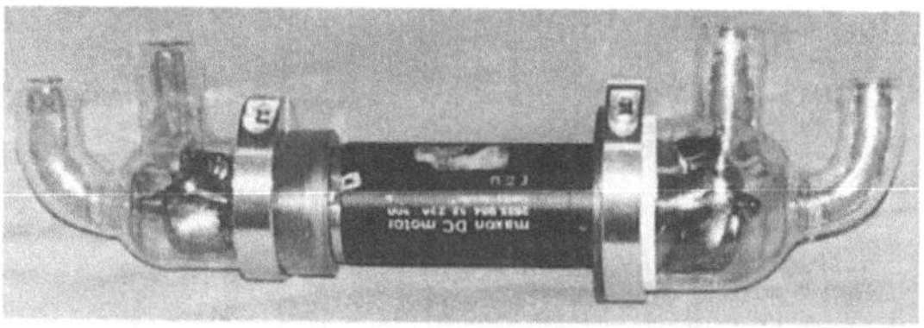

**Fig. 13.** In the impeller total heart, i.e., biventricular assist impeller pumps, two pumps are located on both sides of, and driven by, a single DC motor

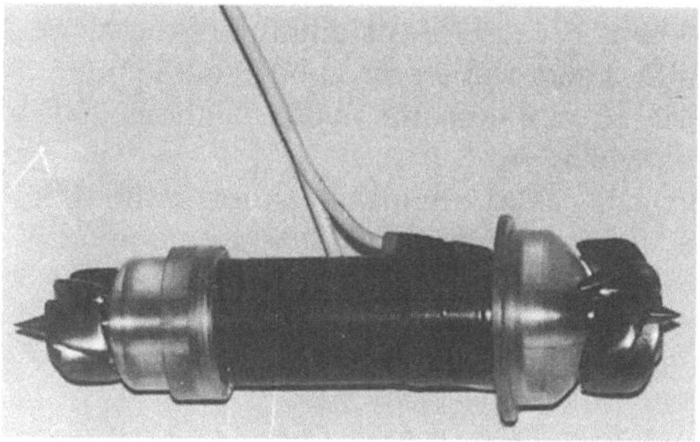

**Fig. 14.** To meet with the requirements that both pumps deliver the same volume of work against different pressure, the left impeller (*right*) and the right impeller (*left*) have the same vane and shroud forms but different dimensions

The acute experiments of biventricular assist in pigs were to test the blood compatibility of the device, so as to demonstrate the feasibility of a centrifugal-type impeller total heart. Four pigs weighing 30–50 kg were used for these experiments. The left pump delivered the blood from the left atrium to the aorta and the right pump from the right atrium to the pulmonary artery (Fig. 12). The bypass flow on both sides was measured by a noninvasive transonic volume flow meter and was adjusted to 1.5~2.0 l/min, about 40–50% of the total flow. The systole ratio was fixed at 40% and the frequency at 60/min. In case of heart failure, the circulation was maintained principally by the pulsation of the pump (Fig. 15, top; a case of left ventricular failure); during normal heart function, the perfusion was done by the natural and artificial hearts; thus, the blood pressure

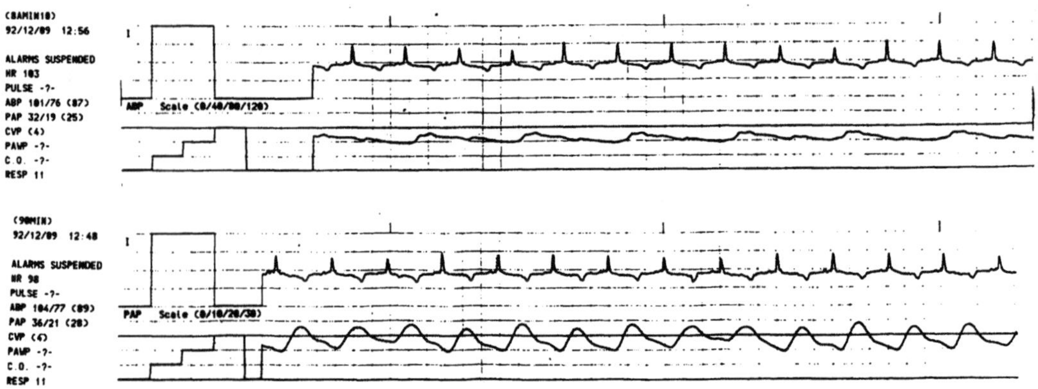


**Fig. 15.** A case of left ventricular failure (*top*) with normal right ventricular function (*bottom*) during biventricular assistance in pigs with impeller total heart

tracing has a complicated form, overlapped by the blood flow from both natural and artificial hearts (Fig. 15, bottom; the same case with normal right ventricular function).

Each experiment lasted 6 h; blood samples, were taken preoperatively, at the beginning of the pumping, and every 2 h for hematological measurements. In Table 3, the values of RBC, WBC, PLT, HCT, HGB, FHB, and LDH are listed. All these parameters remained in the normal range. From the 4th to the 6th hour, most parameters dropped slightly, perhaps because of the dilution of the blood due to the intravenous infusion of saline. There was no thrombosis in the pump, in spite of the low dosage of heparin to maintain the ACT at about 200", approximately 1.5–2.0 times the normal value.

The acute experiments with biventricular assist pumps have proven that this device is ready to be used in chronic survival experiments. It is a unique total heart at present, driven by a single motor; both pumps eject the blood simultaneously, and the flow equilibrium of two pumps is achieved automatically. Conclusively, this device merits further development.

## Control Experiments with Rollers

For control, the same experiments were done with three pigs, employing clinically used SARNS Rollers (Fig. 16). All the experimental conditions were strictly controlled to be as equal as possible to those in experiments with biventricular assist impeller pumps. The roller pumps were operated meticulously to achieve optimal results. The hematological measurements listed in Table 4 indicate that the blood biochemical parameters from experimental pigs with roller pumps remained in the normal range during biventricular assistance lasting 6 h.

**Table 3.** Hematological variations in pigs ($n$ = 4) during acute experiments of biventricular assistance with the impeller total heart

| | RBC ($10^6/\mu l$) | WBC ($10^3/\mu l$) | PLT ($10^3/\mu l$) | HGB (g/dl) | HCT (%) | Fr.Hb. (mg/dl) | LDH (U/l) |
|---|---|---|---|---|---|---|---|
| Preoperative | 6.45 ± 1.37 | 14.23 ± 3.63 | 777.3 ± 485.7 | 7.92 ± 3.52 | 30.88 ± 7.04 | 3.79 ± 0.59 | 804.0 ± 477.2 |
| Pump on | 7.07 ± 1.28 | 15.88 ± 5.03 | 801.8 ± 440.5 | 10.75 ± 2.10 | 34.40 ± 7.28 | 4.39 ± 1.12 | 1102.5 ± 569.3 |
| 2 h | 5.26 ± 1.54 | 11.15 ± 5.73 | 602.0 ± 510.8 | 8.03 ± 2.90 | 27.90 ± 11.80 | 3.33 ± 0.68 | 1171.8 ± 716.3 |
| 4 h | 5.62 ± 2.01 | 13.58 ± 7.02 | 447.7 ± 422.4 | 8.53 ± 3.50 | 27.00 ± 9.07 | 5.30 ± 2.15 | 1532.3 ± 538.3 |
| 6 h | 4.47 ± 2.51 | 10.18 ± 7.36 | 529.3 ± 474.3 | 6.78 ± 4.36 | 21.58 ± 12.42 | 5.46 ± 2.18 | 1149.5 ± 406.0 |

**Table 4.** Hematological variations of pigs ($n$ = 3) during control experiments of biventricular assistance with clinically used roller pumps

| | RBC ($10^6/\mu l$) | WBC ($10^3/\mu l$) | PLT ($10^3/\mu l$) | HGB (g/dl) | HCT (%) | Fr.Hb. (mg/dl) | LDH (U/l) |
|---|---|---|---|---|---|---|---|
| Preoperative | 6.30 ± 0.74 | 13.00 ± 2.66 | 376.5 ± 240.8 | 11.38 ± 1.66 | 35.30 ± 0.52 | 9.68 ± 8.76 | 586.8 ± 304.1 |
| Pump on | 7.00 ± 0.65 | 15.20 ± 5.34 | 375.8 ± 230.8 | 11.86 ± 2.25 | 39.50 ± 7.78 | 5.63 ± 4.06 | 734.8 ± 311.8 |
| 1 h | 6.50 ± 0.75 | 9.64 ± 4.12 | 285.6 ± 138.4 | 11.54 ± 1.81 | 36.62 ± 4.11 | 5.53 ± 3.16 | 658.0 ± 343.4 |
| 2 h | 6.80 ± 0.59 | 6.74 ± 2.93 | 259.4 ± 111.9 | 11.78 ± 1.63 | 37.66 ± 0.86 | 6.13 ± 3.43 | 751.4 ± 331.0 |
| 3 h | 6.70 ± 0.97 | 8.32 ± 2.55 | 288.6 ± 123.5 | 11.62 ± 1.97 | 36.98 ± 1.57 | 7.79 ± 5.07 | 891.8 ± 295.8 |
| 4 h | 6.60 ± 1.11 | 9.84 ± 2.45 | 245.6 ± 127.9 | 11.46 ± 2.59 | 36.74 ± 2.67 | 8.43 ± 7.83 | 1094.6 ± 342.1 |
| 5 h | 6.00 ± 1.62 | 10.46 ± 3.69 | 250.0 ± 120.2 | 10.24 ± 3.06 | 33.38 ± 7.13 | 7.69 ± 5.93 | 1142.6 ± 428.6 |
| 6 h | 5.50 ± 1.65 | 12.14 ± 4.75 | 220.4 ± 117.5 | 9.80 ± 3.25 | 31.92 ± 10.72 | 6.75 ± 4.89 | 1025.4 ± 607.8 |

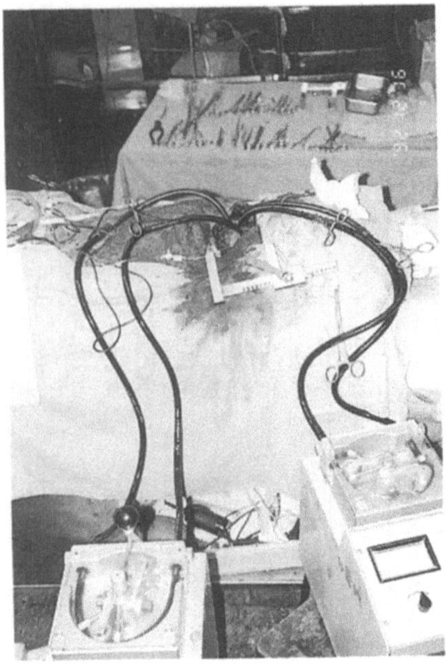

**Fig. 16.** The control experiments of biventricular assistance in pigs with roller pump

## Dynamic Sealing of Impeller Pumps

The sealing problem of the centrifugal pump has puzzled us for more than two decades. Until now, only the traditional passive sealing has been considered, which keeps the blood from entering the motor or the pump bearing. If this resistance function fails, then the sealing is destroyed.

In the author's impeller pumps, an active sealing has been applied. There are two impellers in a single pump, one for pumping, another for sealing (Fig. 17). The latter establishes a pressure gradient along the radius, namely a pressure difference between the motor rotating shaft and the periphery, preventing the blood from permeating the motor. In other words, the sealing impeller pushes any blood that may leak from the pump chamber back again into the pump. This dynamic sealing is safer and more reliable than any passive sealing.

## Magnetohydrodynamic Centrifugal Pump – an Alternative to the Problematic Mechanical Heart

The present artificial heart has been called a mechanical heart, and assisted circulation has been mechanical circulation. This means that our ideas, experiences, and activities have been largely limited until now. This is probably the reason why we have contributed much more than we have achieved in the past.

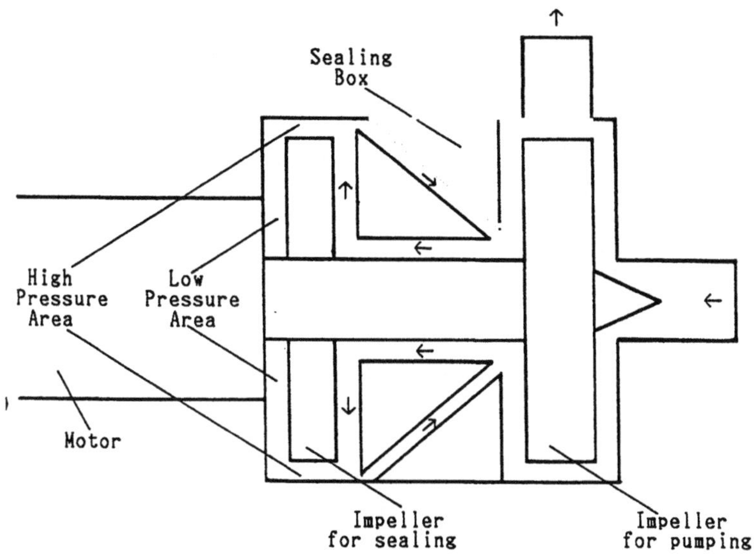


**Fig. 17.** A dynamic sealing of the impeller pump, which has two impellers, one for pumping, another for sealing; the latter establishes a pressure gradient along the radius, namely, a pressure difference between the rotating center and the periphery, to prevent the blood from entering the motor and to push the blood, if it leaks from the pump, back to the pump again

Therefore, in the further development of the artificial heart, we should turn our strategy from improving the available device to investigating the new pumping principle.

The magnetohydrodynamic (MHD) pump, for example, is much more suitable for blood circulation than the present displacement-type diaphragm pump or centrifugal-type impeller pump. In an MHD pump, the fluid is delivered by electromagnetic force. There are no mechanical moving parts in the MHD pump, either for rotation or for reciprocation. As the main problems of the present artificial heart, such as mechanical realiability or blood compatibility are related to mechanical moving parts in the pump, the MHD pump without any mechanical moving parts promises to have long-term applications for circulation.

The MHD pump has been used in industry for decades, to deliver fluid metal or other conductive liquid. No one has tried, however, to use an MHD pump for blood circulation, because according to traditional ideas, the blood is nonconductive [8, 9].

The author has discovered, to the contrary, that blood is a good conductor under a sufficiently strong electric field [10]. Furthermore, the electromagnetic force in an MHD pump is proportional to the magnetic field strength, proportional to the electric field voltage, and proportional to the pump dimension (Fig. 18). To achieve the physiologically required blood pressure and volume, the magnetic field strength should be 20 Tesla or more. Such a strong magnetic field can be realized only with the use of a superconductor [11].

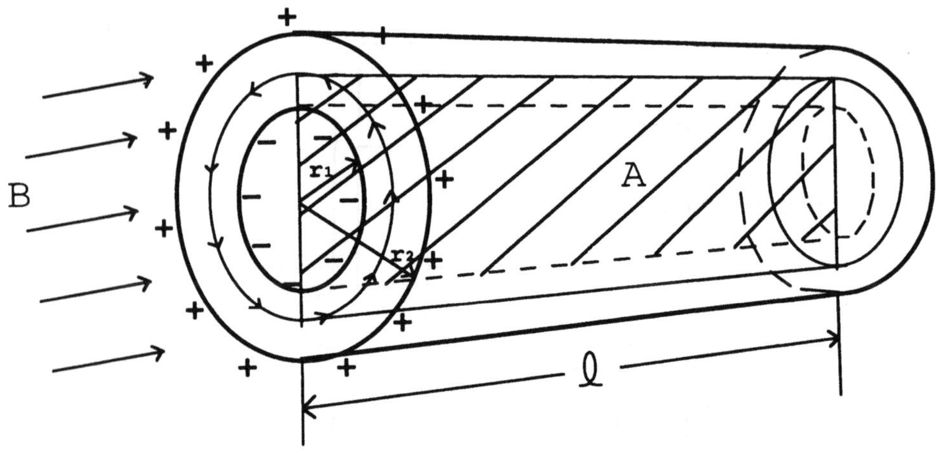


**Fig. 18.** The MHD Centrifugal pump. Two conductive cone-shaped concentric cylinders serve as pump housings and electrodes. As a current passes the blood between the inner and outer housings, the blood will rotate under the action of a magnetic field, to obtain a centrifugal force like that in an impeller pump, in which the rotation of the blood is driven by a rotating impeller. The Lorenz force in the MHD pump is proportional to the magnetic field strength, to the electric field voltage, and to the pump dimension and inversely proportional to the resistivity of the blood. That is to say, $F = nBVA/\sigma$, where $B$ is a magnetic field strength, V is the electric field volt, $A$ is the area of pump cross section, and $\sigma$ is the resistivity of the blood (see [10])

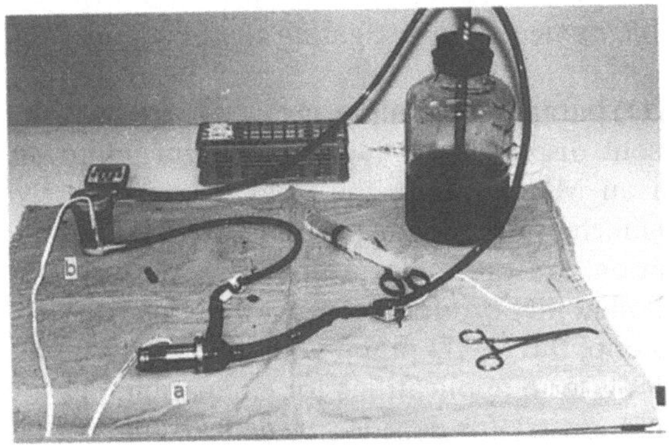


**Fig. 19.** Hematological experiments with the MHD pump. Blood circulation is maintained by an impeller pump (*a*), and the MHD (*b*) serves only as electrodes. Comparing the first half period with electric current of 1A in MHD pump and second half period without current, the blood damage caused by current passing through the blood directly was determined (see [10])

Most people are concerned about whether the electric current, passing through the blood directly, will result in blood damage. The author's experiments have demonstrated that the blood damage caused by current is acceptable (Fig. 19). More experiments should be made, after a strong enough magnetic field is established, to confirm this result.

It is clear by now that (a) blood is a good conductor under certain conditions; (b) the current passing through the blood causes no serious blood damage; (c) with a superconductor, a magnetic field could be made as strong as 20 Tesla or more; and thus (d) an MHD blood pump is feasible.

**Table 5.** Comparison of MHD pump with diaphragm pump and impeller pump with regard to mechanical moving parts and energy transformation

| | Pneumatic- or electric-powered diaphragm pump | Electromechanical impeller pump | MHD centrifugal pump |
|---|---|---|---|
| Mechanical moving parts ($n$) | >3 | 1 | 0 |
| Energy transformations ($n$) | >2 | 2 | 1 |

The advantages of the MHD pump are clear from a comparison of the energy transformation periods with the mechanical moving parts of the mechanical diaphragm pump and the impeller pump (Table 5). The MHD pump, a new concept, may usher in a new generation of artificial hearts.

## References


1. Qian KX (1989) Progress in impeller pumps in China. In: Unger F (ed) Assisted circulation, vol 3. Springer, Berlin Heideberg New York
2. Qian KX et al. (1989) The realization of a pulsatile implantable impeller pump with low hemolysis. Artif Organs J ISAO 13(2):162–169
3. Qian KX et al. (1989) Low hemolysis pulsatile impeller pump: design concept and experimental results. J Biomed Eng 11(6):112–116
4. Qian KX (1987) The development of the left ventricular bypass pumps for adults and children. Chin J Biomed Eng 6(2):80–82
5. Qian KX (1990) A linear motor and compact cylinder-piston driver for left ventricular bypass. J Biomed Eng 12(1):106–112
6. Qian KX (1990) A new total heart design via implantable impeller pumps. J Biomater Appl 4(4):12
7. Qian KX et al. (1987) Toward an implantable total impeller heart. ASAIO Trans 33(3)
8. Branover H (1978) Magnetohydrodynamic flow in ducts. Wiley, New York
9. Backer RS et al. (1987) Handbook of electromagnetic pump technology. Elsevier Science, New York
10. Qian KX et al. (1993) A superconductive electromagnetic pump without any mechanical moving parts. ASAIO Trans 39(3):649–653
11. Schuch L et al. (1988) Ein neuer Werkstoff erobert die Welt. Eine Beschreibung des Phänomens, elektrischen Strom ohne Widerstand zu leiten. Markt and Technik, Munich

# Part IV
# Biologic Assistance and Energy Sources

# Introduction

F. Unger

Cardiomyoplasty brought a new element into the discussion of the whole concept of cardiac assistance. After preparation of the M. trapecius the muscle is wrapped over the left ventricle for chronic assistance. It is stimulated according to the ECG by a special pacemaker (Medtronic). This basic concept, developed by Carpentier, was reported extensively in the last issue. It shows the principle feasibility of using a chronic energy source. This muscle can be used as a pouch to drive a compliance chamber, as is reported by Stephenson and others. In this context, Liotta and Aluarez demonstrate a clinical concept of chronic heart assistance based on clinical work.

# Skeletal Muscle Ventricles for Biologic Cardiac Assistance*

H. LU, R.L. HAMMOND, G.A. THOMAS, and L.W. STEPHENSON

## Historical Background

### Development of Muscle Grafts Applied to the Heart

Skeletal muscle was first introduced to cardiac surgery between 1930 and 1940. In 1931, De Jesus used pectoralis muscle to repair a penetrating cardiac injury in a young man [1]. Two years later, Leriche and Fontaine applied a pectoralis major muscle graft to the surface of infarcted canine myocardium in order to reinforce the myocardial scar [2]. After a few months, the grafts were found to be viable and well incorporated into the surrounding myocardial tissue. In 1935, Beck experimentally demonstrated the development of collateral blood flow from muscle grafts to the canine epicardium [3]. In his study, after application of the muscle graft to the myocardium, both coronary arteries were gradually occluded. Over a period of weeks, communication between the skeletal muscle and coronary circulations formed. After that Beck and others applied nonstimulated muscle grafts and other tissues to the ischemic hearts of human beings for the treatment of coronary artery disease [4, 5].

In 1959, Petrovsky reported favorable results with the use of diaphragmatic pedicle grafts in the treatment of left ventricular aneurysms in man [6, 7]. He sutured the muscle grafts directly to the epicardial surface and over the aneurysm of the left ventricle. He attempted to apply the diaphragmatic graft with sufficient tension to flatten out and obliterate the aneurysm. The grafts were well tolerated, became firmly adhered to the myocardium, reinforced the scarred tissue, and also may have improved the myocardial blood supply. About 30% of these patients were freed from their symptoms of chest pain and dyspnea. The operative mortality was approximately 20%.

In the same year, Kantrowitz and McKinnon wrapped pedicle grafts of canine left hemidiaphragm around the heart and stimulated the grafts via the phrenic nerve in synchrony with cardiac systole [8, 9]. They observed active contraction of the muscle grafts but no hemodynamic changes. In a later experiment, Kantrowitz and Kusaba showed that a stimulated diaphragmatic graft wrapped around the heart was able to increase left ventricular pressure, peak femoral artery pressure, and aortic blood flow in an animal with failing heart [10]. This effect lasted for only 15 min, owing to muscle fatigue.

* Supported by NIH Grant HL 34778

In 1964, Nakamura and Glenn enlarged the right canine atrium with a hemidiaphragm pedicle graft to about twice its original size [11]. After stimulating the graft via the phrenic nerve, contraction of the transposed graft produced an increase in intra-atrial pressure. In another experiment they wrapped the hemidiaphragm graft directly around both ventricles [11]. Similarly, contraction of the graft wrapped around both ventricles produced an increase in aortic pressure. Repeated stimulation after 11 months showed nearly the same results. Two years later, Termet wrapped canine latissimus dorsi muscle around the heart [12]. After 8 months, he stimulated the grafts via the thoracodorsal nerve after inducing cardiac fibrillation. He reported an aortic systolic pressure of 80 mmHg with each muscle graft contraction during ventricular fibrillation. Termet stated that this effect lasted 10–15 min, until the muscle fatigued. After applying inlay and onlay grafts of diaphragm to the canine right ventricle, Scheperd found, in 1969, that denervation atrophy occurred despite an intact blood supply [13]. She noted that this effect was less severe if the nerve supply was maintained and the grafts were electrically stimulated on a long-term basis.

In 1980, Drinkwater and Chiu constructed left ventricular inlay grafts from vascularized canine rectus abdominis muscle [14]. There was an acute increase of up to 30 mmHg in the left ventricular pressure with each graft stimulation while the dog was maintained on cardiopulmonary bypass. The same year, Macoviak replaced full-thickness portions of the right ventricular free wall with pedicled grafts of canine diaphragm [15]. These grafts were stimulated directly or through the intact phrenic nerve [16–18]. With supramaximal voltage stimulation, direct stimulation of the graft also resulted in right ventricular capture and synchronous graft-cardiac contraction. Graft thickening concurrent with each muscle graft contraction was documented by echogram [16]. Weeks after implantation, the muscle grafts showed active tension development when stimulated by an implantable R-wave synchronous pacemaker [18]. Collateral blood flow between the muscle graft and the adjoining myocardium was documented after 1 month.

In 1982, Schaff reported the use of pectoralis to treat patients with infected false aneurysms of the left ventricle [19]. In 1985 and 1986, respectively, Carpentier in Paris and Magovern in Pittsburgh reported improvement in cardiac performance after applying pedicle grafts of latissimus dorsi muscle to the hearts of human beings suffering from various cardiac maladies [20, 21]. The grafts were originally stimulated with an implantable R-wave synchronous (DDD) pulse generator, with the ventricular lead diverted to the skeletal muscle. Later, a pulse generator capable of delivering trains of stimuli to the latisimuss dorsi muscle were substituted for the DDD pulse generators. The operation has become known as cardiomyoplasty. To date, almost 500 patients in the world have undergone cardiomyoplasty. Currently, phase-II clinical trials are being conducted under the supervision of the Food and Drug Administration in the United States, and phase-III clinical trials are expected to start soon.

Despite the growing enthusiasm for cardiomyoplasty, the precise mechanism by which most patients are benefitted is still not fully understood. It is clear in some patients that the stimulated skeletal muscle wrap actually assists left ventricular systolic ejection, as witnessed by improvements in left ventricular ejection fraction with stimulator On vs. Off and improvements in cardiac output with stimulator On vs. Off. Most patients who undergo cardiomyoplasty and survive the procedure improve one or more NYHA functional classes for heart failure. They feel better and frequently experience dramatic improvements in their physical activity.

## Development of Skeletal Muscle Pumping Chambers or Ventricles

The construction of pumping chambers or ventricles is another, potentially more important, application of skeletal muscle for cardiac assistance. In 1959, Kantrowitz, working on the concept of diastolic counterpulsation, wrapped left canine diaphragm muscle around the descending aorta [8, 9]. The muscle graft was stimulated during diastole through the intact phrenic nerve by an external stimulator. Kantrowitz showed an increase in diastolic aortic pressure of about 26% until the muscle fatigued several seconds later. Subsequent experiments by Von Recum showed that skeletal muscle pouches generated pressure when wrapped around a latex bladder but failed after several hours due to fatigue [22]. In 1964, Kusserow used quadriceps femoris muscle to power an external bellows-type blood pump [22]. The pump worked for several hours.

Ten years later, Spotnitz constructed skeletal muscle pouches from the canine rectus muscle [23]. He found the physical characteristics to be similar to those of the heart described by Frank and Starling. This observation should not have been too surprising, because Otto Frank, a German physiologist, had recognized in 1895 that the response of isolated frog heart to alteration in tension just prior to contraction was similar to that of skeletal muscle [24]. Spotnitz noted an increase of the transmural pressure in conjunction with an increase of the resting wall tension (preload developed during active tension). With filling pressures of 50–150 mmHg, systolic pressures of greater than 500 mmHg could be obtained. However, because Spotnitz's rectus muscle pump was relatively noncompliant, it is unlikely that it could have been used even if it had not fatigued rapidly.

In 1978, Juffe used gluteus maximus muscle to construct pouch-like pumping chambers [25]. The gluteus muscle was dissected free from its insertions and formed into a pouch. A balloon transducer was then introduced into the pouch, and the muscle was stimulated via the gluteal nerve by a pacemaker. Initially, pressures as high as 170 mmHg were recorded. Juffe reported some degree of muscle contraction for up to 26 days. Failure of this muscle pump may have been due to nerve damage or ischemic damage.

During the past few years, skeletal muscle ventricles have been further developed by a series of investigators in Dr. Stephenson's group and connected to the circulation for cardiac assist in a variey of configurations. Effective cardiac assistance has been demonstrated in each configuration. One skeletal muscle ventricle in an aorta-to-aorta configuration as a diastolic counter pulsator pumped blood effectively for 836 days; to the authors' knowledge, this represents the longest living laboratory animal or human being with a functioning heart-assist device [26].

# Physiology of Heart and Skeletal Muscle

## Comparison of Heart and Skeletal Muscle

Heart muscle and skeletal muscle share many features. However, due to varying functional requirements, they differ in several important physiologic and histologic properties. Both muscle types have the ability to convert chemical energy into mechanical work and resemble each other in their basic ultrastructure. The sarcomere, the contractile unit, is similar in structure. The myofibrils of the heart and skeletal muscle are arranged longitudinally. Both muscle types have a sarcoplasmic reticulum and similar transverse tubular systems [27].

The metabolic demands of heart and skeletal muscle are different. The cardiac muscle must contract rhythmically and relentlessly throughout an entire lifetime without developing fatigue. On the other hand, skeletal muscles are generally required to perform mechanical work for relatively short periods of time with intervening periods of rest.

Histologically, cardiac muscle cells are relatively uniform, whereas skeletal muscle consists, basically of two types of fibers: slow-twitch fibers and fast-twitch fibers, albeit with some intermediate forms. Slow-twitch (type I) fibers, like cardiac muscle fibers, are relatively fatigue resistant. Fast-twich (type II) fibers are more prone to fatigue. Most muscles are made up of a mixture of both fiber types, the relative number and distribution of each fiber type varying with the function a particular muscle must perform. A muscle that contains mostly fast-twitch fibers is called fast muscle. This type of muscle has a short-twitch duration and is specialized for fine, skilled movement, such as some extraocular muscles and some of the muscles of the hand.

Only a few muscles consist solely of slow-twitch fibers and hence are called slow muscle. They respond slowly, have a long latency, and are adapted for long, slow posture-maintaining contractions, such as the soleus muscle. The metabolism of type-I fibers (slow-twitch) relies primarily on aerobic, oxidative phosphorylation pathways, whereas that of the type-II fibers (fast-twitch) relies predominantly on the anaerobic, glycolytic pathways. Type-I fibers have less sarcoplasmic reticulum and a larger mitochondrial volume than type-II fibers. Each fiber type carries specific myosin isotypes (contractile proteins). Type-I fibers have "slow" myosin isoforms, whereas type-II fibers have "fast" myosin isoforms. The myosin isotypes differ in the efficiency of energy utilization [28, 29].

In comparison to skeletal muscle, heart muscle has a highly developed aerobic metabolism, with a large mitochondrial volume. Unlike skeletal muscle, which contains 2–5% mitochondria by volume, cardiac muscle contains approximately 30% mitochondria by volume [27].

The amount of active tension that can be achieved by each muscle differs. Skeletal muscle can generate an active tension of 1–5 kg/cm$^2$, whereas cardiac muscle generates active tension of only about 0.5 kg/cm$^2$ [30].

The neuroelectrical properties of the two muscle tissues are also different. Cardiac muscle works as an electrical syncytium. Intercalated disks are thought to facilitate the flow of current between cells by functioning as low-resistance pathways. In this way, the entire myocardium contracts nearly simultaneously as an "all-or-none" unit in response to a solitary electrical stimulus. In contrast, skeletal muscle cells are organized into motor units, each containing its own nerve ending. These individual motor units can be activated independently. Therefore, the entire muscle does not necessarily contract simultaneously.

Successful application of skeletal muscle as a cardiac assist device requires some important manipulation of its characteristics. The problem of muscle fatigue has been solved by transforming the type-II fatigue-prone fibers into type-I fatigue-resistant fibers. This is achieved by chronic electrostimulation of the motor nerve.

## Skeletal Muscle Transformation

In 1960, Eccles and Eccles investigated whether the twitch property of a muscle (fast or slow) was determined by the muscle fiber itself or by its motor neuron [31]. They conducted a cross-innervation experiment in cats [32]. The motor nerve to the soleus muscle (a predominantly slow-twitch type-I muscle) was switched surgically with the motor nerve to the flexor digitorum longus (a predominantly fast-twitch type-II muscle). After the nerves regenerated, the contraction rate of the soleus, reinnervated by the nerve to the flexor digitorum longus, was accelerated, whereas the contraction rate of the reinnervated flexor digitorum longus muscle was slowed.

In 1969, Salmons and Vrbova found that it was actually the stimulation pattern of the motor nerve that determined the muscle fiber type [33]. They transformed a fast-twitch muscle into a slow-twitch muscle by delivering exogenous electrical stimuli (using an implantable electrical stimulator) to the nerve of the fast-twitch muscle, with a stimulation frequency pattern similar to that observed in the nerve of a slow-twitch muscle. After several weeks of stimulation, the transformation was complete.

In the following years, groups led by Salmons and Pette further investigated the effect of electrical stimulation upon skeletal muscle [34–36]. They found that the muscle fibers undergo profound physiologic, biochemical, and morphological changes, particularly with regard to resistance to fatigue. In the development of skeletal muscle power for cardiac assist, this process is termed electrical conditioning or preconditioning.

## Burst Stimulation and Electrical Conditioning

A single electrical stimulus, which results in a single muscle twitch, is not sufficient for a skeletal muscle to generate cardiao-type work. It is necessary to use a group of appropriately timed stimuli. This type of stimulation is called burst stimulation. It leads to a rapid mechanical summation of motor units and generation of substantial contractile force [37–43].

A burst consists of a series of electrical pulses. The pulses can vary in amplitude, duration, and number, but are usually constant in frequency within one burst. The magnitude of the contractile force achieved by a skeletal muscle may be influenced by varying the duration of a single burst (burst duration), the time between two bursts, the frequency of the pulses within a burst (burst frequency), and the amplitude of the pulses.

Burst frequency is typically set between 25 and 50 Hz. (Strictly speaking, Hertz refers to a number of cyclic waveforms of a sinusoidal nature occurring in 1 s. The correct descriptor should be pulses per second, in that the individual stimuli are monopolar square wave pulses. However, Hz continues in common use in the literature.) An increase of the burst frequency produces an increase in the contractile force (until tetanus occurs). During stimulation of skeletal muscle, the burst duration usually lasts 25–33% of the duty cycle. During the remaining 67–75% of the duty cycle, there is no stimulation.

The application of an exogenous electrical stimulation pattern to a skeletal muscle motor nerve over an extended period of time is referred to as electrical (pre)conditioning. It enables skeletal muscle to adapt to new work patterns by the processes studied by the basic muscle physiologist mentioned above. Low-frequency electrical stimulation (2 Hz) of a muscle results in transformation to a slow-twich muscle (type I). The fiber composition of the muscle is transformed from the native mixture of types to a uniform slow-fiber population, and the muscle becomes more fatigue resistant. Quantitative and qualitative changes occur in the histologic, histochemical, and physiologic properties of the skeletal muscle [34, 35]. The changes take place in an apparently well-coordinated sequence and are progressive during the duration of stimulation, until a new steady state is reached.

As a first step, the energy metabolism begins to change [35]. Due to an increased mitochondrial volume density, the activities of the enzymes involved in aerobic substrate oxidation increase. In contrast, the activities of the anaerobic enzymes decrease. Simultaneously, cytosolic $Ca^{2+}$-binding and sequestration are reduced by a decrease in parvalbumin and a transformation of the sarcoplasmic reticulum membranes [35]. Chronic electrostimulation also induces progressive changes in the contractile properties. The isometric twitch contraction time as well as the relaxation time increase. A relatively rapid change occurs during the first 2 weeks because of changes in the $Ca^{2+}$ transport. The remaining changes in contraction time which occur later are caused by alterations in myosin composition [34, 35].

The transformation from fast to slow fibers is accompanied by morphological changes. The muscle fibers change from a mixture of large and small fibers to a population of uniformly small fibers [35]. At the same time, an increase in capillary density occurs in some species [34].

Profound quantitative and qualitative changes in the protein profile of the muscle are caused by electrical stimulation. There is an increase in protein synthesis, as well as in protein breakdown, with a net reduction in muscle weight and cross-sectional area. The transformation from a fast-twitch to a slow-twitch muscle is completed by a change in the expression of fast-type in favor of slow-type myosin isoforms. In the canine latissimus dorsi muscle, conditioning is usually complete at 6 weeks. It should be noted that further changes may occur if the stimulation pattern or workload is altered.

Changes caused by electrical stimulation have been found to be reversible once the stimulation is discontinued [21, 34]. The time course of the recovery is more prolonged than that of the original transformation in terms of metabolism and capillary density, but more rapid for myosin isoform transitions, following a "last in, first out" pattern.

## Experimental Studies with Conditioned Skeletal Muscle

### Continuous Low-frequency Stimulation

Following the basic studies of muscle plasticity performed by Pette, Salmons, and others [28, 29, 33–35, 44–48], later investigators began to re-evaluate muscle with a view to redirecting skeletal muscle power for cardiac assist. Macoviak et al. directly stimulated the canine diaphragm at 10 Hz for 5 weeks [49]. This stimulation resulted in a transition of muscle fibers within a few centimeters of the stimulating electrode to a nearly uniform population of fatigue-resistant type-I fibers. More importantly, Macoviak found that conditioning could also be accomplished at a stimulation frequency of 2 Hz. That lower frequency is similar to that of the normal canine heart rate. Armenti was able to transform the entire hemidiaphragm using similar stimulation patterns, but by stimulating the phrenic nerve instead of stimulating the muscle directly [50].

In 1985, Bitto demonstrated transformation of the rectus abdominis and pectoralis muscles, which was technically more difficult, owing to the innervation by multiple nerves [51].

In another study, Mannion showed that a significant slowing of the rate of fatigue also occurred after stimulation of the canine latissimus dorsi muscle at either 2 or 10 Hz frequencies for 6 weeks [52]. The two stimulation frequencies generated similar increases in fatigue resistance, although the development of intramuscular fibrous tissue and the diminution of muscle fiber diameter were less in the muscles stimulated at 2 Hz.

Clark and Acker used phosphorous nuclear magnetic resonance($^{31}$P-NMR) to show that the conditioned latissimus dorsi muscle has an improved capacity for oxidative phosphorylation similar to that of the heart [53]. In a companion study, Acker measured the oxygen consumption of a conditioned latissimus dorsi muscle while performing isometric work [54]. The conditioned muscle was more efficient in using oxygen than the contralateral control.

### Burst Stimulation over 1 Year

In our laboratory, the effects of burst stimulation on the histochemical and physiologic characteristics of the latissimus dorsi muscle have been studied in muscle which was stimulated in situ for over 1 year [55]. Stimulation was carried out at two different muscle contraction rates, a high rate of 120 contractions/min and a low rate of 54 contractions/min. The different rates were obtained by varying the burst duration and the time between the bursts. The burst frequency was kept constant at 25 Hz. After 1 year, there was no evidence of muscle fiber damage, no abnormality of nerve conduction time, and no loss in the acquired fatigue resistance. The nerve stimulation threshold changed only slightly over the experimental time. A comparison between the two contraction rates showed that the muscle contracted at the rate of 120/min had developed low isometric tension. So far, it has not been determined whether a skeletal muscle contracting at 120/min for a prolonged period will remain strong enough to perform cardiac-type work.

## Skeletal Muscle Ventricles

### Muscle Selection

Several skeletal muscles that have been considered for cardiac assistance are noncritical muscles, in that they can be diverted to another use without causing major physical impairment to the patient. We prefer the latissimus dorsi muscle. It is a powerful, large, flat, and broad-based muscle that can be formed into various shapes. In addition, the latissimus dorsi muscle has only one main blood supply and is innervated by a single nerve, which makes the surgical techniques of dissection and isolation of the neurovascular supply relatively easy.

### Skeletal Muscle Ventricle Construction

We have constructed skeletal muscle ventricles (SMVs) in dogs. After the animal is anesthetized, the left or right latissimus dorsi muscle is mobilized through a flank incision extending from the axilla to the tip of the 11th rib. All attachments, with the exception of the thoracodorsal neurovascular pedicle and the tendinous insertion to the humerus, are divided. The mobilized muscle is then wrapped around a mandrel. The size and shape of the mandrel may vary according to the size of the animal and the experimental protocol. Generally, the muscle is wrapped about 1.5 times around the mandrel. After suturing of the muscle layers to each other, the muscle wrap is attached to the mandrel by means of a Dacron felt collar. SMV construction may vary slightly for different SMV circulatory configurations or uses.

In order to stimulate the skeletal muscle ventricle, an electrode is placed around the proximal thoracodorsal nerve and connected to an implantable pacemaker. This pacemaker is different from those routinely used to pace the heart, given that a skeletal muscle requires a burst pattern of stimuli to elicit the forceful and sustained contractions for cardiac-type work.

The skeletal muscle ventricle, placed either inside the thoracic cavity or on the chest wall under the skin and the subcutaneous tissue, is sutured to the surrounding tissue in order to prevent migration of the SMV or kinking of its neurovascular pedicle. The operation is completed by closing the subcutaneous tissue and the skin over the skeletal muscle ventricle.

Before the skeletal muscle ventricle is able to perform work, the mandrel has to be removed, which is done after a delay period of a few days to several weeks. This delay allows adhesions to form between the muscle layers and helps the normal resting and exercise-induced blood flow to recover in the muscle layers [32, 37, 56]. The delay period also allows for the muscle to adhere to the felt sewing ring by fibrous tissue.

## Skeletal Muscle Ventricles in Mock Circulation

Acker studied the pumping function of skeletal muscle ventricles by measuring and manipulating the preload and afterload in a mock circulation device [38]. For this purpose, two similar polyurethane bladders were connected by a rigid conduit. One of the bladders was placed inside the skeletal muscle ventricle; the other one was placed in a hermetically sealed rigid Plexiglas canister. The bladders and the connecting conduit were filled with saline. The canister was pressurized with air. The pressure in the resting skeletal muscle ventricle represented the preload pressure (Fig. 1). Likewise, the canister pressure represented the systemic afterload. The skeletal muscle ventricles pumped continuously against an afterload of 80 mmHg with a preload of 40–50 mmHg. At the initiation of pumping, the mean systolic pressure was 134 mmHg, and flow was 464 ml/min. After 2 weeks of continuous pumping, the systolic pressure was 104 mmHg and flow was 206 ml/min. Two skeletal muscle ventricles pumped for 5 and 9 weeks, respectively.

In a subsequent study, skeletal muscle ventricles were constructed and then underwent a 3-week vascular delay period, but without conditioning [42]. Using the same preload and afterload in a mock circulation device, the mean stroke work of these SMVs was $400 \times 10^3$ erg after 2 weeks of continuous pumping. This stroke work was intermediate between that of the canine left and right ventricles. Two dogs continued to produce significant stroke work after 2 months. Stevens

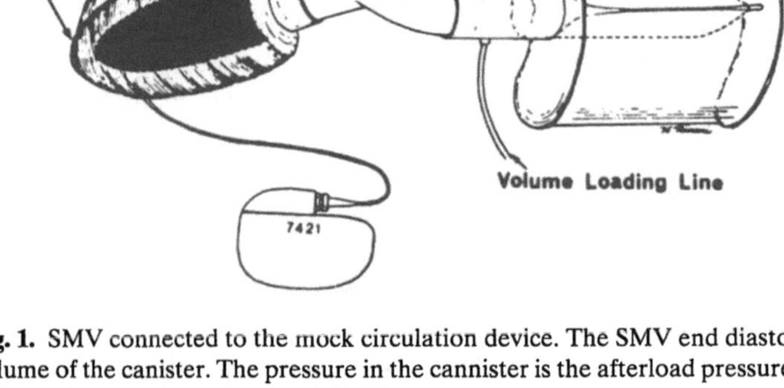


**Fig. 1.** SMV connected to the mock circulation device. The SMV end diastole is diagramed. $V_l$ is the volume of the canister. The pressure in the cannister is the afterload pressure($P_l$). The pressure of the saline column is the preload and SMV pressure

and Brown have also measured similar heart and SMV work outputs using canine rectus abdominis muscle during acute studies [57].

## Different SMV Configurations in Circulation

### SMV for Right Heart Assistance

Bridges et al. studied the function of SMVs designed for complete right heart bypass and partial right heart bypass [58–60]. He connected a skeletal muscle ventricle to the superior and inferior vena cava and pulmonary artery. In the case of complete right-heart bypass (group I), both the superior vena cava and the inferior vena cava were ligated and all blood was directed to the skeletal muscle ventricle. In the case of partial right-heart bypass (group II), only the inferior vena cava was ligated and the blood flow could go either to the skeletal muscle ventricle or to the right atrium. In group I, after 4 h of continuous complete right-heart bypass, stroke work was 163% of canine right ventricular stroke work. Skeletal muscle ventricle output was 1.14 l/min, central venous pressure was 13 mmHg, and systemic systolic blood pressure was 95 mmHg. SMV peak pressure was 37–54 mmHg. Bridges showed in his study that a skeletal muscle ventricle is capable of performing the work of the right ventricle with near-physiologic filling pressures for up to several hours. At the initiation of complete right-heart bypass, the systemic arterial blood pressure was 100–110 mmHg. After 4 h, the systemic arterial blood pressure was still greater than 100 mmHg.

Another configuration for right heart assist with skeletal muscle ventricle involved an SMV placed between the right ventricle and the pulmonary artery with two porcine valved conduits. The pulmonary artery was ligated between the two limbs of the conduits [61] (Fig. 2A,B). In this study, SMVs were constructed from the right latissimus dorsi muscle of eight dogs. After connection to the circulation, the SMVs were stimulated to contract in a 1:2 diastolic mode with a 33 Hz burst frequency. Cardiac output increased by 22%, systemic systolic arterial pressure by 9%, and peak pulmonary artery pressure by 31% at the initiation of this study. In six dogs, effective right heart assist was sustained for periods of between 1 and 12 weeks. Two dogs survived for longer than 3 months.

### Aorta–SMV–Aorta Configuration

We have had the most extensive experience with SMVs connected to the systemic circulation in an aorto-aorta configuration. In early acute studies, Mannion connected SMVs to the descending thoracic aorta by incorporating a T-system and a valve, which allowed control of the skeletal muscle ventricle filling pressure [37, 39]. In this study, the SMV was able to function well in the circulation. After 4 h, the generated stroke work was $0.68 \times 10^3$ ergs, which is about three times that of the native canine right ventricle.

Acker et al. constructed a tube-shaped skeletal muscle ventricle from latissimus dorsi muscle [40]. This geometry allowed through-and-through blood

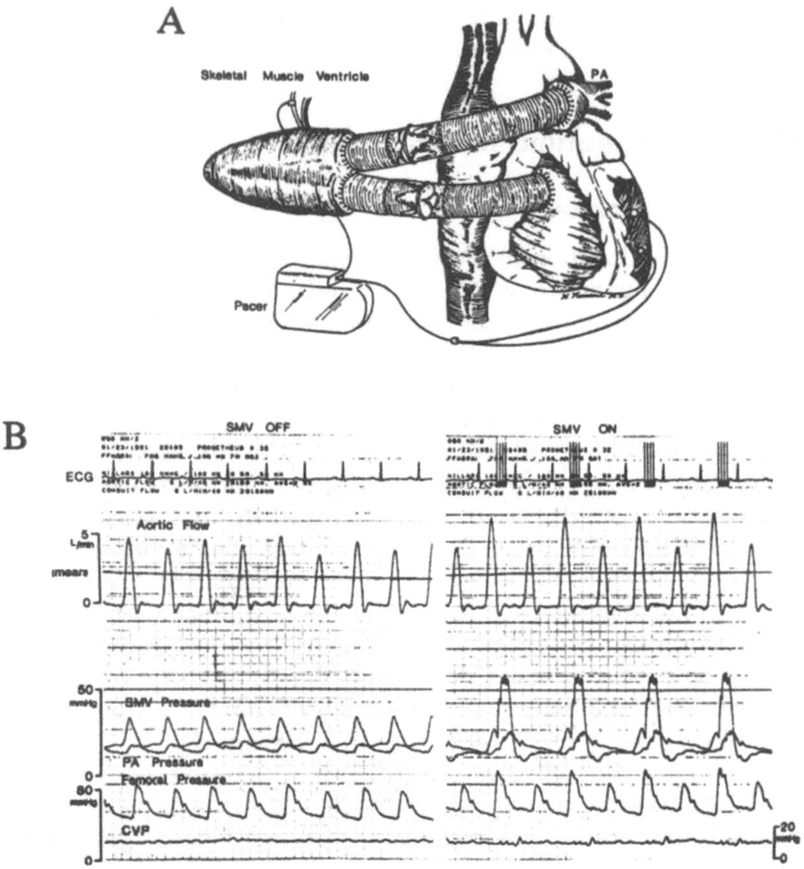


**Fig. 2.** **A** The skeletal muscle ventricle is connected from RV to PA. The main pulmonary artery (*PA*) has been ligated proximal to the anastomosis. **B** Representative hemodynamic tracings recorded during stimulation of the skeletal muscle ventricle (*SMV*) with 33 Hz burst stimulation and without stimulation of the SMV

flow. The device was connected to the circulation by dividing the descending thoracic aorta and re-establishing flow through a Gore-Tex bladder-conduit device. Two-dimensional short-axis echocardiograms of the SMV obtained from one dog after 12 days of continuous counterpulsation demonstrated a 70%, 90%, and 100% decrease in cross-sectional area at the midpoint of the SMV at 25 Hz, 43 Hz, and 85 Hz stimulation, respectively, during SMV contraction. Pulsed Doppler blood flow measurements, just distal to the outlet end of the SMV, during a normal cardiac cycle were compared with those during an assisted cardiac cycle. The forward blood flow was 29%, 40%, and 63% greater during the assisted cardiac cycle than during the unassisted normal cardiac cycle at 25 Hz, 43 Hz, and 85 Hz stimulation, respectively.

Anderson subsequently constructed SMVs in 15 dogs (Fig. 3A–C) [62]. After a 4-week vascular delay period, the SMVs were connected to the descending

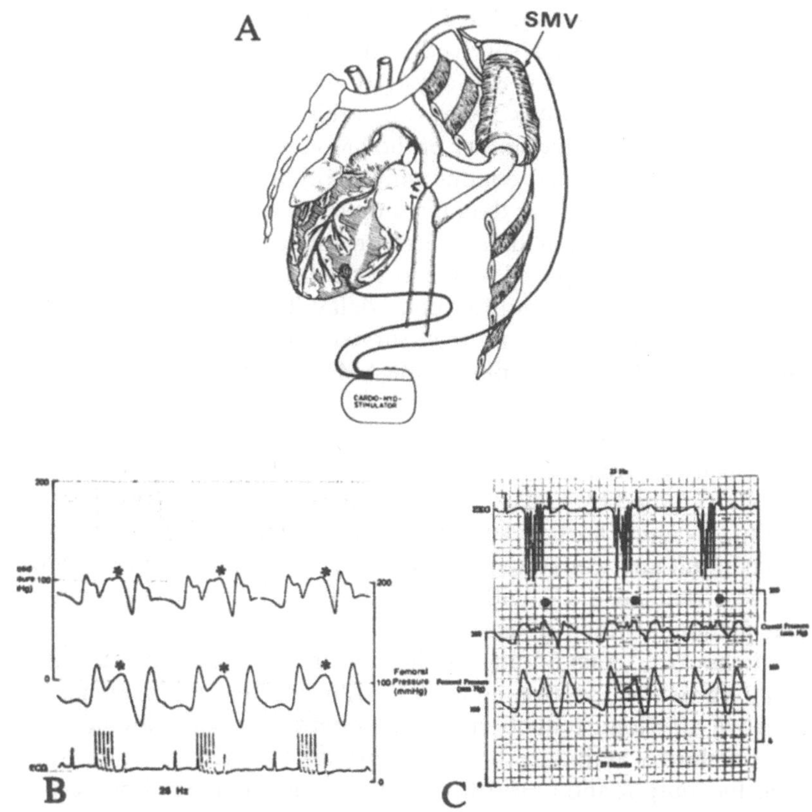


**Fig. 3. A** Skeletal muscle ventricle (*SMV*) is connected in circulation for left heart assist via a bifurcated polytetrafluorethylene graft. The descending thoracic aorta is tied off between the anastomosis of the two grafts, completely diverting the blood flow through the SMV. **B** Pressure tracings from the dog at 1 year. **C** Pressure tracings from the dog at 27 months. *Black circles* mark peak diastolic pressure augmented by SMV

thoracic aorta using bifurcated PTFE grafts. With the aorta ligated between the two limbs of the grafts, obligatory blood flow through the SMV was obtained. Six of these SMVs had a lining induced by the fibrous reaction from the mandrel that had been in the SMV prior to connection to the circulation. Nine were lined with autogenous pleura or pericardium in an effort to reduce thromboembolic complications. Twelve of the 15 SMVs eventually showed some thrombus in the ventricular cavity, but no evidence of thromboembolic complication was detected in any of the animals. These SMVs were used as diastolic counterpulsators; substantial augmentation of diastolic blood pressure was documented. Femoral arterial diastolic pressure increased by 35% during the SMV contraction at operation, and maintained this value at 40 weeks when SMVs contracted at a 1:2 ratio with the heart at 33 Hz stimulation frequency. In the aorta, distal to the SMV, blood flow increased during the operation by 34% at 25 Hz burst, 48% at 43 Hz, and 53% at 85 Hz. However, when the reflux of blood back into the SMV was taken into account, the net increase declined to 3.5%. Ten animals survived between 1 week and 9 months. One animal survived and remained healthy with good diastolic pressure augmentation for 836 days [26, 63, 64]. Hemodynamic measurements obtained at the 27 months' follow-up in this dog are shown in Fig. 3C.

Pochettino et al. changed the geometry of the SMVs and used a longer vascular delay without muscle electrical conditioning [65]. Dogs were studied in an aorta-SMV-aorta configuration. The data from up to 28 weeks in the circulation demonstrated that a long vascular delay period resulted in an improvement of initial SMV function when compared with shorter delays, but no difference was detected between 10 weeks' delay and 18 weeks' delay. Thromboembolic complications were not detected in animals that survived 1 or more weeks. Also, thrombus was not noted by echography in the SMVs of those dogs while they were alive or at autopsy.

For prevention of reflux fo blood from the distal aorta back into the SMV during SMV relaxation, skeletal muscle ventricles with efferent valved homografts have been studied by Fietsam et al. in an extrathoracic, aorta-to-aorta configuration [66]. A canine aortic root homograft with aortic valve served as an efferent valved conduit and was connected between descending aorta and SMV. This study showed that an SMV with a valved efferent limb using an aortic homograft can maintain effective diastolic pressure augmentation for greater than 4 months. Echocardiogram findings of the dogs in this study showed that the aortic homograft valve was functioning at POD 126, and that the presence of a valve may improve afterload reduction. In the longest-surviving animal, acute reversible heart failure was induced with propranolol at 126 days. A 61.3% reduction in cardiac output and a 37.6% reduction in mean arterial blood pressure were induced by beta-blockade. During profound low cardiac output, SMV stimulation with 33 Hz improved cardiac output by 16.9%, improved the tension tiem index by 14.9%, and improved the endocardial viability ratio by 34.1%. Utilizing the same valve configuration, Nakajima et al. [80] connected intrathoracic SMVs to the circulation, and the longest survival is 369 days at this writing.

## Left Atrial–SMV–Aorta Configuration

In early mock circulation studies, the SMV was able to generate a pressure of 105 mmHg at a preload of 10 mmHg and against an afterload of 80 mmHg. These results encouraged us to connect SMVs to the systemic circulation or pulmonary circulation at atrial preloads. Dogs were used to study a left atrial-SMV-aorta configuration by Hooper et al. (Fig. 4A,B) [67]. Skeletal muscle ventricles were constructed from the latissimus dorsi muscle and placed in the left hemithorax. After a 3-week vascular delay period, SMVs were electrically preconditioned with 2-Hz stimulation for 6 weeks. At a second operation, SMVs were connected between the left atrium and thoracic aorta by afferent and efferent aortic root homografts, and stimulated to contract in a 1:2 diastolic counterpulsation mode. At a mean left atrial pressure of 12.4 mmHg and a burst stimulation frequency of 33 Hz, SMV stroke volume was initially 43% of that of the native left ventricle,

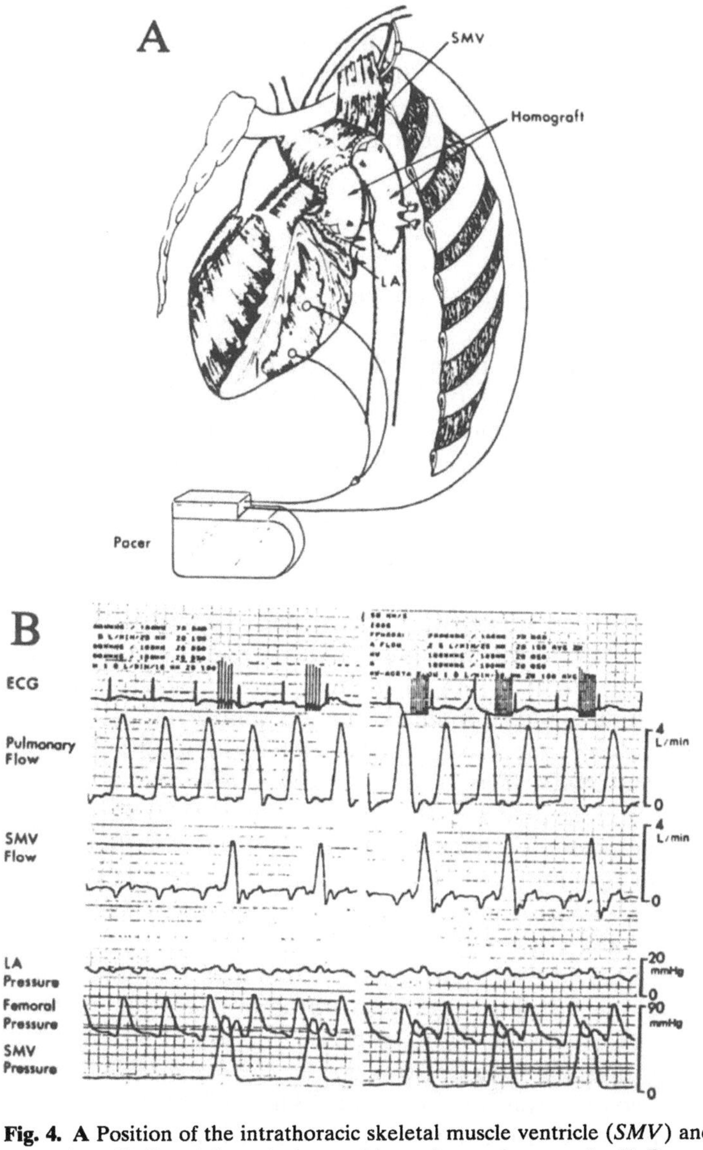


**Fig. 4.** **A** Position of the intrathoracic skeletal muscle ventricle (*SMV*) and connection to left atrial appendage (*LA*) and thoracic aorta with aortic root homografts. **B** Recordings from one animal at 33 Hz (*left*) and 50 Hz (*right*). Mean skeletal muscle ventricle (*SMV*) flow was 253 ml/min and 391 ml/min at the respective burst frequencies

achieving a flow equivalent to 21% of cardiac output. At 50-Hz stimulation, the SMV fraction rose to 27% of the cardiac output. Skeletal muscle ventricle power output at 33 Hz was 0.016 W, increasing to 0.024 W at 50 Hz, corresponding to 14% and 22%, respectively, of left ventricular power output. After 4 h of continuous pumping, the SMVs were still generating flows of more than 70% of starting values and more than 60% of initial power output. This study demonstrated that

SMVs can function in the systemic circulation at physiologic left atrial preloads. However, the maximum peak developed SMV pressure was 70.6 ± 2.3 mmHg during this actue experiment. Therefore, the diastolic augmentation was no better than the aorta-SMV-aorta configuration. The lower augmentation seen in the LA-SMV-Aorta configuration may be related to the lower filling pressures in this model [23, 38].

## LV Apex–SMV–Aorta Configuration

The SMV configuration from left ventricle apex to thoracic aorta for left-heart assist was recently described by Huiping Lu [68] (Fig. 5A–C). Skeletal muscle ventricles were constructed from left latissimus dorsi muscle in 12 dogs; in group I ($n = 6$), SMVs were placed in the apex of the left hemithorax, in group II ($n = 6$), SMVs were positioned extrathoracically on the chest wall in subcutaneous tissue. After a 3-week vascular delay period, SMVs were electrically preconditioned with 2 Hz continuous stimulation for 6 weeks. At a second operation, the heart was exposed through a median sternotomy in group I (for 3-h acute studies) and a left thoracotomy in group II (the longer-term studies). The plastic mandrel was removed from the SMV. After incising the pericardium, two myocardial leads were placed on the right and left ventricle for sensing. Two valved conduits were used to connect the SMV to the circulation. The conduits consisted of a woven Dacron tube with a 12- to 14-mm diameter porcine valve (Hancock, Medtronic Inc.). The afferent conduit connected the left ventricular apex to the SMV, and the efferent conduit connected the SMV to the thoracic aorta, without cardiopulmonary bypass. A circular piece of Gore-Tex (W.L.Gore & Associates, Inc., Flagstaff, Arizona) was used to cap the base of the SMV. Two circular openings of 12- to 14-mm diameter each were made for inflow and outflow. Each conduit was sutured to an opening in the Gore-Tex base cap. The valves were placed 1.5 cm from the SMV base. A left ventrcular apex connector was used to couple the LV apex to the afferent conduit.

The functions of intrathoracid SMV (group I, $n = 6$) and extrathoracic SMV (group II, $n = 6$) were evaluated during surgery. The peak pressure generated by the intrathoracic versus extrathoracic SMVs was 91 ± 10 vs. 93 ± 10 mmHg, respectively, and the end-diastolic pressure was 8 ± 3 vs. 9 ± 5 mmHg, respectively. The SMV stroke volume was 13.2 ± 5.4 vs. 13.6 ± 4.3 ml, respectively. When the SMVs were stimulated at 1:2 ratio with the heart, 47% of the systemic blood flow was pumped by the SMV in group I (0.73 ± 0.23 vs. 1.54 ± 0.42 l/min, $p < 0.05$; SMV output vs. total systemic blood flow) and 51% in group II (0.78 ± 0.19 vs. 1.53 ± 0.42 l/min, $p < 0.05$) (see Table 1).

Systemic hemodynamic data of both groups were compared between control and stimulation (1:2, SMV to heart). In both groups, significant changes occurred in diastolic blood pressure (52 ± 9 vs. 82 ± 11 mmHg, $p < 0.05$, in group I; 50 ± 6 vs. 79 ± 7 mmHg, $p = 0.05$, in group II), in left ventricle systolic tension-time index (16.9 ± 2.7 vs. 12.5 ± 3.3 mmHg/s, $p < 0.05$, in group I; 14.0 ± 0.8 vs. 9.9 ± 1.1 mmHg/s, $p < 0.05$, in group II), and in left ventricle +dp/dt (1140 ± 152 vs. 864 ± 131 mmHg/s, $p < 0.05$, in group I; 1002 ± 155 vs. 668 ± 147 mmHg/s, $p < 0.05$, in

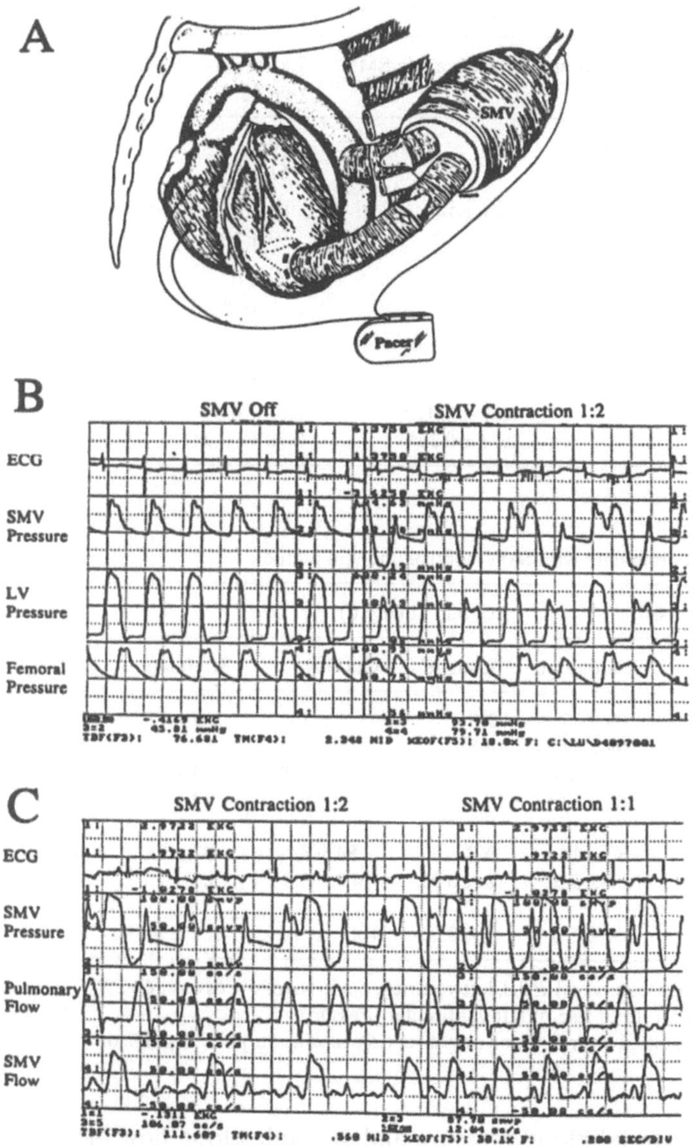


**Fig. 5.** **A** Skeletal muscle ventricle (*SMV*) in the circulation for cardiac assistance: LV apex-to-aorta configuration (extrathoracic SMV position) with two valved conduits. The afferent conduit connects the LV apex to the SMV, and the efferent conduit connects the SMV to the descending thoracic aorta. **B** Pressure traces obtained from an extrathoracic SMV at the time of surgery with SMV contraction Off (*left*) and contraction On (*right*) at 1:2 ratio with the heart (*right*). Channels: *1*, ECG; *2*, SMV pressure; *3*, left ventricular pressure; *4*, femoral arterial pressure. During SMV assist of the heart, mean arterial pressure increased (channel 4) and left ventricle tension-time decreased (channel 3). **C** Flow traces (channels 3,4) obtained from the same SMV at the same time as in Fig. 4A. SMV contraction at 1:2 (*left*) and 1:1 (*right*) ratio with the heart. The SMV performed native heart function at both ratios. Channels: *1*, ECG; *2*, SMV pressure; *3* pulmonary arterial pressure; *4*, SMV blood flow output

**Table 1.** Function of intrathoracic and extrathoracic SMVs in the systemic circulation

| Variable | SMV contraction Off or on | Intrathoracic SMV ($n = 6$) | Extrathoracic SMV ($n = 6$) | $p$ value* |
|---|---|---|---|---|
| SMV contraction | Off | 0 | 0 | |
| (beats/min) | On | 55 ± 7 | 61 ± 7 | NS |
| Intra-SMV peak | Off | 87 ± 14 | 84 ± 8 | NS |
| pressure (mmHg) | On | 91 ± 10 | 93 ± 10 | NS |
| Intra-SMV diastolic | Off | 52 ± 9 | 50 ± 6 | NS |
| pressure (mmHg) | On | 8 ± 3* | 9 ± 5* | NS |
| SMV stroke volume | Off | 0 | 0 | |
| (ml) | On | 13.2 ± 5.4 | 13.6 ± 4.3 | NS |
| SMV flow | Off | 0.09 ± 0.03 | 0.01 ± 0.06 | NS |
| (l/min) | On | 0.73 ± 0.23* | 0.78 ± 0.19* | NS |

* Significance was accepted at $p < 0.05$.

**Table 2.** Systemic hemodynamic data with SMV control and stimulated

| Parameter | Group I ($n = 6$) | | | Group II ($n = 6$) | | |
|---|---|---|---|---|---|---|
| | Control | Stimulation | Change | Control | Stimulation | Change |
| HR | 110 ± 13 | 109 ± 12 | NS | 116 ± 13 | 115 ± 11 | NS |
| MABP | 69 ± 9 | 69 ± 11 | NS | 61 ± 5 | 62 ± 7 | NS |
| CO (l/min) | 1.43 ± 0.46 | 15.4 ± 0.42 | NS | 1.46 ± 0.37 | 1.53 ± 0.42 | NS |
| BPdia (mmHg) | 52 ± 9 | 82 ± 11* | $p < 0.05$ | 50 ± 6 | 79 ± 7* | $p < 0.05$ |
| LVPBP | 87 ± 14 | 80 ± 13 | NS | 84 ± 8 | 72 ± 7* | $p < 0.05$ |
| LVsTTI (mmHg/s) | 16.9 ± 2.7 | 12.5 ± 3.3* | $p < 0.05$ | 14.0 ± 0.8 | 9.9 ± 1.1* | $p < 0.05$ |
| LVdp/dt | 1140 ± 152 | 864 ± 131* | $p < 0.05$ | 1002 ± 155 | 668 ± 147* | $p < 0.05$ |

*BPdia*, mean diastolic artery pressure; *LVPBP*, left ventricle peak systolic pressure; *LVsTTI*, systolic tension time index; *LVdp/dt*, rate of rise of left ventricular pressure
*HR*, Heart rate/min; *MABP*, mean arterial blood pressure; *CO*, cardiac output; * Significance: $p < 0.05$ by unpaired $t$-test.

group II). The mean arterial blood pressure and systemic blood flow increased slightly with SMV on, but these changes were not statistically significant (see Table 2).

In group I, SMV function and systemic hemodynamic changes were measured over 3 h (see Table 3). The SMVs peak pressure, stroke volume, and output maintained 97%, 80%, and 82% of their initial values, respectively, after 3 h. SMV contraction resulted in a 58% increase in the mean diastolic pressure initially (52 ± 9 to 82 ± 11 mmHg; $p < 0.05$) and in a 73% increase (45 ± 7 to 78 ± 8 mmHg; $p < 0.05$) after 3 h of continuous pumping. This was associated with a 26% decrease in the systolic tension-time index initially (16.9 ± 2.7 versus 12.5 ± 3.3 mmHg/s; $p < 0.05$) and with a 25% decrease (14.5 ± 2.3 versus 10.9 ±

**Table 3.** Hemodynamic parameters during 3-h study with stimulation OFF and ON

| Stimulation | Start | | 1-h | | 2-h | | 3-h | |
|---|---|---|---|---|---|---|---|---|
| | Off | On | Off | On | Off | On | Off | On |
| HR (l/min) | 109 ± 13 | 109 ± 13 | 111 ± 12 | 111 ± 12 | 110 ± 11 | 110 ± 11 | 109 ± 11 | 109 ± 11 |
| SV (ml) | 13.1 ± 4.8 | 14.3 ± 4.6 | 13.6 ± 1.8 | 14.5 ± 2.6 | 13.5 ± 4.6 | 14.3 ± 4.8 | 13.5 ± 5.5 | 15.7 ± 6.2 |
| $BP_{sys}$ (mmHg) | 92 ± 11 | 82 ± 10* | 89 ± 8 | 81 ± 9* | 91 ± 5 | 83 ± 6* | 89 ± 6 | 80 ± 7* |
| $\overline{BP}_{dia}$ (mmHg) | 52 ± 9 | 82 ± 11* | 50 ± 8 | 81 ± 9* | 44 ± 7 | 73 ± 11* | 45 ± 7 | 78 ± 8* |
| MAP (mmHg) | 66 ± 9 | 69 ± 11* | 64 ± 7 | 67 ± 9 | 59 ± 6 | 64 ± 10* | 60 ± 7 | 64 ± 8* |
| LVp | 87 ± 14 | 80 ± 13* | 85 ± 10 | 78 ± 11* | 82 ± 8 | 76 ± 7* | 84 ± 9 | 75 ± 6* |
| LVedp (mmHg) | 5.3 ± 1.8 | 5.1 ± 1.5 | 0.2 ± 2.5 | 4.6 ± 1.9 | 4.8 ± 2.6 | 4.4 ± 2.3 | 5.3 ± 2.1 | 5.6 ± 1.3 |
| CO (l/min) | 1.43 ± 0.46 | 1.54 ± 0.42* | 1.49 ± 0.19 | 1.63 ± 0.26* | 1.49 ± 0.48 | 1.54 ± 0.52 | 1.45 ± 0.56 | 1.52 ± 0.62 |
| TTI (mmHg/s) | 16.9 ± 2.7 | 12.5 ± 3.3* | 16.7 ± 1.8 | 13.2 ± 2.1* | 15.1 ± 1.3 | 12.3 ± 1.1* | 14.5 ± 2.3 | 10.9 ± 2.0* |
| EVR | 1.12 ± 0.08 | 1.88 ± 0.15* | 1.06 ± 0.05 | 1.76 ± 0.17* | 0.92 ± 0.18 | 1.49 ± 0.32* | 1.06 ± 0.16 | 1.73 ± 0.22* |

*HR*, Heart rate; *SV*, stroke volume; $BP_{sys}$, systolic carotid artery blood pressure; $\overline{BP}_{dia}$, mean diastolic carotid artery pressure; *MAP*, mean carotid artery pressure; *LVp*, left ventricle peak pressure; *LVedp*, left ventricle end-diastolic pressure; *CO*, cardiac output; *TTI*, systolic tension time index; *EVR*, endocardial viability ratio

* $p < 0.05$ (paired *t*-test).

2.0 mmHg/s; $p < 0.05$) at 3 h. In these studies, left ventricular endocardial viability ratio (EVR) was significantly increased during SMV contraction and indicated that SMV contraction improved subendocardial blood flow. Measurements in one animal were made for over 10 h. The SMV stroke volume and stroke work were comparable to those of the native canine heart (12.4 ± 0.9 ml vs. 12.3 ± 1.6 ml ($p$ = NS) and 0.81 ± 0.04 × $10^6$ ergs vs. 0.8 ± 0.03 × $10^6$ ergs ($p$ = NS), respectively). In the longer-term study (group II), the dogs tolerated LV-SMV-aorta counterpulsation well and were able to move about freely. Dog 5 had an SMV stroke volume 94% of the native heart initially (13.5 ± 1.2 versus 14.3 ± 1.1 ml), and 71% of this value was maintained on postoperative day 3. The diastolic arterial pressure augmentation, with SMV stimulation, was 27 mmHg during surgery (40 ± 2 versus 67 ± 2 mmHg; $p < 0.05$) and 35 mmHg on postoperative day 3 (60 ± 2 versus 95 ± 2 mmHg; $p < 0.05$). In group II, mean length of survival was 7.5 days. The primary complications were valve dysfunction and thrombus within the conduits and SMVs.

The results from this configuration demonstrate that in an LV apex-to-aorta configuration SMV stroke volume and stroke work were equal to or better than those of the native heart; the SMV pumped 47–51% of systemic flow after connection to the circulation at 1:2 ratio contracting with the heart. Intrathoracic and extrathoracic SMVs functioned equally well.

Using an SMV to pump blood between the left ventricle and the aorta, such as was done in this experiment, might overcome some of the potential problems encountered with other SMV configurations. Since the SMV with the LV-to-aorta configuration predominantly fills during left ventricular systole, the potential problem of inadequate filling pressures with the left atrium to aorta configuration is overcome. Additionally, since during a portion of the SMV pumping cycle the pressure in the SMV cavity is equal to the left ventricular end-diastolic pressure, there is likely to be improved blood flow in the muscle layers of the SMV when compared with the aortic diastolic counterpulsator configuration [69, 70]. Other potential problems of continuous high pressure in the aorta-to-aorta configuration might also be avoided.

Earlier, both Brister and Stevens used unconditioned rectus muscle to pump blood from the left ventricle to the aorta [71–73]. Muscle was wrapped around a bladder with a single valve. Brister's model used a valve in the afferent conduit and Stevens' model used a valve in the efferent limb of the conduit. Brister apparently did not measure flow but did observe augmentation of diastolic aortic pressures. In Stevens' model, during propranolol-induced acute heart failure the cardiac output was initially increased 31% over control during SMV contraction, but only 8% over control at 1 h. In our current experiment, cardiac output increased only slightly with the SMV functioning. This may have been because our animals had normal hearts, whereas Stevens' animals were in heart failure. Although the cardiac output in the current experiment improved only slightly with the SMV pumping, 47% of the systemic blood flow was pumped by the SMV rather than the left ventricle. Even though the percent of blood pumped by the SMV compared with the left ventricle did decrease slightly over the 3-h study (47% initially to 40% at 3 h) the deterioration in function was not nearly as rapid as occurred in Stevens' study. This is most likely because Stevens' used unconditioned muscle, whereas the muscle in our study had been electrically conditioned to make it fatigue resistant. Electrical conditioning of a muscle also causes the muscle to lose some strength. This could explain why the initial increase in cardiac output seen in Stevens' study was greater than that seen in our current study. The fact that Stevens used a different muscle, i.e., rectus vs. latissimus, may also account for this difference.

Platt et al. used computer modeling to study left ventricular assist devices in the systemic circulation [74]. Their data indicated that synchronous diastolic counterpulsation in an LV apex-to-aorta configuration provided maximal assistance; ventricular uptake of blood provided increased oxygen availability by 78% and decreased oxygen consumption by 27% when compared with an atrial-aortic model. Additionally, synchronous pulsatile flow was superior to nonpulsatile and asynchronous flow methods. Voytik used electronics to compare an LV apex-to-aorta configuration with atrial-aortic and aorto-aorto designs [75]. Greater increases in cardiac output and SMV power and a greater reduction in LV power were obtained with the LV-aorta design than with any other model configuration.

## Complications: SMV Thrombus and Rupture

Since the first attempts at using skeletal muscle to augment cardiac performance, many obstacles have been overcome. The first problem, muscle fatigue, has for the most part been solved by the process of electrical conditioning, as well as by the practice of allowing for a vascular delay period.

Skeletal muscle ventricle thrombus formation and rupture presently are problems in some SMV configurations [68], but not in others [65]. However, the incidences of both SMV thrombus and rupture have dropped considerably in current studies, and it has been uncommon for any thrombus that forms in the SMVs to embolize.

According to Acker and co-workers' first report of SMVs functioning chronically in circulation, two of six dogs died of renal failure from thromboembolism [40]. The inner surface of those SMVs was lined by polytetrafluoroethylene (PTFE). In an attempt to decrease the incidence of thromboembolism, Anderson lined the surface of SMVs with either pleura or pericardium. In nine dogs, three of the SMVs lined wiht pleura were found to be thrombus free postoperatively at 2, 12, and 40 weeks, respectively.

While the efforts to decrease thrombosis were directed towards blood-surface interactions, the rate and characteristics of blood flow into and out of the SMVs also may contribute to thrombus formation. Pochettino significantly decreased the rate of thrombosis by modifying the design of the mandrel, using an ovoid shape to improve the blood flow characteristics inside the SMVs. These SMVs were not lined with separate tissue, but only by the reactive fibrous tissue formed around the mandrel, similar to the unlined group in Anderson's study [65]. Although the incidence of thrombosis is still high, this represents the lowest rate that we have been able to achieve to date.

A dose of 1–1.5 ml heparin sodium was usually administered intravenously during the second operation (phase II). After connection of the SMVs to the circulation, the dogs were given aspirin 75 mg/day as an antithrombotic agent.

Recent efforts have been directed again towards the inner surface of the SMV as a blood-contacting surface. The presence of an endothelial lining has been shown to improve the thromboresistance of vascular grafts. Over the past 15 years, much work has been done on the endothelialization of vascular grafts [76, 77]. We have investigated seeding endothelial cells into SMVs. In preliminary experiments, we have been able to document the presence of an endothelial monolayer on the luminal surface of SMVs after seeding with endothelial cells. However, it remains to be seen whether this type of lining will decrease the current incidence of thrombosis and thromboembolism associated with SMVs in the circulation. Other investigators are attemping to seed the inner surfaces of cardiac assist devices and artificial hearts with endothelial cells [78, 79].

After connection of SMVs to the circulation, rupture of skeletal muscle ventricle has occurred more frequently in the aorta-to-aorta configuration. Rupture of the SMV is probably related to the high SMV preloads in this configuration. In the earlier studies on SMVs with an aorta-to-aorta configuration, the incidence of rupture was 34% within 39 days postoperatively [80]. However, we have had several long-term animals with SMVs in the circulation, and one animal with an aorta-aorta SMV pumped blood effectively as an aortic diastolic counterpulsator during the entire 2-year period.

Most ruptures of the SMVs were located at the sutrue line between the SMV and the vascular graft. One of the reasons may have been the unsuitable anatomosis between the vascular grafts and the base of the SMV. After direct suturing of two vascular grafts to the base of the SMV, the round shape of the SMV base became a figure-eight shape. The two corners of the figure-eight shaped SMV base may lead to rupture over time, and the SMV inlet and outlet obstruction could have occurred.

In current studies, a circular piece of Gore-Tex cardiovascular material has been used to cap the base of the SMV. First, two circular openings which match the two vascular grafts are made for the SMV inflow and outflow. Then, each vascular graft is sutured to an opening in the Gore-Tex base cap before surgery [68]. During the phase-II operation, the Gore-Tex base cap is connected to the base of the SMV with continuous suture. With this method, the round-shaped base of the SMV is maintained, and SMV inflow and outflow obstruction are avoided. Recently, using this technique in the aorta-to-aorta configuration, there were no ruptures within 9 months. We believe that the problems of SMV thrombsis and rupture will both be overcome in the near future.

## References


1. de Jesus FR (1931) Breve consideraciones sobre un case de herida penetrante del corazon. Bol Assoc Med P R 23:380–382
2. Leriche R (1933) Essai experimental de traitement de certains infarctus du myocarde et de l'aneurisme de coeur par une graffe muscle strie. Bull Soc Nat Chir 9:229–232

3. Beck CS (1935) A new blood supply to the heart by operation. Surg Gynecol Obstet 61:407–410
4. Beck CS (1937) Coronary sclerosis and angina pectoris: treatment by grafting a new blood supply upon the myocardium. Surg Gynecol Obstet 64:270–272
5. Beck CS (1936) Further data on the establishment of a new blood supply to the heart by operation. J Thorac Surg 5:604–611
6. Petrovsky BV (1961) The use of the diaphragm graft for plastic operations in thoracic surgery. J Thorac Cardiovasc Surg 41:348–355
7. Petrovsky BV (1959) The use of diaphragmatic flaps for plastic purpose in thoracic surgery. Chest Surgery (Moscow) 51:73–80
8. Kantrowitz A, McKinnon W (1959) The experimental use of the diaphragm as an auxillary myocardium. Surg Forum 9:266–268
9. Kantrowitz A (1960) Functioning autogenous muscle used experimentally as an auxillary ventricle. Trans Am Soc Artif Intern Organs 68:305–307
10. Kusaba E, Schraut W, Sawatani S (1973) A diaphragmatic graft for augmenting left ventricular function: a feasibility study. Trans Am Soc Artif Intern Organs 19:251–257
11. Nakamura K, Glenn WWL (1964) Graft of the diaphragm as a functioning substitute for the myocardium. J Surg Res 4:435–439
12. Termet H, Chalencon JL, Estour E et al. (1966) Transplantation sur le myocarde d'un muscle strie excit' pace maker. Ann Chir Thorac Cardiovasc 5:568
13. Scheperd MP (1969) Diaphragmatic muscle and cardiac surgery. Ann R Coll Surg Engl 45:212–231
14. Drinkwater DC, Chiu RC-J, Modry D et al. (1980) Cardiac assist and myocardial repair with synchronously stimulated skeletal muscle. Surg Forum 31:271–273
15. Macoviak JA, Stephenson LW, Spielman S et al. (1980) Electrophysiologic and mechanical characteristics of diaphragmatic autograft used to enlarge right ventricle. Surg Forum 31:270–271
16. Macoviak JA, Stephenson LW, Spielman S et al. (1981) Replacement of ventricular myocardium with diaphragmatic skeletal muscle. J Thorac Cardiovasc Surg 81:519–527
17. Macoviak JA, Stephenson LW, Alavi A, Kelly AM, Edmunds LH Jr (1981) Effect of electrical stimulation on diaphragmatic muscle used to enlarge right ventricle. Surgery 90:271–277
18. Macoviak JA, Stephenson LW, Kelly AM, Likoff MJ, Riechek N, Edmunds LH Jr (1981) Partial replacement of the right ventricle with a synchronously contracting diaphragmatic skeletal muscle autograft. Proceedings of the 3rd Meeting of the International Society for Artif Organs, 1981, vol 5, suppl, pp 550–555
19. Schaff HV, Arnold PG, Reeder GS (1982) Late mediastinal infection and pseudoaneurysm following left ventricular aneurysmectomy repair utilizing pectoralis major muscle flap. J Thorac Cardiovasc Surg 84:912–916
20. Carpentier A, Chachques JC (1985) Myocardial substitution with a stimulated skeletal muscle: first successful clinical case. Lancet i:1267
21. Magovern GJ, Park SB, Magovern GJ Jr et al. (1986) Latissimus dorsi as a functioning synchronously paced muscle component in the repair of a left ventricular aneurysm. Ann Thorac Surg 41:116
22. von Recum A, Stule JP, Hamada O et al. (1977) Long-term stimulation of diaphragm muscle pouch. J Surg Res 23:422–427
23. Spotnitz HM, Merker C, Malm JR (1974) Applied physiology of the canine rectus abdominis: force-length curves correlated with functional characteristics of a rectus-powered "ventricle": potential for cardiac assistance. Trans Am Soc Artif Intern Organs 20:747–756
24. Frank O (1895) Zur Dynamik des Herzmuskels. Z Biol 32:370–447
25. Juffe A, Ricoy JR et al. (1978) Cardialization: a new source of energy for circulatory assistance. Vasc Surg 12:10–17
26. Mocek FW, Anderson DR, Pochettino A et al. (1992) Skeletal muscle ventricles in circulation long-term: one hundred ninety-one to eight hundred thirty-six days. J Heart Lung Transplant 11:S334–S340
27. Adams FR, Schwartz A (1980) Comparative mechanisms for contraction of cardiac and skeletal muscle. Chest 78:123–139

28. Pette D, Muller W, Leisner E, Vrbova G (1976) Time-dependent effects on contractile properties, fibre population, myosin light chain and enzymes of energy metabolism in intermittently and continuously stimulated fast-twitch muscle of the rabbit. Pflugers Arch 364:103
29. Pette D, Vrbova G (1992) Adaptation of mammalian skeletal muscle fibers to chronic electrical stimulation. Rev Physiol Biochem Pharmacol 120:115–202
30. Mommaerts WFHM (1982) Heart muscle. In: Fishman AP, Richards DW (eds) Circulation of the blood, man and ideas. American Physiological Society, Bethesda, pp 127–198
31. Buller JC, Eccles JC, Eccles RM (1960) Differentiation of fast and slow muscles in the cat hind limb. J Physiol 150:399–416
32. Mannion JD, Velchik M, Acker MA, Hammond RL, Alavi A, Stephenson LW (1986) Transmural blood flow to multi-layered latissimus dorsi skeletal muscle ventricles during circulatory assistance. Trans Am Soc Artif Intern Organs 32:454–460
33. Salmons S, Vrbova G (1969) The influence of activity on some contractile characteristics of mammalian fast and slow muscles. J Physiol 210:535–549
34. Salmons S, Henriksson J (1981) The adaptive response of skeletal muscle to increased use. Muscle Nerve 4:94–105
35. Pette D (1984) Activity-induced fast to slow transitions in mammalian muscle. Med Sci Sports Exerc 16:517–528
36. Chi MMY, Hintz CS, Henriksson J et al. (1986) Chronic stimulation of mammalian muscle: enzyme changes in individual fibers. J Physiol 251:C633–C642
37. Mannion J, Hammond RL, Stephenson LW (1986) Hydraulic pouches of canine latissimus dorsi: potential for left ventricular assistance. J Thorac Cardiovasc Surg 91:534–544
38. Acker MA, Hammond RL, Mannion JD, Salmons S, Stephenson LW (1986) An autologous biologic pump motor. J Thorac Cardiovasc Surg 94:733–746
39. Mannion JD, Acker MA, Hammond RL, Faltemeyer W, Duckett S, Stephenson LW (1987) Power output of skeletal muscle ventricles in circulation: short-term studies. Circulation 76:155–162
40. Acker MA, Anderson WA, Hammond RL et al. (1987) Skeletal muscle ventricles in circulation: one to eleven weeks' experience. J Thorac Cardiovasc Surg 94:163–174
41. Dewar ML, Drinkwater DC, Wittnich C, Chiu RC-J (1984) Synchronously stimulated skeletal muscle graft for myocardial repair. J Thorac Cardiovasc Surg 87:325–331
42. Acker MA, Hammond RL, Mannion JD, Salmons S, Stephenson LW (1987) Skeletal muscle as the potential power source for a cardiovascular pump: assessment in vivo. Science 236:324–327
43. Chiu RCJ, Garret LW, Dewar LD, De Simon JH, Khalafalla AS, Ianuzzo D (1987) Implantable extra-aortic baloon assist powered by transformed fatigue-resistant skeletal muscle. J Thorac Cardiovasc Surg 94:694–701
44. Salmons S, Stephenson LW (1989) Adaptive capacity of skeletal muscle and its therapeutic applications. In: Neuromuscular. Maple-Vail, New York
45. Salmons S, Sreter FA (1976) Significance of impulse activity in the transformation of skeletal muscle type. Nature 263:30–34
46. Salmons S, Jarvis JC (1990) Cardiomyoplasty: the basic issues. Cardiac Chronicle 4:1–6
47. Leberer E, Seedorf U, Pette D (1986) Neural control of gene expression in skeletal muscle. Calcium-sequestering proteins in developing and chronically stimulated rabbit skeletal muscles. Biochem J 239:295–300
48. Pette DL, Vrbova G (1985) Neural control of phenotype expression in mammalian muscle fibers. Muscle Nerve 8:676–689
49. Macoviak JA, Stephenson LW, Armenti F et al. (1982) Electrical conditioning of in situ skeletal muscle for replacement of myocardium. J Surg Res 32:429–439
50. Armenti FR, Bitto T, Macoviak JA et al. (1984) Transformation of canine diaphragm to fatigue-resistant muscle by phrenic nerve stimulation. Surg Forum 35:258–269
51. Bitto T, Mannion JD, Hammond RL et al. (1986) Pectoralis and rectus abdominus muscle for potential correction of congenital heart defect. Proceedings of the 2nd World Congress on Pediatric Cardiology, pp 609–612
52. Mannion JD, Bitto T, Hammond RL, Rubinstein N, Stephenson LW (1986) Histochemical and fatigue characteristics of conditioned latissimus dorsi muscle. Circ Res 58:298–304

53. Clark BJ, Acker MA, Subramanian H et al. (1988) In vivo $^{31}$P-NMR spectroscopy of chronically stimulated canine skeletal muscle. Am J Physiol 2545:C258–C266
54. Acker MA, Anderson WA, Hammond RL, Stephenson LW (1987) Oxygen consumption of faitigue-resistant muscle. J Thorac Cardiovasc Surg 94:702–709
55. Acker MA, Mannion JD, Brown WE et al. (1987) Canine diaphragm muscle after one year of continuous electrical stimulation: its potential as a myocardial substitute. J Appl Physiol 62:1264–1270
56. Mannion JD, Velchik M, Hammond RL et al. (1989) Effects of collateral blood vessel ligation and electrical conditioning on blood flow in dog latissimus dorsi muscle. J Surg Res 47:332–340
57. Stevens L, Brown J (1986) Can noncardiac muscle provide useful cardiac assistance? Am Surg 52:423–427
58. Bridges CR Jr, Brown WE, Hammond RL et al. (1989) Skeletal muscle ventricles: improved performance at physiologic preloads. Surgery 106:275–282
59. Bridges CR Jr, Woodford EJ, Mora G, Anderson DR, Stephenson LW, Norwood WI (1990) Use of skeletal muscle power to augment the pulmonary circulation. Surg Forum 41:267–271
60. Bridges CR Jr, Hammond RL, DiMeo F, Stephenson LW (1989) Functional right heart replacement with a skeletal muscle ventricle. Circulation 80[Suppl III]:183–191
61. Niinami H, Hooper TL, Hammond RL et al. (1992) Skeletal muscle ventricles in the pulmonary circulation: up to sixteen weeks' experience. Ann Thorac Surg 53:750–757
62. Anderson DR, Pochettino A, Hammond RL et al. (1991) Autogenously lined skeletal muscle ventricles in circulation: up to nine months' experience. J Thorac Cardiovasc Surg 101:661–670
63. Ruggiero R, Niinami H, Pochettino A et al. (1991) Skeletal muscle ventricles: update after 18 months in circulation. Artif Organs 15:350–354
64. Ruggiero R, Anderson DR, Niinami H et al. (1991) Skeletal muscle ventricles in circulation: 24-month update. BAM 1:129–137
65. Pochettino A, Lu H, Hammond RL et al. (1992) Skeletal muscle ventricles in circulation with improved thromboresistance: up to 28 weeks' experience. Ann Thorac Surg 53:1025–1032
66. Fietsam R Jr, Huiping Lu, Hammond BA, Gregory AT, Nakajima H, Stephenson LW (1993) Skeletal muscle ventricles with efferent valved homograft. J Card Surg 8:184–194
67. Hooper TL, Niinami H, Hammond RL et al. (1992) Skeletal muscle ventricles as left atrial-aortic pumps: short-term studies. Ann Thorac Surg 54:316–322
68. Lu H, Fietsam R Jr, Hammond RL et al. (1993) Skeletal muscle ventricles: left ventricular apex to aorta configuration. Ann Thorac Surg 55:78–85
69. Zweifach BW (1974) Quantitation studies of microcirculation structure and function. I. Analysis of pressure distribution in terminal vascular bed in cat mesentry. Circ Res 34:843–857
70. Renkin EM (1984) Control microcirculation and blood-tissue exchange. In: Handbook of physiology, sect 2: the cardiovascular system – microcirculation. American Physiological Society, Bethesda
71. Stevens L, Badylak SF, Janas W, Gray MH, Geddes LA, Voorhees WD III (1989) A skeletal muscle ventricle made from rectus abdominis muscle in the dog. J Surg Res 46:84–89
72. Neilson IR, Brister SJ, Khalafalla AS, Chiu RC-J (1985) Left ventricular assistance in dogs using a skeletal muscle-powered device for diastolic augmentation. J Heart Trans 4:343–347
73. Brister S, Fradet G, Dewar M, Wittnich C, Lough J, Chiu RC-J (1985) Transforming skeletal muscle for myocardial assist: a feasibility study. Can J Surg 28:341–344
74. Platt KL, Moore TW, Barnea O, Dubin SE, Jaron D (1993) Performance optimization of left ventricular assistance. A computer model study. ASAIO 39:29–38
75. Voytik SL, Babbs CF, Badylak SF (1990) Simple electrical model of the circulation of explore design parameters for a skeletal muscle ventricle. J Heart Trans 9:160–174
76. Herring MB, Baughman S, Glover JL (1985) Endothelium develops on seeded human arterial prosthesis: a brief clinical report. J Vasc Surg 2:727–730
77. Ortenwall P, Wadenvik H, Kutti J, Risberg B (1990) Endothelial cell seeding reduces thrombogenicity of Dacron grafts in humans. J Vasc Surg 11:403–410
78. Bernhard WF (1988) A fibrillar blood prosthetic interface for both temporary and permanent ventricular assist devices: experimental and clinical observations. Artif Organs 12:89–111

79. Lelkes PI, Samet MM (1991) Endothelialization of the luminal sac in artificial cardiac prosthesis: a challenge for both biologists and engineers. J Biomech Eng 113:132–142
80. Nakajima H, Nakajima HO, Gregory AT et al. (1993) Chronic morphologic changes of skeletal muscle ventricles in circulation. Ann Thorac Surg (in press)

# Chronic Heart Assist System*

D. Liotta and C.B. Alvarez and CONICET-PROCOAR Investigators

## Introduction

Chronic heart failure (CHF) is the end of most heart diseases: ischemic heart disease, valvular disease, congenital heart disease, hypertension, etc. It has been defined as the physiopathological state where an abnormality of the heart function is responsible for the fall of the cardiac output necessary to mantain the metabolic requirements. This definition is not entirely correct, as there are situations where one can see that there is no variation in the cardiac output. The correct definition should be: systolic or diastolic dysfunction, or both, accompanied by a reduced tolerance to exercise, a high incidence of ventricular arrythmias, and a shortened life expectancy [1].

CHF is produced by coronary disease in two thirds of cases. Causes, in order of importance, are: primary myocardiopathy; hypertension, which is declining as an etiologic factor; Chagas' disease; frequent endemic pathology in South America; and, finally, congenital heart disease [2].

The prevalence of CHF in the population of the USA is estimated at approximately 1% (almost 3 million people): this incidence increases with age. Observations in Framingham's study show an increase in the annual rate of 3% from 35 to 64 years of age and of up to 10% in individuals over 65 years old [3].

Undoubtedly, CHF is now the most common hospital discharge diagnosis in people over 65 years old. Around 400 000 patients develop CHF every year in the USA. While the incidence of other cardiac diseases is decreasing, that of CHF is increasing due first to an increase in the proportion of individuals of advanced age in the population, and second to the major survival of acute myocardial infarction patients followed by left ventricular enlargement.

In Framingham's study, mortality of CHF within the first 4 years after diagnosis was 51% in men and 34% in women. The same study showed that mortality attributed to moderate and severe CHF ranged from 30% to 50% in the first year.

The mortality among CHF patients is reported to range between 10 and 20% a year; i.e., 200 000–400 000 deaths a year are caused by CHF in the United States, and from 1 million to 2 million a year [4, 5] worldwide.

*This study was funded by the *Consejo Nacional de Ciencia y Tecnologia*, CONICET, Argentina.

There are also regions where other negative factors are added to these diseases. In South America, chagasic cardiomyopathy is frequently due to trypanosomiasis (Chagas disease); 16 to 18 million people worldwide are likely to be infected by *Trypanosoma cruzi*, and 30–40% of these persons will ultimately have some degree of cardiac involvement. It is important to point out that 40% of patients with chagasic cardiomyopathy die suddenly, and 90% of patients with this syndrome have severe episodes of multiform ventricular extrasystole [6].

The prognostic factors of CHF are, first and most important, left ventricular dysfunction, second, the conjunction of coronary disease. The incidence of arrythmias and the decreasing tolerance to exercise add to the high levels of plasmatic norepinephrine [7], and a low level of sodium in plasma [8] is an additional index that helps to determine the prognosis of patients with severe CHF.

Undoubtedly, a separate chapter must be reserved for patients with refractory CHF, in functional class IV or with oxygen consumption ($VO_2$) lower than 10 ml/kg/min, who may be included in the list for transplantation [9]. Unfortunately, due to the scarcity of donors the possibilities are greatly reduced.

Furthermore, although medical treatment with ACE inhibitors reduces the mortality, it does not help to achieve a good and long survival [10].

## Background from the Surgical Point of View

Treatment of end-stage CHF is still a major challenge for physicians. This is why scientists all over the world have been devoted for many years to the development of mechanical aid systems for the circulation of blood. Thus, in 1960 Kolff and co-workers [11], Liotta and co-workers [12], and other researchers developed a family of devices to manage acute heart failure (AHF).

On July 18, 1963, for the first time, Liotta et al. [13, 14] employed a left ventricular assist device (LVAD) for the treatment of a patient with acute heart dysfunction during the early postoperative period of aortic valve surgery.

On April 4, 1969, and for the first time in the history of medicine, Cooley, Liotta et al. [15] implanted a total artificial heart (TAH) in a patient, introducing the concept of staged heart transplantation. The technique was expanded worldwide and is used at a large number of clinical centers [16]; thus mechanical devices in aid of blood circulation and used as bridges to heart transplantation are at present general medical practice. Nevertheless, the main challenge of modern cardiology, the management of end-stage CHF, remains unsolved.

Several researchers have developed devices for long-term treatment of CHF. Thus:

- Pierce et al. [17] introduced a brushless DC motor-driven total artificial heart.
- Portner and his associates [18] developed an electrically powered spring-decoupled pulsed solenoid energy converter coupled to a dual pusher-plate, sac-type blood pump.

- A belt skin transformer provides transmission of primary power across the intact skin for a period of time [19].
- White [20] tested a thermal-powered system comprised by a Stirling engine/hydraulic converter attached to a ventricular assist device.
- Liotta et al. [21, 22] used a brushless DC motor-driven single pusher plate at the animal laboratory in the early days of artificial heart research.

The limitation to these devices is the need for an external power source through a percutaneous access port. Quality of life is severely restricted, and patients are subject to serious complications such as infections. Furthermore, the transmission of electrical power through intact skin requires constant recharging of internal batteries.

Investigations on remodeling the outstanding properties of skeletal muscle plasticity have led to cardiomyoplasty to treat CHF in man [23–28]. The pacing of skeletal muscle grafts with a train of pulses from a muscle stimulator may transform a high-powered but fatigable skeletal muscle into a somewhat lower powered but fatigue-resistant muscle which will match the work output of the cardiac muscle on a gram-per-gram basis.

The concept of using autologous skeletal muscle for cardiac assistance is not new. The first documented attempt was disclosed by Kantrowitz and McKinnon [29] in 1959. They wrapped the left hemidiaphragm of a dog to a segment of the descending thoracic aorta and stimulated the diaphragm contraction during diastole.

In addition to dynamic cardiomyoplasty, Stephenson et al. [30] reported on the use of muscle energy as an aid in blood pumping. Thus the latissimus dorsi (LD) muscle is detached from all of its insertion and is wrapped around a conical mandrel to create a ventricular shaped skeletal muscle pouch. In addition, Chiu et al. [31] have developed a skeletal muscle-powered implantable chamber counterpulsator.

Liotta et al. [32] have reported on the advantages of using the force and displacement of the natural linear contraction of LD muscle, thus avoiding a major anatomical disruption.

Spitzer [33] proposed the attachment of a 200-ml piston implanted in the thigh to the lower insertion of the rectus femoris muscle. The contraction creates physiological pressures capable of driving an artificial heart in the chest.

Ugolini [34] reported that a fluid energy collector should be capable of storing energy from the contraction of the psoas major muscle and of transferring it to an artificial heart pump by a hydraulic conduit.

Farrar and Hill [35] disclosed a muscle-powered two-stage mechanical convertor to a hydraulic energy convertor which could be applied to a circulatory blood pump [36].

At the animal laboratory (dogs and calves), Liotta et al. [37, 38] reported on physiological studies concerning the linear-pull force and displacement of the LD muscle.

Undoubtedly, an endogenous source of power employing skeletal muscle for cardiac assist devices should be of great advantage. Problems related to the use of energizing systems (electrical, pneumatic, hydraulic) outside the body are thus avoided [39].

## Material and Methods

Configuration and anatomic placement of the ProCor chronic heart system are illustrated in Figs. 1–3. The major implanted subsystems included are:

1. A biomechanical coupling. A special prosthesis has been developed to serve at the interface of the tendon muscles with the mechanical unit.
2. A muscle-force multiplier. It transmits the muscle power to the blood pump lever actuator system. It has two entries, one for the left LD and teres major

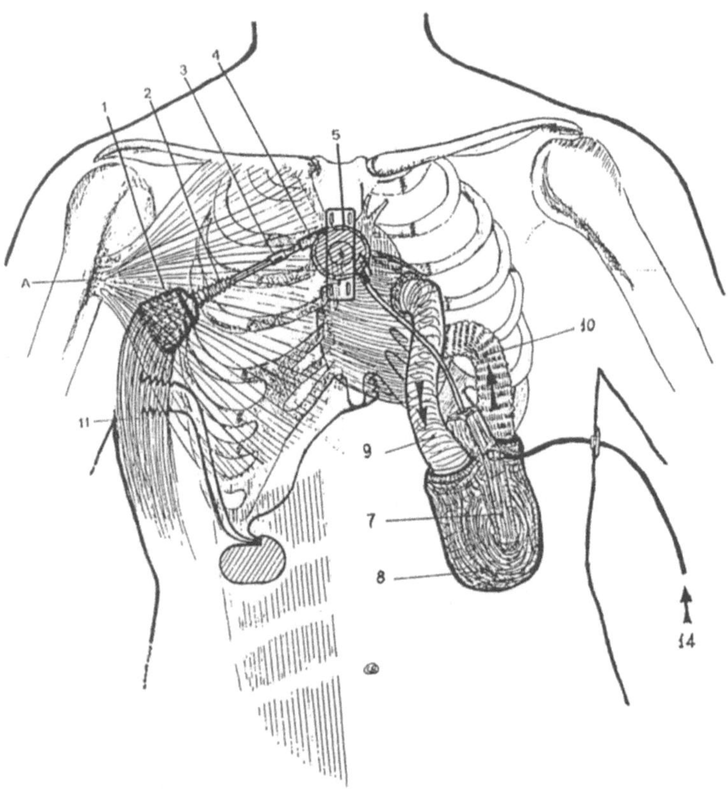


**Fig. 1.** Front view of ProCor chronic heart assist system. *1*, Right LD-TM muscles mechanical interface; *2*, sliding segment of tension guide; *3*, junction of tension guide with muscle-force multiplier; *4*, muscle elastic stop; *5*, retrosternal muscle-force multiplier; *6*, tension guide between muscle-force multiplier and actuator; *7*, blood pump actuator; *8*, dual pusher-plate blood pump; *9*, LA inflow pump connector; *10*, descending thoracic aorta outflow pump connector; *11*, LD-TM intramuscular leads; *12*, line of external pneumatic system; *14*, input line; *15*, insertion to $^7/_8$; *A*, LD-TM humeral insertion surgically removed; *5th*, fifth rib projection

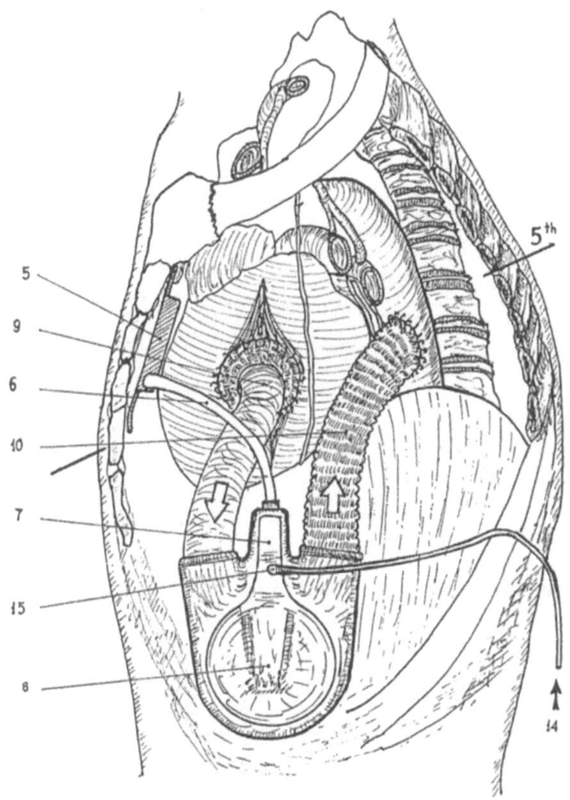


**Fig. 2.** Left chest: lateral view of ProCor Chronic Heart System (see Fig. 1 for the explanation of numbers). Description of blood pump connection LV apex and ascending aorta has been published elsewhere [39]

(TM) muscles and another for the right LD and TM muscles. The muscle-force multiplier has been set to work independently with one group, either right or left muscle. Furthermore, it can work with both groups of muscles, that is, i.e. right and left acting together.

3. A lever actuator system that drives a blood pump.
4. A dual pusher-plate blood pump.
5. A tension guide that transmits the force and displacement from the muscle to the blood pump lever actuator system directly. The muscle-force multiplier is interposed at a point in the guide's path.
6. A variable volume compensator.
7. A muscle stimulator (cardiomyostimulator, model MYOS, Biotronik).

In addition, an external hydraulic-pneumatic power source is connected to the energy convertor attached to the lever actuator system. The external hydraulic-pneumatic pump is joined with convertor through a percutaneous access port by means of a 3-mm ID polyamide tube.

The blood pump with the lever actuator system unit is implanted within the abdominal wall, in the left upper quadrant, anterior to the posterior rectus sheath and between the costal margin and iliac crest. Inflow and outflow conduits, of

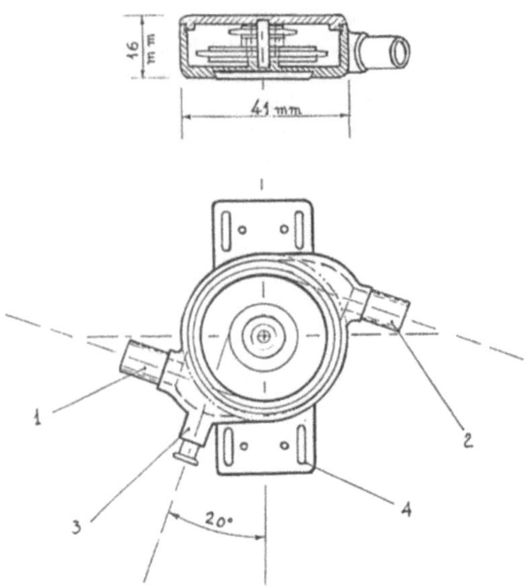


**Fig 3.** Two entries, LD-TM muscle-force multiplier. *1*, Input connector for left LD-TM muscles; *2*, input connector for right LD-TM muscles; *3*, output connector for blood pump actuator; *4*, titanium plate to be sutured to the sternum

either low-porosity Dacron or Goretex (Gore Laboratory) with external reinforcement, penetrate the diaphragm at the costal margin and connect the blood pump between either the left ventricular apex or the left atrium to either the ascending or the descending aorta. The variable volume compensator is placed in the left pleural cavity and joins the lever actuator unit through a polyamide tube that penetrates the diaphragm at the costal margin.

The muscle-force multiplier is secured by suturing it in a retrosternal position. The tension guides for the left and right LD biomechanical coupling are placed in the pleural space, from where they emerge to the external chest wall between the anterior and median axillary lines.

## Preconditioning of LD and TM Muscles

The humeral insertions of the LD and TM muscles are surgically removed in a block, including a longitudinal segment of periosteum. The skin incision is made from a point 1–2 cm superior to the humeral insertion of the LD muscle; inferior to it, the incision reaches the 7th rib. The vertical incision follows the posterior axillary line at the anterior edge of the LD muscle. The patient is in a supine position and is anesthetized whithout curariform drugs. The tension force (passive stretching force) is measured with a dynamometer; the tendons of the LD and TM muscles are pulled to thc point of normal humeral insertion to register this measurement.

The LD and TM muscle neurovascular bundles are exposed. A pair of intramuscular leads (Biotronik) are inserted. The proximal cathodic lead is woven near the nerve branches; the anodic lead is located 6–8 cm distally, in the mass of the LD and TM muscles. An analyzer is used to measure acute threshold and resistances of the muscles and leads. The muscle stimulator in the sheath of the right abdominal rectus muscle is implanted. The sensing wire for the heart is fixed in the myocardium.

## Major Subsystems

The ProCor pump drive/unit comprises a dual pusher-plate seamless sac-type blood pump. The sac, fabricated with bioSpan (Polymer Technology Group, Emeryville, CA) segmented polyurethane, is bonded to a pair of symmetrically opposed pusher plates and fixed to a skeletal aluminium frame that incorporates fittings for 25-mm custom bileaflet heart valves (ATS). The lever actuator allows efficient transmission of mechanical energy from the muscle-force multiplier to the pusher-plate assembly.

With a nominal maximum stroke volume of 60 ml (BS-2), a dp/dt from 1600 (50 ms) to 1800 (45 ms) mmHg/s, pump frequency 40 beats/min, and systemic pressure of 100 mmHg, the ProCor system can pump outputs of 2–2.5 l/min. The system is synchronized with the ECG to pump during the diastolic period of the natural cardiac cycle. Blood pump systolic time is an important consideration. In vitro testing with a specially designed muscle simulator has been of great help in understanding this point:

- Systolic time of 400 ms requires 2.30 kg of muscle force.
- Systolic time of 350 ms requires 2.5 kg of muscle force.
- Systolic time of 300 ms requires 2.95 kg of muscle force.
- Systolic time of 200 ms requires 3.27 kg of muscle force.

Consequently, the muscle force must increase 40% from 400 ms to 200 ms, 30% from 350 ms to 200 ms, and 11% from 300 ms to 200 ms.

Briefly, the ProCor skeletal muscle-powered implantable blood pump requires 3 kg of muscle power and 2–2.5 cm muscle displacement. The blood pump functional parameters are systolic time 300 ms, dp/dt 1800 (45 ms) mmHg/s, pump rate 40 beats/min, and systemic blood pressure 100 mmHg (1/2 synchronous counterpulsation) in order to have a basic minimum of 2–2.5 l/min pump output.

A special graft has been developed for the biologic-to-mechanical system interface. An 8-mm-diameter high-porosity medical-grade Dacron graft is incorporated into the body of the muscle tendons. The LD and TM muscle tendons, with their flat, anatomical configuration, are wrapped around and carefully sutured to the Dacron graft. A titanium-machined piece incorporated in the composite graft provides solid interlocking for the traction guide.

The muscle-force multiplier is firmly sutured retrosternally. The basic purpose of a force multiplier is to save muscular mass energy. For example, from a required maximal muscle force of 3 kg and 2–2.5 cm of displacement the multiplier increases the muscle force to 6 kg and decreases the displacement to 1.25 cm. This is possible due to the unique design of the actuator, coupled with the dual pusher plate; only 9 mm displacement for each pusher plate is necessary to obtain the maximum pumping efficiency of the system. The motion of the dual pusher-plate unit is 18 mm. The required pulling force of 3 kg of the LD and TM muscles and a displacement of 2–2.5 cm can be easily attained. Furthermore, the calculated force of the right and left LD and TM muscles acting together should be 6 kg and the muscle multiplier output should be 12 kg.

## Console-based System

During and immediately after surgery, the ProCor power and control electronics must be externalized within an extracorporeal console with a modular design, wherein all console circuits are redundant (Fig. 4). The external hydraulic-pneu-

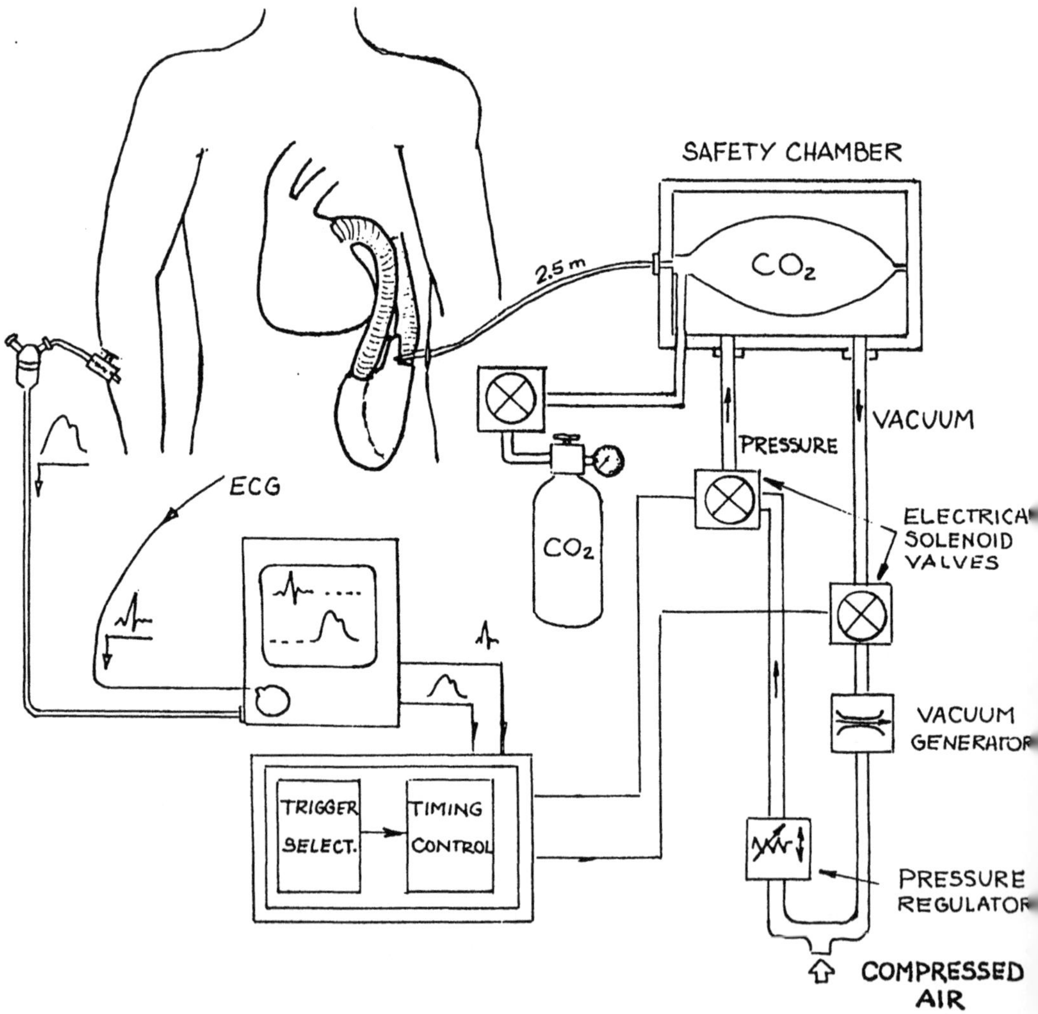


**Fig. 4.** External pneumatic-based console

matic system is connected through a percutaneous access port located in the left lateral abdomen, distant from the operative area. While the muscle power and displacement are closely monitored during the postoperative period, the external driving system remains on standby.

Severely ill patients may require cardiac assistance without delay. During skeletal muscle remodeling (2–4 weeks) the ProCor LVAD must be powered by the external pneumatic unit.

## Case History

*J.B., age: 60 years*: Arterial hypertension for the past 15 years; diabetes; nicotinism (a smoker since 15 years of age); high digestive hemorrhage in 1988, (erosive gastritis by endoscopic diagnosis); dyspnea for the past 15 years; five previous hospitalizations due to heart failure, one of these hospitalizations being especially severe, due to acute pulmonary edema, and another one due to supraventricular tachyarrythmia.

*Presumptive diagnosis*: Dilated myocardiopathy of unknown origin.

*Reason for hospitalization*: Two months before his present hospitalization he experienced an increase in his dyspnea from functional class (FC) II to the present FC III–IV, with periodic episodes of paroxysmal nocturnal dyspnea and orthopnea. The patient was medicated with digitalis, diuretics, enalapril, amiodarone, and oral hypoglycemics without significant clinical improvement. For this reason he was referred to our institute for the diagnosis of his myocardiopathy and for further treatment.

*May 24, 1993:* The patient was admitted with dyspnea; FC III–IV; heart rate 110/min; arterial blood pressure 100/70, intermittent protodiastolic gallop, rales at the bases of the lungs; sinus rhythm, heart frequency 110, PR 0.20, QRS 0.15 s, left bundle-branch block, frequent monofocal ventricular extrasystoles.

Laboratory: hematocrit 48%; white cells 9800; glycemia 130 mg/%; BUN 91 mg/%; creatinine 1.49 mg/%; sodium 141 mEq/l; potassium 4.5 mEq/l; total cholesterol 289 mg/%; test for Chagas' disease: negative. The patient received furosemide 60 mg/day; enalapril 5 mg/day; digital amiodorone 600 mg/day. Chest X-ray: severe cardiomegaly; echocardiography: dilated myocardiopathy with severe depression of the systolic function; 24-h Holter: heart rate varies from 70 beats/min to sinus rhythm tachycardia of 130/min, frequent polymorphous PVC; amiodarone 800 mg/day was prescribed.

*May 27, 1993:* Dyspnea FC II, tolerance to the supine position. Radionuclide ventriculogram, severe impairment of the systolic function. Ejection fraction at rest, 30%; during exercise, 39%; increase at the end of the diastolic volume. It is understood that the relatively high percentage of the ejection fraction is due primarily to the extremely augmented left ventricular volume. Cardiac catheterization, severe myocardial dysfunction, pulmonary hypertension, normal coronary arteries. Pressures: RAP 16, RVP 70/18, PAP 70, WCP 35, LVP 110/40, Ao 110/70.

Endomyocardic biopsy: Swollen myocytes with big quadrangular hyperchromatic nuclei are observed, thus showing evidence of severe myocardial cell hypertrophy. The intramyocardic arterioles are normal.

Briefly, findings are: (a) cardiac hypertrophy secondary to systemic hypertension; (b) cellular infiltration suggestive of previous myocarditis; (c) vast deposits of hemosiderin in myocardial cells.

*May 31, 1993*: FC II; patient discharged.

*June 22, 1993*: The patient was readmitted with severe heart failure. Rales in both lungs, third heart sound, elevated jugular venous presure, peripheral hypoperfusion, painful hepatomegaly. Cardiopulmonary exercise test: a minimum tolerance to exercise; $VO_2$ max. 12.4 ml/kg/min, anaerobic threshold undefined during test. A self-limited ventricular tachycardia developed during maximum effort. Intravenous treatment with diuretics, nitroglycerin; dopamine was instituted. A medical (surgical – clinical) consultation takes place, in which heart transplantation is advised. The patient and his relatives refuse heart transplantation. Instead, a program of chronic mechanical circulatory assistance is suggested, to which patient and relatives agree. Patient is discharged from hospital.

*July 9, 1993*: Patient was hospitalized once more with FC-IV dyspnea. A few minutes following his admission he suffered a cardiac arrest with ventricular fibrillation that lasted 90 min; he received external cardiac massage, drugs, electrical shock; VF reverted. Phase I of the chronic heart assist system was decided.

*July 20, 1993*: The first phase of the program was carried out. The tendons of the LD and TM muscles were surgically removed from their humeral insertions and the biomechanical coupling was implanted. Excellent tolerance to the procedure. A training program of the LD and TM muscles was inmediately started.

*July 25, 1993*: Patient suddenly developed acute pulmonary edema.

*August 10, 1993*: Patient clinically stable, good tolerance to the LD and TM muscle stimulation without pain or discomfort at the muscle contractions (Figs. 5–7).

*August 15, 1993*: Patient in pulmonary edema.

*October 16–December 11, 1993:* In severe left ventricular failure with periodic crises of pulmonary edema, patient required permanent i.v. vasoactive drugs (dopamine, dobutamine, amrinone).

*December 11, 1993*: Patient developed cardiac arrest. After 20 min external cardiac massage he recovered with good neurological responses.

*December 14, 1993*: Cardiac surgery with ECC; the heart assist system was implanted. The blood pump between the LV apex and the ascending aorta was placed. The muscle-force multiplier retrosternally was firmly sutured. Following surgery, the patient mantained a systolic arterial pressure of 90 mmHg and excellent diuretic rhythm. However, after a few hours severe acute RV dysfunction was observed (RAP 20 mmHg, PAP 18 mmHg, WCP 5 mmHg, cardiac output 3.2 l/min). RV assistance was considered. However, the patient's neurological state precluded further surgical circulatory assistance.

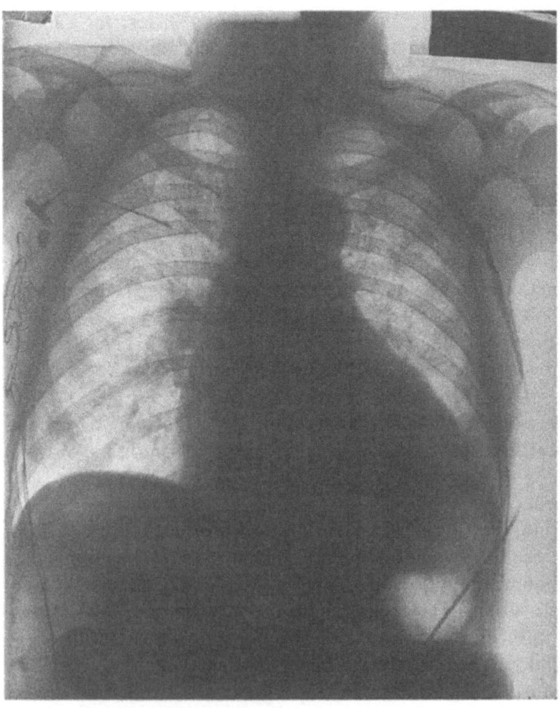

**Fig. 5.** Chest X-ray of patient J.B. The right LD-MT biomechanical junction can be seen (*upper left*). The cardiomyostimulator and LD-TM intramuscular leads are visualized in the right upper abdomen

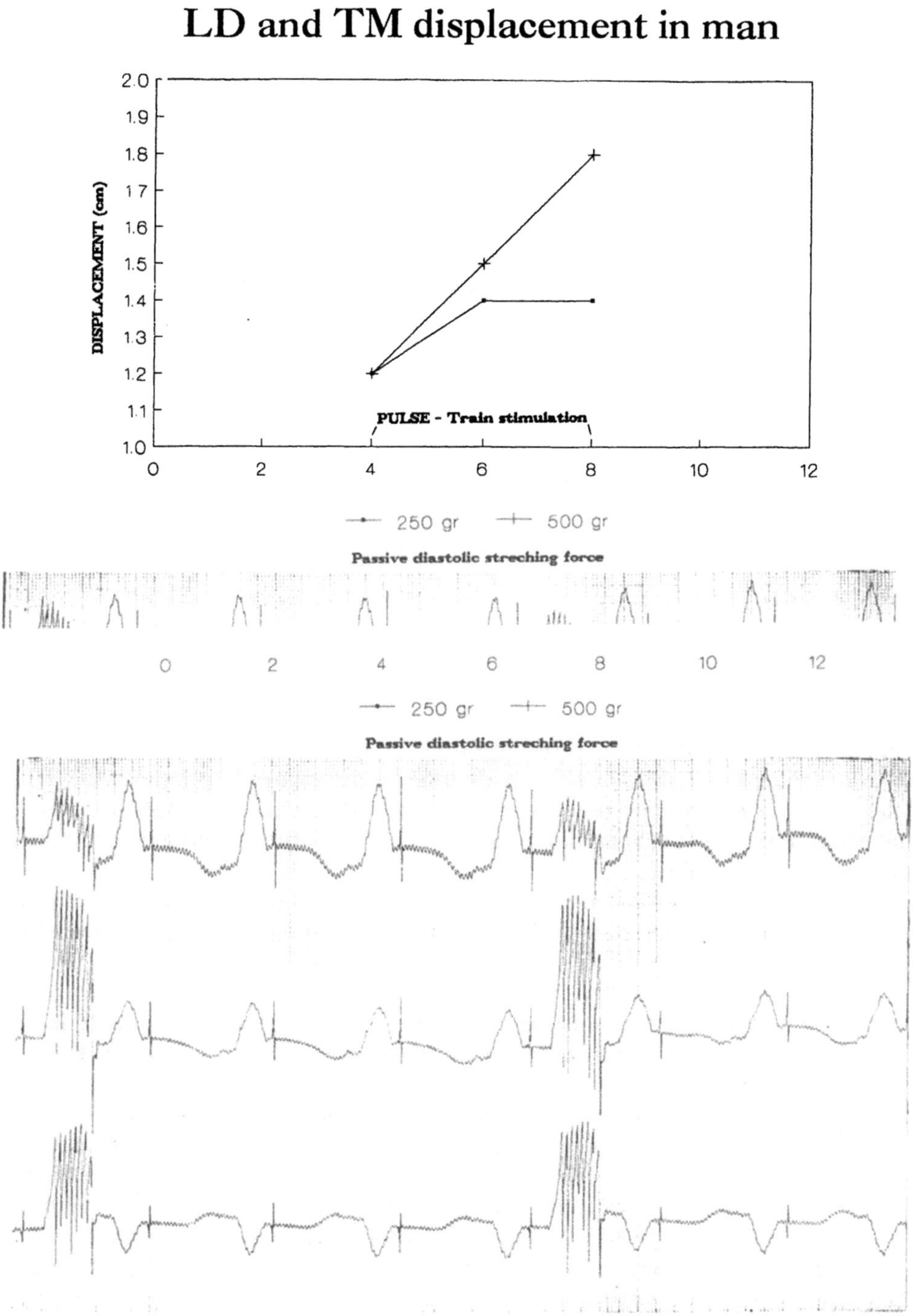


**Fig. 6.** Physiological studies on LD-TM muscle displacement in patient J.B. *Upper drawing*: LD-TM muscle displacement and its relationship with LD-TM passive diastolic streching force (muscle tension force) and with the muscle pulse-train stimulation (4–8 pulses). *Lower drawing*: LD-TM muscle stimulation with a pulse-train of 8 pulses. The muscle stimulation $^1/_4$ during diastole has been synchronized. ECG pacemaker rhythm)

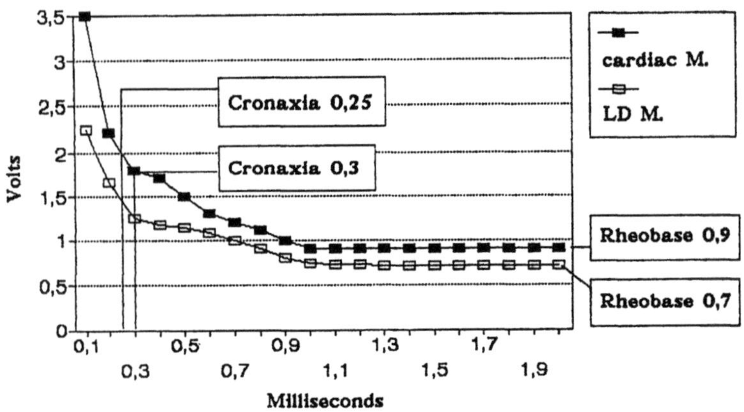


**Fig. 7.** Comparative cronaxia studies on LD-TM muscles and the myocardium in patient J.B.

## Discussion

Selecting patients for cardiac chronic mechanical assistance is not an easy task. The broad range of variability in the NYHA FC III is well recognized. Furthermore, for not very well understood reasons, patients in FC IV may have a sudden stabilization without further progression of the symptomatology.

More than 40 variables have been identified as predictors of prognosis in CHF, and these can be grouped broadly into clinical and electrocardiographic criteria, hemodynamic and echocardiographic indices, or biochemical and neurohormonal abnormalities.

Clinical criteria are based particularly on the duration and level of symptomatic dyspnea (NYHA class) relative to prognosis. Furthermore, the need for hospitalization with worsening symptoms of heart failure is associated with a higher subsequent mortality. The etiology of heart failure has a bearing on prognosis. Many (but not all) studies have shown that heart failure due to ischemic heart disease carries a worse prognosis than that due to dilated cardiomyopathy.

Many of the hemodynamic and echocardiographic prognostic indices relate to the underlying level of left ventricular dysfunction and dilatation. Numerous studies have shown that the left ventricular ejection fraction is the most powerful independent predictor of outcome in patients, particularly those with a myocardial infarction, in whom there is an exponential increase in mortality with decreasing ejection fraction (ejection fraction >40%: 2-year mortality 7%; ejection fraction <20%: 2-year mortality 50%).

Exercise capacity, maximal oxygen consumption ($VO_2$ max), and other hemodynamic indices of functional cardiac reserve provide further important prognostic information. The 1-year mortality for patients with a $VO_2$ max lower than 10 ml/kg/m was near 80%, compared with 20% for those with a $VO_2$ max of 10–18 ml/kg/min.

The degree of activation of the two main neuroendocrine compensation mechanisms (the renin-angiotensin axis and the sympathetic nervous system) also have been shown to correlate with prognosis. The activity of the renin-angiotensin system, as reflected by levels of plasma renin or angiotensin II or the presence of hyponatremia, has a discriminating prognostic value, whereas plasma norepinephrine levels have defined higher-risk groups of patients in a number of studies.

The predictive value of ventricular arrhythmia is less well defined, although some studies have demonstrated the importance of ventricular arrythmias relative to mortality.

Of the many prognostic variables described, NYHA functional class, cardiothoracic ratio, and left ventricular ejection fraction are the most clinically applicable. Many of the recent trials have used one or more of these variables as patient selection criteria and combinations of various prognostic indices to stratify and identify groups of patients at high, medium, and low risk.

Nevertheless, the changing criteria and the progression of the disease, characterized clinically by cardiac pump failure, are the most important clinical points of view in deciding the indication for chronic circulation assistance.

ProCor, the chronic univentricular-designed support for CHF patients in FC IV, is at an advanced stage of development. The unique system combines an endogenous source of power – the skeletal muscle – and an external hydraulic-pneumatic driving unit.

The development of a mechanical system to study the physiological parameters of skeletal muscle has been of great help. This artificial skeletal muscle driven by a pneumatic source of power helps us to comprehed many specific points, for example, the relationship between amount of muscular force and systolic contracting time, or that between skeletal muscle dp/dt and pump output. The performance of the pump system driven by the artificial skeletal muscle has been carefully studied.

The ProCor LVAD provides a variable load to the patient's heart with early decompression to facilitate myocardial function recovery.

During this early period, the ProCor LVAD is driven by the external hydraulic-pneumatic unit, with pump rate 80/min and pump output 4–5 l/min. Chronic stabilization is obtained when the pump is driven by the skeletal muscle, pump rate 40/min, ½ synchronous counterpulsation, pump output 2–2.5 l/min; it prevents heart decompensation secondary to chronic unloading, and the skeletal muscle biologic motor is preserved.

The lethal outcome of our patient was due primarily to severe acute RV failure, a common observation in terminally ill cardiac patients with multiorgan failure under LVAD. Concomitant RVAD support was considered, but the patient rapidly deteriorated from the neurological point of view. Bleeding/coagulopathy, a common complication after surgery, was not observed in our patient. Terminal cardiac patients are better candidates for a total artificial heart procedure.

One encouraging clinical observation regarding neuromuscular stimulation must be pointed out. Our patient was under electrical pacing of LD and TM muscles day and night, and he did not refer to any discomfort whatsoever due to muscle displacement.

*Acknowledgements.* We are indebted to a large number of professionals who, over a period of 2 years, have been of great help to the CONICET-Procoar program.

We wish to thank Ricardo Dalton, MD, for having gathered the clinical data of patient J.B., and Mrs. Maria Leonor Arguello and Mrs. Silvana Tidoni for their expert technical assistance in the preparation of this manuscript.

## References

1. Cohn JN (1988) Current therapy of the failing heart. Circulation 78:1099–1107
2. Alvarez CB et al. (1987) Enalapril en la insuficiencia cardiaca congestiva – estudio cooperativo. Rev Argent Cardiol 55:134–143
3. Kannel WB, Plehn JF, Couples LA (1988) Cardiac failure and sudden death in the Framingham study. Am Heart J 115:869–875
4. Cohn JN, Archibal DG, Francis GS et al. (1987) Veterans Administration cooperative study. Circulation 75:IV49–IV54
5. Woosley RL, Echt DS, Roden DM (1986) Effects of congestive heart failure on the pharmacokinetics and pharmacodynamics of antiarrythmic agents. M J Cardiol 57:25B
6. Hagar JM, Rahimtoola SH (1991) Chagas' heart disease in the United States. N Engl J Med 325:763–768
7. Cohn JN, Levine TB, Olivari MT, Garberg W, Lura D, Francis GS, Simon A (1984) Plasma norepinephrine as a guide to prognosis in patients with chronic congestive heart failure. N Engl J Med 311:819–823
8. Levine TB, Franciosa JA, Urobel T, Cohn JN (1982) Hyponatraemia as a marker for high renin heart failure. Br Heart J 47:161–166
9. Jennings GL, Esler MD (1990) Circulatory regulation at rest and exercise and the functional assesment of patients with congestive heart failure. Circulation 81:II5–II13
10. Consensus Trial Study Group (1987) Effects of enalapril on mortality in severe congestive heart failure. N Engl J Med 316:1429
11. Kolff WJ (1983) Artificial organ forty years and beyond. Trans Am Soc Artif Intern Organs 29:6–24
12. Liotta D, Crawford ES, Cooley DA, De Bakey ME, Urquia M, Feldman L (1962) Prolonged partial left ventricular bypass by means of intrathoracic pump implanted in the left chest. Trans Am Soc Artif Intern Organs 8:90
13. Liotta D, Hall CW, Henly WS, Beall AC, Cooley DA, De Bakey M (1963) Prolonged assisted circulation during and after cardiac or aortic surgery. I. Prolonged left ventricular bypass by means of an intrathoracic circulatory pump. II. Diastolic pulsation of the descending thoracic aorta. Trans Am Soc Artif Intern Organs 9:182
14. Liotta D, Hall CW, Henly WS, Cooley DA, Crawford ES, De Bakey ME (1963) Prolonged assisted circulation after cardiac or aortic surgery. Prolonged partial left ventricular bypass by means of intracorporeal circulation. Am J Cardiol 12:399
15. Cooley CA, Liotta D, Hallman GL, Bloodwell RD, Leachman RD, Nora JD, Fernbach DJ, Milan JD (1969) Orthotopic cardiac prosthesis for two-staged cardiac replacement. Am J Cardiol 24:723–730
16. Farrar DJ, Hill JD, Gray LA et al. (1988) Heterotopic prosthetic ventricles as a bridge to cardiac transplantation: a multi-center study in 29 patients. N Engl J Med 318:330–340.
17. Rosenberg G, Pierce WS, Landis DL, Snyder AJ, Richenbacher WE, Weiss W, Felder G, (1984) Progress in the development of the Pennsylvania State University motor-driven artificial heart. In: Unger F (ed) Assisted circulation, vol 2. Springer, Berlin Heidelberg New York, pp 270–284

18. Portner PM, Oyer PE, Jassawalla JS, Chen H, Miller PJ, LaForge DH, Green GF, Shumway NE (1984) A totally implantable ventricular assist device for end-stage heart disease In: Unger F (ed) Assisted circulation. Springer, Berlin Heidelberg New York, pp 115–141
19. Portner PM, LaForge DH, Pitzele S, Maeder PA, Lee J (1979) Transcutaneous energy for an implanted electrical circulatory support system using distributive inductive coupling. Proc Eur Soc Artif Organs 6:109–112
20. White MA (1986) Implantable energy source for artificial heart. In: Akutsu T (ed) Artificial heart. Springer, Berlin Heidelberg New York, chap 4
21. Liotta D, Taliani T, Giffonielo AH, Sarria Deheza F, Liotta S, Lizarraga R, Tolocka L, Pagano J, Bincciotti E (1961) Artificial heart in the chest: preliminary report. Trans Am Soc Intern Organs 7:318
22. Liotta D, DelRio M, Cooley D (1986) The artificial heart. In: Cheng TO (ed) Comprehensive cardiology. Pergamon, New York, pp 1164–1181
23. Salmons S, Streter EA (1976) Significance of impulse activity in the transformation of skeletal muscle type. Nature 263:30–34
24. Salmons S, Vrbova G (1969) The influence of activity on some contractile characteristics of mammalian fast and slow muscle. Physiol J (Lond) 210:535–549
25. Salmons S, Jarvis J (1990) The working capacity of skeletal muscle transformed for use in cardiac assist role. In: Chiu RCJ et al. (eds) Transformed muscle for cardiac assist and repair. Futura, Mount Kisco, pp 89–104
26. Carpentier A, Chachques JC (1985) Myocardial substitution with a stimulated skeletal muscle: first successful clinical case Lancet 1:1267
27. Stephenson LW (1991) 4th World Symposium on Transformed Skeletal Muscle of Cardiac Assist. J Card Surg 6 (1) Suppl
28. Chiu RC, Bourgeois LM (1990) Transformed muscle for cardiac assist and repair. Futura, Mount Kisco
29. Kantrowitz A, McKinnon W (1959) The experimental use of the diaphragm as an auxiliary myocardium. Surg Forum 9:266
30. Stephenson LW, Ruggiero R, Niinami H, Pochettino A, Hammond RL, Hooper TL, Huiping L, Anderson DR, Spanta AD (1991) Skeletal muscle ventricles; update after 18 months in circulation. Artif Organs 15:350
31. Chiu R, Walsh GL, Dewar MI et al. (1987) Implantable extra-aortic balloon assist powered by transformed, fatigue-resistant skeletal muscle. J Thorac Cardiovasc Surg 94:694–701
32. Liotta D, Ortolan E, DeCarli, Sancineto, Liotta CA, Alvarez CB (1990) Linear contraction LD muscle–powered LVAD. Biomation in 21st Century, International Symposium May 12–15. Nihon University School of Medicine, Tokyo
33. Spitzer DE (1984) Apparatus for powering a body implant device. (US patent 4, 453, 537)
34. Ugolini F (1986) Skeletal muscle for artificial heart drive: theory and in vivo experiment. In: Chiu RCJ (ed) Biomechanical cardiac assist: cardiomyoplasty and muscle–powered devices. Futura, Mount Kisko, pp 193–210
35. Farrar DJ, Hill JD (1992) A new skeletal linear-pull energy convertor as a power source for prosthetic circulatory support devices. J Heart Lung Transplant 11:341–350
36. Laura P et al. (1991) Estudios de un sistema hidraulico aplicado a una bomba de sangre para la asistencia circulatoria. Proc CONICET, Bueuos Aires
37. Pisarello J, Zeuli S, Galetar J, Ponzone C, Godia J, Liotta CA, Peschi M, Pinchete C, Liotta D (1992) Desarrollo de un dispositivo de asistencia ventricular izquierda implantable con fuente de energia endogena para el tratamiento de pacientes con insuficiencia cardiaca cronica terminal. (Programa PROCOAR), XIII Congreso Nacional de Cardiologia, Mar del Plata, Argentina, Oct 8–12
38. Liotta D, Ponzone C, Godia J, Pisarello J, Galetar J, Liotta CA, Alvarez CB (1993) Autologous skeletal muscle-driven implantable assist blood pump for chronic refractory heart failure. International Society of Cardio-Thoracic Surgeons. Third World Congress, Salzburg, 25–27, Jan 1993
39. Liotta D and CONICET-PROCOAR investigators (1993) Direct linear-pull skeletal muscle-powered chronic implantable assist blood pump for end-stage heart failure. In: D'Alessandro LC (ed) Heart Surgery 1993. CONICET-PROCOAR, Rome, pp 229–240

# Appendix

CONICET is a Federal Agency of Scientific Research (Argentina) President: Professor Domingo Liotta, MD
CONICET – PROCOAR investigators:
National Director: Domingo Liotta, MD

- Engineers: Daniel F. Sanchez, Laureano Nava, Luis A. Pinchete, Teresita Cuadrado, Santos Zeuli, Roberto J.J. Williams, Marcelo Peschi.
- Assistant Engs.: Mr. R. Gil Roy, Mr. R.G. Luayza Mr. G. Abraham.
- Instituto de las Clinicas Cardiovasculares, Buenos Aires.
- Cardiology: Carlos B. Alvarez, MD, Ricardo Dalton, MD, Ricardo Tuda, MD, Bernardo Lozada, MD, Carlos Killinger, MD, Sergio Nijenshon, MD.
- Surgery: Carlos Ponzone, MD, Jose Godia, MD, Juan Carlos Vazquez, MD, Mariano E. Brizzio, MD, Domingo Liotta, MD.
- Hospital Italiano, Buenos Aires.
- Orthopedic Surgery Service: E.G. Ortolan, MD, C.F. Sancineto, MD, P. De Carli, MD, Carlos A. Liotta, MD.
- Audiovisual Recording: Mr. Noe Olivera.
- Private Industry:
  Uretec SA, Bahia Blanca: Mr. Roberto G. Luayza.
- Cientifica Argentina: Mr. Felix O. Caivano, Mr Mario Michalick.
- Biomedica Argentina SA: Mr. B. Lozada, MD, Mr. R. Garillo, MD
- Cycla S.A.: Mr. Jose Caporelli, Mr Sergio Jaremko.
- Emeclar: Mrs. Magdalena Clar.
- Bioingenieria Mecanica: Mr. A.M. Blason.

# Part V
# Total Artificial Heart

# Introduction

F. UNGER

The total artificial heart is at the present time no longer an object of discussion. Basic research on it is nevertheless still very important for developing a new understanding of the overall regulation of circulation. These devices are designed for biological testing as well as for developing implantable driving devices. Based on my own personal experience with total artificial hearts, we must keep in mind that it is much easier to drive an artificial heart as an assist device. The total artificial heart will become an object of discussion again when assist devices show reliability in long-term use. At present, research on special driving systems is under way. Rosenberg reports on the experience using a total implantable mechanical heart at Penn State, and Kaufmann reports on a motor-gear unit whose components can be also used for assisted circulation.

# In Vivo Testing of a Clinical-size Totally Implantable Artificial Heart

G. Rosenberg, A.J. Snyder, W.J. Weiss, J.S. Sapirstein, and W.S. Pierce

## Introduction

In 1984, work was begun on a 100-ml stroke volume roller-screw-type electric motor-driven total artificial heart at the Pennsylvania State University. The pumping system utilized two seam-free segmented polyurethane sacs housed within semi-rigid polysulfone cases. Size 25-mm outlet and 29-mm inlet Delrin disk Bjork-Shiley convexo-concave valves were used in both the left and right blood pumps. Screw-on quick connects for the atria and great vessels were employed to facilitate implantation of the device. The blood pumps were attached to either end of the energy converter. The energy converter used a brushless DC motor to drive a roller-screw mechanism. Attached to the ends of the screw portion of the roller-screw mechanism were two pusher plates, which alternately compressed the blood sacs. This roller-screw system employed an external electronic automatic control system in all experiments. The system has been described extensively elsewhere [1–5]. This 100-cc stroke volume roller-screw total artificial heart was implanted in 12 calves; one calf survived for 388 days [6, 7]. After the initial postoperative period, this animal thrived; it was eventually killed due to inadequate cardiac output. The results of these initial experiments were extremely encouraging, and work was begun on a 70-cc stroke volume device that would be capable of being orthotopically placed in a human patient.

The present system utilizes the same basic design, scaled in size for clinical use. Figures 1 and 2 show the completely implanted total artificial heart system as it will be employed clinically. The system includes both external and implanted components. The battery pack is shown over the patient's left shoulder. Connected to this battery pack is the transcutaneous energy transmission system electronics and primary coil. The electronics are clipped to the patient's belt, while the primary coil is held around the patient's chest by a lightweight harness. Direct current from the battery pack is delivered to the transcutaneous energy transmission primary oscillator. There, this direct current is converted into 158 kHz RF current, which is inductively coupled across the intact skin to the implanted TETS secondary coil that supplies current to the implanted electronics assembly. The electronics assembly consists of a hermetically sealed titanium enclosure which houses the control electronics, an implanted battery capable of running the system for approximately 30 min, and the telemetry transmitter and receiver electronics. Energy is taken from the electronics assembly and delivered

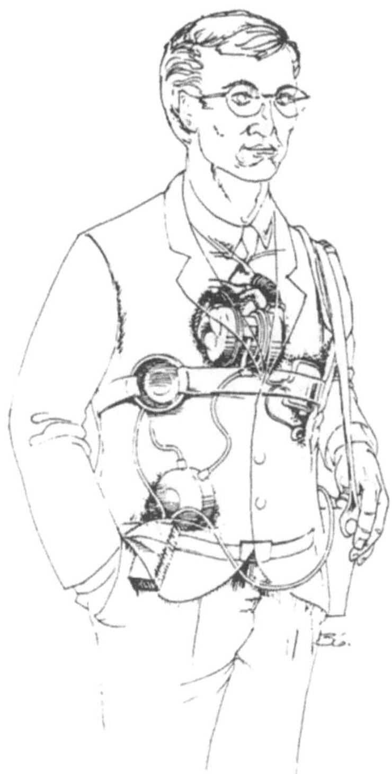

**Fig. 1.** Completely implanted TAH system as it will be employed clinically

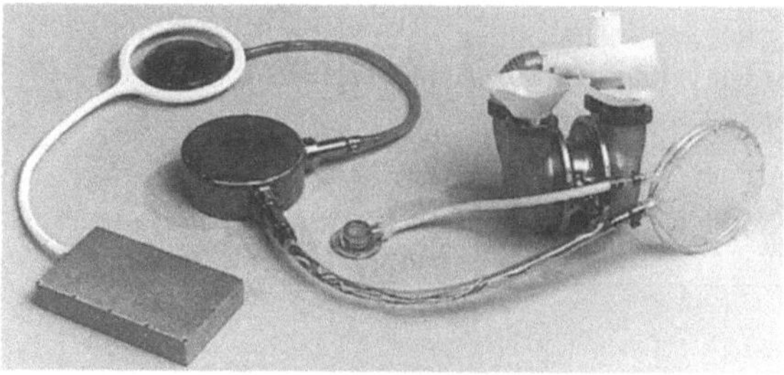

**Fig. 2.** Total artificial heart system showing TETS primary, TETS secondary, implanted electronics, blood pumps and energy converter, compliance chamber, and subcutaneous access port

directly to the energy converter to power the blood pump. Other implanted components are the compliance chamber and the subcutaneous access port used for replenishment of gases that diffuse from the system. The system specifications are given in Tables 1 and 2.

## Control

### Maintaining Left-Right Balance

Analysis of motor voltage and speed permits estimation of the end-diastolic volume and afterload of the left pump [8]. The left end-diastolic volume is

**Table 1.** System specifications of the 70-cc total artificial heart

| | |
|---|---|
| Energy converter | Dual pusher-plate roller-screw drive<br>Brushless DC motor<br>14-pole, 3-phase, 12-volt, NdFeB magnets<br>Position sensing<br>3 Hall-effect sensors and magnet ring<br>No other sensors<br>Stroke length: 1.9 cm |
| Blood pumps | Static stroke volume: 70 cc<br>Dynamic stroke volume: 55–60 cc<br>Valves: Bjork-Shiley monostrut Delrin disk<br>27-mm inlet, 25-mm outlet |
| Maximum cardiac output | 9 l/min at 150 beats/min into 100 mmHg AoP<br>@ CVP = 15 mmHg and LAP = 13 mmHg |
| Cardiac output control | Adjustable for RAP sensitivity or AoP inverse sensitivity |
| Left-right balance control | Left full-empty, right limited fill<br>LAP <15 mmHg for 15 mmHg CVP |
| Internal battery | 9-cell NiCd, 600 m amp-hr, 2/3 Af size<br>Maximum operating time (at 40°C)<br>30 min at 5 l/min into 90 mmHg mean AoP<br>Full recharge time: 14 h |
| External battery | Two 10-cell NiCd packs, 4.0 amp-hr, D size<br>Maximum operating time<br>6 h at 6 l/min into 100 mmHg mean AOP |
| Energy-transmission system | 158 kHz modified ThermoCardiosystems type<br>maximum efficiency (DC in to DC out):<br>78% at 62 watts output<br>output voltage: 13.5–14.2 volts, regulated<br>input voltage: 11–16 volts DC |
| Telemetry (two-way) | Ingoing: TETS carrier FSK at 300 baud<br>Outgoing: 32.77 MHz FSK at 300/1200 baud<br>Two-way error rate: typically $<10^{-4}$ errors/bit |

the only measurement needed to achieve balance between the left and right cardiac outputs, thus preventing the development of unphysiological left atrial pressures. Left-right balance is actively maintained by the preload control. Left systolic duration is the major determinant of the right diastolic time. The preload control continually searches for the right diastolic time necessary to keep the left pump just on the verge of complete filling. The controller reduces the right diastolic time ($T_{RD}$) in small increments until a decrease in left end-diastolic volume (EDV) is detected, indicating that the effective (dynamic) right pump stroke volume has fallen below that which the left pump can accommodate. $T_{RD}$ is then increased in increments, restoring left pump filling, until no further increase in left EDV is observed. The result is that the system hovers around a stable point at which, for some range of right atrial pressure (RAP),

**Table 2.** Components of the 70-cc total artificial heart system

| Components | Dimensions (cm maximum) | Volume (cc) | Mass (g) |
|---|---|---|---|
| Energy converter | 3.1 w × 8.3 dia | 120 | 510 |
| Blood pumps (case, sacs, valves) | 3.0 w × 9.4 ht | 190 × 2 | 100 × 2 |
| Electronics assembly (incl. batterties) | 3.7 w × 9.7 dia | 280 | 650 |
| TETS secondary coil | 1.9 w × 7.1 dia | 60 | 120 |
| Compliance chamber | 1.1 w × 10.9 dia | 70 | 70 |
| Total implanted components | | 910 | 1550 |
| TETS primary electronics | 7.6 × 12.7 × 2.3 | 220 | 315 |
| Patient battery pack | 19 × 15.2 × 10.2 | 2934 | 4600 |
| Total external components | | 3154 | 4915 |

1. The left pump fills completely, or nearly completely, on every cycle
2. The right pump remains in a limited-fill state
3. The right dynamic stroke volume (SV) equals the left dynamic SV, minus the bronchial flow per beat
4. The required right diastolic time depends upon RAP; higher RAP requires shorter $T_{RD}$ to maintain the same right SV
5. The left atrial pressure (LAP) is the pressure necessary to fill the left pump completely at the current beat rate

At very high RAP, it becomes impossible for the energy converter to make right diastole sufficiently short to keep the right pump in a limited-fill state, and left atrial pressure will begin to rise more rapidly with rising RAP.

## Varying Cardiac Output with Metabolic Demand

The preload control, as a side effect of maintaining left-right balance, provides cardiac output that is dependent upon central venous pressure. As RAP rises, shorter right diastolic times are necessary to maintain left-right balance. If no other changes in timing are made, the pump rate will therefore rise as RAP rises. Since left SV remains constant, cardiac output (CO) also rises with RAP, as shown in Fig. 3. Our control method allows amplification or suppression of this Starling effect through variation of the left diastolic time ($T_{LD}$) [9]. If, as right diastolic time is decreased, left diastolic time is decreased also, CO becomes quite sensitive to RAP. The initial slope of the cardiac function curve is nearly as large as that of the "textbook" natural heart, although the curve is displaced to the right.

Variation in total peripheral resistance, as measured by changes in afterload, is more often used as the primary indicator of metabolic demand. As estimated arterial pressure falls below its nominal resting value, the left diastolic time used for a given right diastolic time is reduced, thus raising the pump rate (Fig. 4).

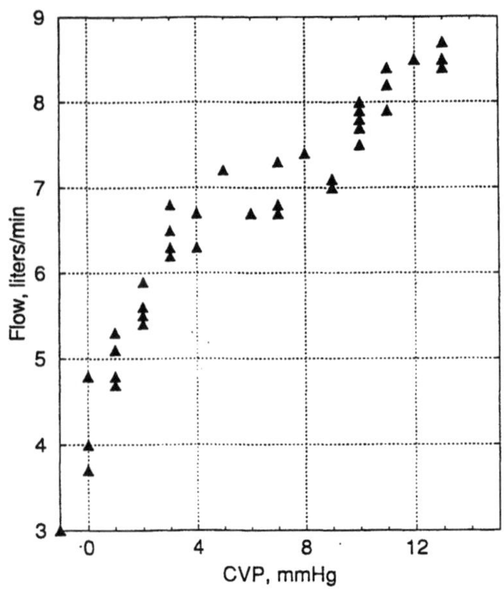


**Fig. 3.** Cardiac output vs. CVP (RAP) at constant AoP, with the controller set for moderate preload sensitivity

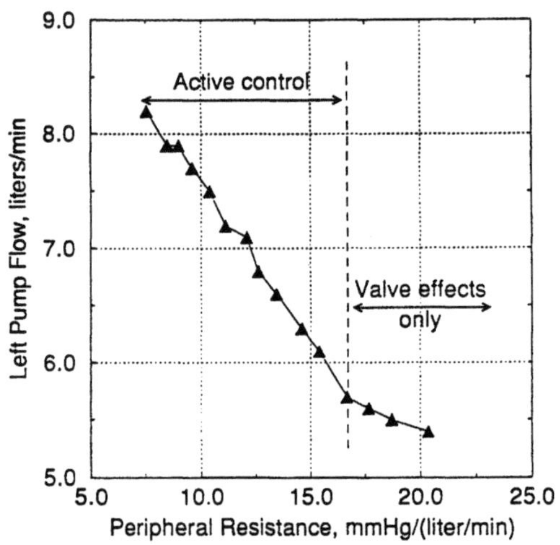


**Fig. 4.** Cardiac output vs. peripheral resistance at constant RAP (~10 mmHg), with the afterload control enabled. (Valve effect is regurgitation and backflow)

## Energy Transmission Methods

The transcutaneous energy-transmission system (TETS) delivers power to the implanted electronics for driving the energy converter and for charging the internal battery [10, 11]. The energy is transferred by inductive coupling between a closely spaced coil pair, the implanted, or "secondary", coil forming a raised mound around which the external, or "primary", coil is placed (Fig. 5). The system can deliver up to 63 watts and provides a regulated 13.8- to 14.5-volt source for the implanted controller.

The primary and secondary coils are series tuned to the same frequency using low loss capacitors, which provides a nonreactive load to the external

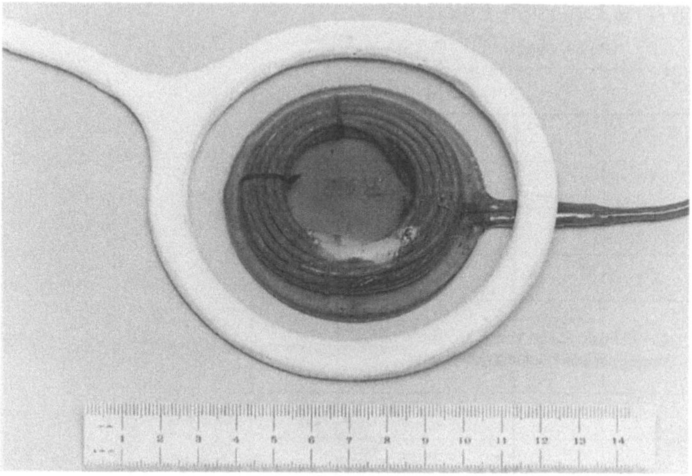

**Fig. 5.** Energy transmission coils. The 5-turn external 'primary' coil is 3.5 inches (8.7 cm) in diameter, and the 18-turn implanted "secondary" coil is 2.9 inches (7.25 cm) in diameter

power oscillator. The primary coil is 3.5 inches (8.7 cm) in diameter and consists of five turns of Litz wire for low loss at high frequencies. The coil is encapsulated with high-strength silicone rubber. The secondary coil is 2.9 inches (7.25 cm) in diameter and consists of 18 turns. The secondary coil is encapsulated with a catalyst-cured polyurethane. The nominal tuned frequency is 158 kHz.

The energy from the secondary coil goes into the internal electronics, where a voltage regulator, rectifier, and filter are located. These components ensure an adequate transfer of energy required to run the blood pump and charge the internal batteries. This system has been stable and provided excellent performance throughout our in vitro and in vivo studies. Figure 6 shows the energy transmission efficiency for two modes of operation (fixed-pulse width, continuously variable pulse width) for the transcutaneous energy-transmission system. The variable-pulse width mode varies the secondary coil current in proportion to load demand. The fixed-pulse width mode delivers current at a constant level but at a duty cycle that varies in proportion to load demand.

## Implanted Battery

The internal battery is required to operate the implanted system for at least 30 min at a flow rate of 6 min. This condition requires a mean power of approximately 9 watts, resulting in the requirement for a minimum of a 0.42 amp-hr pack at 10.8 volts operating at 40°C. Figure 7 shows the mean power demand of the implanted system including the circuit supply current.

We have been able to achieve over 30 min at 5 l/min utilizing a 9-cell pack of 2/3 Af 600 mamp-hr nickel cadmium cells. We continue to perform battery testing in order to track current battery development.

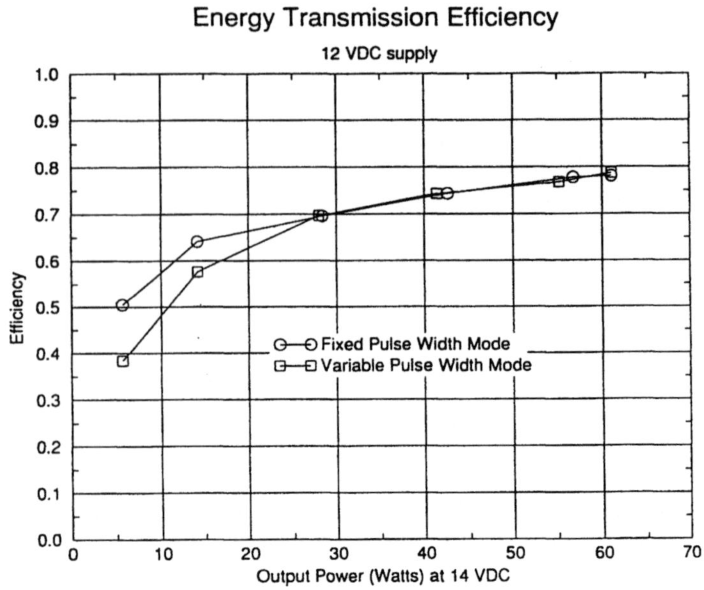


**Fig. 6.** Energy-transmission efficiency vs. power transmitted, for variable- and fixed-pulse width modes

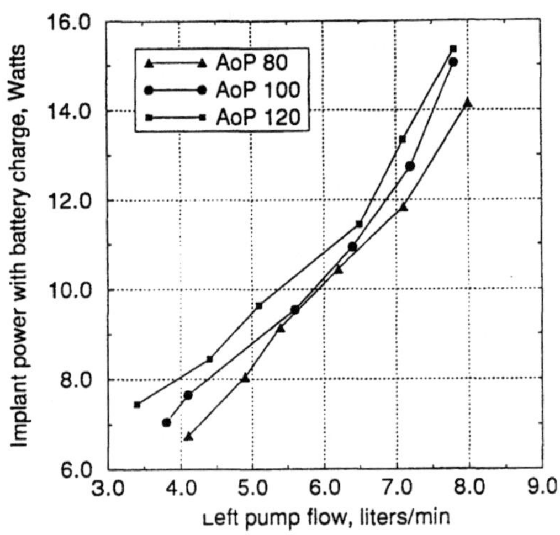


**Fig. 7.** Mean power demand of the implanted system, including battery charging and circuit supply current (pressure in mmHg)

# Implanted Electronics Hardware

The pump control, telemetry, and energy management methods previously described are accomplished on a single six-layer printed circuit board with surface-mounted components on both sides (Fig. 8). The assembled printed circuit board is attached to an aluminum heat-spreader plate that attaches inside the titanium electronics enclosure. The electronics are based on an Intel 87C196KB microcomputer. The use of the device's onboard peripherals has minimized the

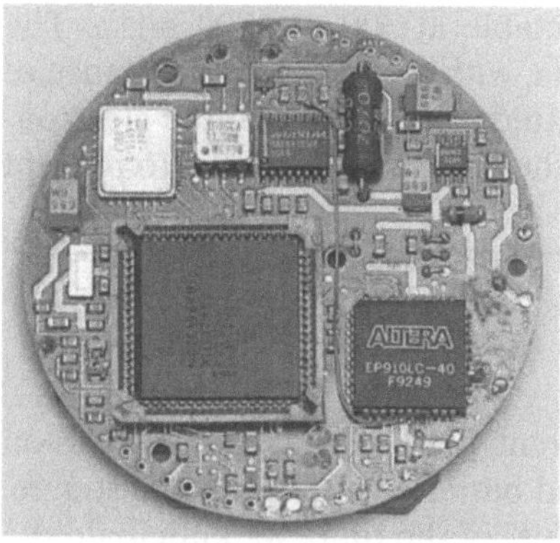

**Fig. 8.** The implanted printed circuit board. The two-sided, six-layer board, with mixed through-hole and surface-mount components, contains all of the electronics needed by the implant. No custom hybrid circuits are required

number of components and interconnects. All motor control and physiologic control algorithms are programmed in software, and a programmable logic device provides high-speed digital functions such as motor commutation and frequency shift-keyed telemetry data demodulation. A standard MOSFET module provides three-phase power to the brushless DC motor of the energy converter. Standard MOSFETs and Schottky diodes are used for battery backup and energy-transmission power switching. A voltage-controlled crystal oscillator provides FM data transmission.

The microcontroller has an onboard watchdog function, which is used to monitor software failure, and an additional hardware monitor is implemented to ensure that the system resets in a timely and proper manner. Integration of all of the implant electronics functions (energy transmission, battery management, communications, motor control) onto a single printed circuit board eliminates board interconnects, which are common failure mechanisms in electronic systems.

## Telemetry

Telemetry is required for the implanted total artificial heart for monitoring the system and for the ability to change control parameters. The methods employed reflect the different requirements for ingoing and outgoing data transmission and the need for tight data security. The abilities to stop the system, to begin pumping slowly, and to alter parameters are required during implantation and during the postoperative period. Parameter changes are required periodically in growing animals; they will rarely be made in clinical cases.

Ingoing telemetry is accomplished by frequency shift keying the energy-transmission oscillator by ±2% at a rate of 300 baud. A sensing circuit on the implanted controller board amplifies, filters, and limits the signal. Demodulation takes place in the programmable logic device. A digital filter removes occasional erroneous samples.

The outgoing telemetry uses a radio frequency carrier, 32.77 MHz, generated by a single chip transmitter on the internal controller board. Frequency shift-key modulation is used, and the baud rate is selectable at 300 or 1200 bits/s. The secondary coil serves as the transmitting antenna, with a transmission distance of approximately 10 m. The information is transmitted from the implanted electronics to the external portable power pack, where the information is used to prompt the user when necessary.

## Portable Power Pack

The portable power pack provides direct current for the energy transmission primary from one of three sources: two attached batteries or an external source. The external battery pack is shown in Fig. 9. Most of the time, we anticipate the patient choosing to remain on battery power, rather than being tethered to a wall supply. The design encourages this because it requires neither the implanted battery, nor temporary use of a wall supply while changing batteries. When going to sleep, the patient will be instructed to connect to a wall source.

Operation on battery power works as follows: in the absence of voltage at the external input, the system draws from one of two batteries. Upon near depletion of the battery in use, a "change battery" condition is triggered, and the system switches automatically to the other battery. A gentle audible indicator prompts the user to remove the nearly depleted battery, move it to the separate charger, and replace it with a freshly charged battery. Accompanying visual indicators identify the audible indicator as "change battery" and clearly show which batteries are to be changed. The appearance of usable voltage at the external input causes both batteries to be disabled and the external source to be used, such as when going to bed plugged into household power. The external power pack has been used only occasionally in in vitro experiments, and as

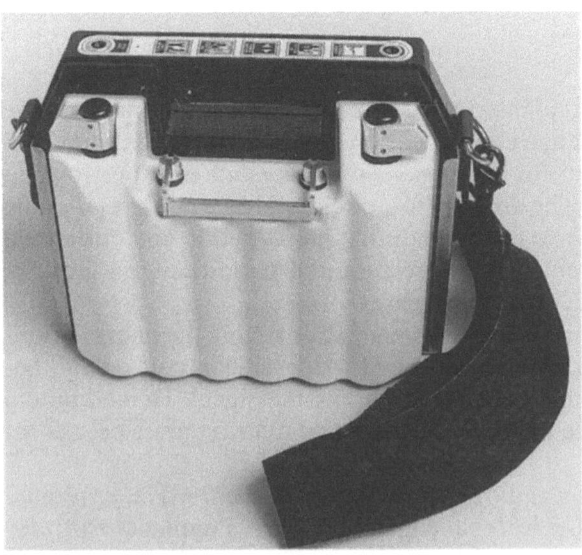

**Fig. 9.** The external battery pack

additional prototypes are manufactured, they will routinely be employed for in vivo experiments.

## In Vivo Studies

A series of 20 calf implants have been performed to evaluate and aid in the development of the 70-cc electric heart [12]. In each instance, a sealed system with implanted compliance chamber and inductively coupled energy transmission has been employed. In general, approximately 3 h of cardiopulmonary bypass time have been required for device implantation. The fit in the chest of a 90-kg Holstein calf has been good. Transition from the heart-lung machine to the electric heart occurs over a 10- to 20-min period. Animals generally stand within a few hours after return to the holding area and have been extubated on the evening of the operative day. Our longest surviving animal using the 70-cc electric artificial heart lived for 5 months (160 days). Major problems in calves who have done poorly relate to postoperative bleeding, pulmonary dysfunction secondary to congestion and pleural effusions, and perioperative infections.

After induction of anesthesia and endotracheal intubation, the animal is maintained on a semi-closed anesthesia system using halothane. After institution of stable cardiopulmonary bypass, the heart is excised. A polyurethane-coated left atrial connector cuff is sutured into place using continuous 4-0 polypropylene suture. Next, the pulmonary artery connector is sutured into place. The aortic connector is then positioned in the field, trimmed to length, and anastomosed using a continuous 4-0 polypropylene suture. The right atrial appendage is excised, and the superior vena cava is opened along its anterior aspect to allow suture of the properly trimmed right atrial connector. Again, continuous suture of 4-0 polypropylene is employed. The electric heart is then brought to the operative field, a subcostal incision is made, and the implanted controller is positioned within the abdominal wall. The secondary coil is positioned over the lower ribs. The atrial and arterial connections to the pump are tightened, and de-airing of the two pumps is accomplished through previously placed catheters. When all air is removed, a pumping is initiated slowly as the heart-lung bypass is weaned. The chest tubes are inserted, and all incisions are closed in a standard fashion.

The animal is then returned to the holding area for immediate postoperative care. The endotracheal tube remains in place until the animal's respiratory function is adequate and hemodynamics are stable. Vital signs and arterial blood gas values are monitored on an hourly basis, and then every 4 h after the animal has stabilized. Once chest tube drainage has fallen below 50 ml/h, a 10% solution of low-molecular-weight dextran is administered. One day after operation, the experimental animal is begun on warfarin sodium sufficient to maintain the prothrombin time at 1.5 times preoperative value. The low-molecular-weight dextran is discontinued after 48 h, but the warfarin sodium is continued for the duration of the experiment. The animal usually begins to eat within the first 24–48 h and is fed a grain mixture as well as ad libitum hay and water.

Experienced personnel observe the experimental animal and administer postoperative care on a 24-h basis. Printouts of total artificial heart system parameters are made at hourly intervals from the system monitor. Other observations, including the time, condition of the animal, and vital signs, are also noted. Complete chemistry and hematology values are entered into a data base using the SAS data management and statistical analysis system.

## In Vivo Results

In general, after the initial postoperative periods, these animals look quite normal. Figure 10 shows calf 98, Lenny, at postoperative day 51. This animal was taken outside on external battery power and then allowed to free roam for 10 min utilizing his internal battery supply. Animal test results for animals surviving greater than 7 days are summarized in Table 3. All animals had sealed systems and were chronically dependent upon energy-transmission systems or implanted batteries. Animals through calf 765 had a percutaneous lead for device monitoring. All subsequent systems have used wireless telemetry. AS can be seen from Table 3, causes of death in the early experience were most often related to failure to recover from the implant procedure. Some of these early deaths may have been related to the use of Jersey calves, which appeared more susceptible to persistant hydrothorax after cardiectomy.

There were five device-related deaths. In one case, valves selected for the left and right pumps were inadvertently switched when the system was packaged for sterilization. Damage at assembly to a controller component prevented the collection of useful diagnostic data in this animal, contributing to his death. In one case, there was corrosion of the stainless screws retaining the hermetic feedthrough to the implanted electronics canister. Leakage currents from the canister were discovered after explant. These currents came from a capacitor whose physical size was larger than that specified by the manufacturer. One

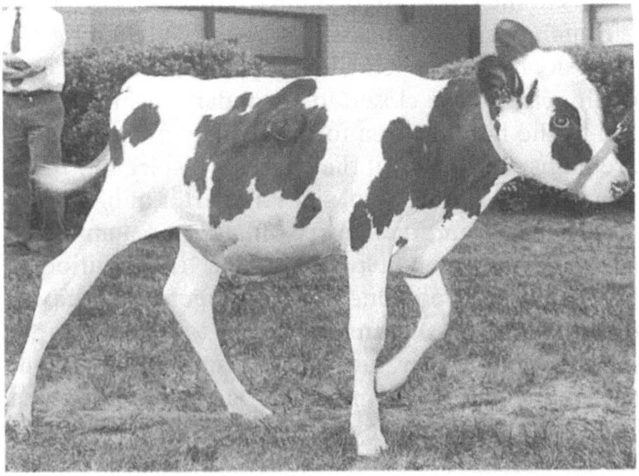

**Fig. 10.** Calf 98, "Lenny", at postoperative day 51 with the totally implanted artificial heart system, running on internal battery

**Table 3.** Total artificial heart implant summary (as of December 17, 1993)

| Calf no. | Operative wt (kg) | Duration (days) | Cause for termination | Necropsy findings |
|---|---|---|---|---|
| 24 | 91 | 8 | Respiratory failure; high PA pressure | Serous fluid in thorax. Adherent valve thrombi × 2. suture line thrombus × 1; small pulmonary embolism |
| B96 | 94 | 13 | Tachypnea, purulent tracheal aspirate | Serous fluid in thorax (lymph); atelectasis; purulence in bronchus |
| 705 | 89 | 15 | Poor caval access, re-operation peripheral nerve damage | Superior vena cava clotted at re-op cannulation site |
| 742 | 103 | 10 | Hemorrhage | LA line dislodged |
| 765 | 91 | 118 | Sepsis | Suture line thrombi × 2; valve junction thrombi × 3; hepatic congestion |
| 18 | 91 | 98 | Perioperative systemic sepsis | Suture line thrombi × 2; right inlet thrombus; vegetation Ao and PA; portal vein thrombus; renal hemorrhagic infarcts |
| 29 | 99 | 160 | Motor stopped | Corrosion, fluid in electronics |
| 86 | 91 | 55 | Multiple resets | Motor conduit disconnected from electronics feedthrough; fluid entered system |
| 98 | 87 | 132 | Multiple resets | Top bearing shifted; rotor magnet deterioration; poor adhesion of conformal coating on stator |
| 118 | 90 | 10 | Respiratory failure | Tracheostomy day 4; atelectasis; necrosis over electronics can |
| 129 | 93 | 10 | Probable CVA | Pulmonary congestion; suture line thrombi |

system had an intraoperative sensor wire failure related to improper system potting. One system was implanted without complete tightening of a conduit clamp; the energy converter wire conduit eventually was dislodged from the canister, permitting body fluid to short sensor connections at the system feedthrough. One system had mechanical rubbing of internal components related to an improperly dimensioned component.

All animals required 21–25 watts at the input to the energy transmission primary in order to provide 8 min of CO. After the initial postoperative period, renal and hepatic function remained well within normal limits. Plasma-free hemoglobin consistently remained below 5 mg/dl. In all of the long-term animals, the central venous pressure became elevated by the 100th postoperative day. This appeared to be a result of CO insufficient for these large animals. Cardiac output indices eventually fell below 50 ml/min/kg.

The in vivo results with the 70-cc electric total artificial heart have been very encouraging. Refinements to manufacturing procedures and assembly procedures have been implemented in an effort to improve device reliability.

## Conclusion

In the past 5 years, a completely implantable 70-cc stroke volume electric total artificial heart has been developed. The complete system, including external battery pack, transcutaneous energy-transmission system, and all sealed implanted components, has been implanted in 20 calves. Four of these animals have survived over 3 months, the longest calf surviving for 160 days. These calves grew normally and maintained normal blood chemistry values throughout the postoperative period. Elevated central venous pressure has been seen in all long-term animals.

Future efforts will be directed towards system refinements and improved manufacturing to provide an extremely reliable device. Extensive reliability testing and expanded in vivo studies are scheduled for the near future.

## References

1. Rosenberg G, Snyder A, Weiss W, Landis D, Geselowitz D, Pierce W (1982) A roller screw drive for implantable blood pumps. Trans Am Soc Artif Intern Organs 28:123
2. Rosenberg G, Cleary T, Snyder A, Landis D, Geselowitz D, Pierce W (1985) A totally implantable artificial heart design. Trans Am Soc Mech Eng 85-WA/DE-11:1–7
3. Pierce W, Rosenberg G, Snyder A, Pae W, Waldhausen J (1990) An electric artificial heart for clinical use. Ann Surg 212:(3)105–110
4. Snyder A, Rosenberg G, Weiss W, Pierce W, Pae W, Marlotte J, Nazarian R, Ford S (1991) A completely implantable total artificial heart system. Trans Am Soc Artif Intern Organs 37:M237–M238
5. Rosenberg G, Pierce W, Landis D, Snyder A, Richenbacher W, Felder G (1984) Progress in the development of the Pennsylvania State University motor-driven artificial heart. In: Unger F (ed) Assisted circulation, vol 2. Springer, Berlin Heidelberg New York, pp 270–285
6. Rosenberg G, Pierce W, Snyder A, Weiss W, Landis D, Pae W, Magovern J (1989) In vivo testing of a roller screw-type electric total artificial heart. In: Unger F (ed) Assisted circulation vol 3. Springer, Berlin Heidelberg New York, pp 385–396
7. Snyder A, Rosenberg G, Reibson J, Donachy J, Prophet G, Arenas J, Daily B, McGary S, Kawaguchi O, Quinn R, Pierce W (1992) An electrically powered total artificial heart: over one year survival in the calf. ASAIO J 38(3):M707–M712
8. Snyder A, Rosenberg G, Landis D (1985) Indirect estimation of circulatory pressures for control of an electric motor-driven total artificial heart. In: Langrana NA (ed) 1985 Advances in bioengineering. The American Society of Mechanical Engineers, New York, pp 87–88
9. Snyder A, Rosenberg G, Pierce W (1992) Non-invasive control of cardiac output for alternately ejecting dual-pusherplate pumps. Artif Organs 16(2):189–194
10. Sherman C, Daly B, Dasse K, Clay W, Szycher M, Handrahan J, Schuder J, Lewis M, Worthington M, Hopkins R, Poirier V (1983) Research and development: systems for transmitting energy through intact skin. Final technical report N01-HV-0-2903-3. Thermo Electron, Waltham
11. Schuder JC, Gold JH, Stephenson HE Jr (1971) An inductively coupled RF system for the transmission of 1 kW of power through the skin. IEEE Trans Biomed Eng BME-18(4)
12. Snyder A, Rosenberg G, Weiss W, Ford S, Nazarian R, Hicks D, Marlotte J, Kawaguchi O, Prophet G, Sapirstein J, Schwartz M, Pierce W (1993) In vivo testing of a completely implanted total artificial heart system. ASAIO J 39:(3) M177–M184

# Total Artificial Heart with High-efficiency Motor-Gear Unit

R. Kaufmann, H. Reul, and G. Rau

## Introduction

Since the first clinical application of a total artificial heart (TAH) by Cooley and Liotta in Houston in 1969 and the subsequent long-term implantations by DeVries in Salt Lake City and Louisville, as well as by Semb in Stockholm in the 1980s about 250 TAHs have been used clinically, mainly in the bridge-to-transplant setting [1]. These pneumatically activated TAHs had a number of potential risk factors such as infection, thromboembolic complications, and bleeding, as well as material degradation. Many of these problems are as yet unsolved. Nevertheless, necessary future development can be clearly outlined: Fully implantable systems including the energy converter have to be developed, fluid mechanics of pump chambers and valves have to be improved, long-term biostability of materials has to be ensured, and adaptive control systems have to be developed. An important step in this direction is currently being undertaken with long-term clinical implants of ventricular assist devices such as those developed by Baxter and Thermo Cardiosystems.

Within an editorial [1] Pantalos developed an optimistic perspective for the TAH by stating that within the next 25 years, carefully designed and controlled clinical trials will demonstrate that the implanted mechanical pumps (both TAH and LVAS) will be as safe, reliable, patient-compatible, and cost-effective as a biological donor heart. In his opinion, clinical trials will bring about reclassification of selected end-stage heart disease patients as cardiac "replacement" candidates rather than cardiac "transplant" candidates. In this scheme, patients will receive either a biological transplant or a mechanical implant.

Despite the fact that world-wide funding in TAH research has decreased over the past 5 years, the spirit and the experience of the pioneers has survived and will help to solve the problems step by step. In this context, our contribution should be regarded as part of an evolutionary process which may hopefully lead to improved patient care and patient survival.

## General Concept

The development of the Helmholtz Total Artificial Heart was initiated in 1990. The target is an orthotopic electromechanical total artificial heart for use as a long-term device for bridging to heart transplantation and, finally, for use as a permanent heart replacement device. The components of this total artificial heart (TAH) system and two main cross sections of the orthotopic pump unit are shown in Fig. 1.

## Transcutaneous Energy Transmitter

The only extracorporeal part is the transcutaneous energy transmitter (TET), which represents known technology [2, 3]. For the TAH a mean power transmission of 20–30 W at 12–15 V is sufficient.

The TET system is fixed by a carrying holster (Fig. 1A) which provides reliable fixation of the DC voltage supply (e.g., NiCd battery packs) and the DC/AC converter. Furthermore, it has to ensure that the primary inductive coupling coil is exactly positioned on the skin surface. Below this position a small implanted secondary coil receives the electrical energy and distributes it to the TAH and the

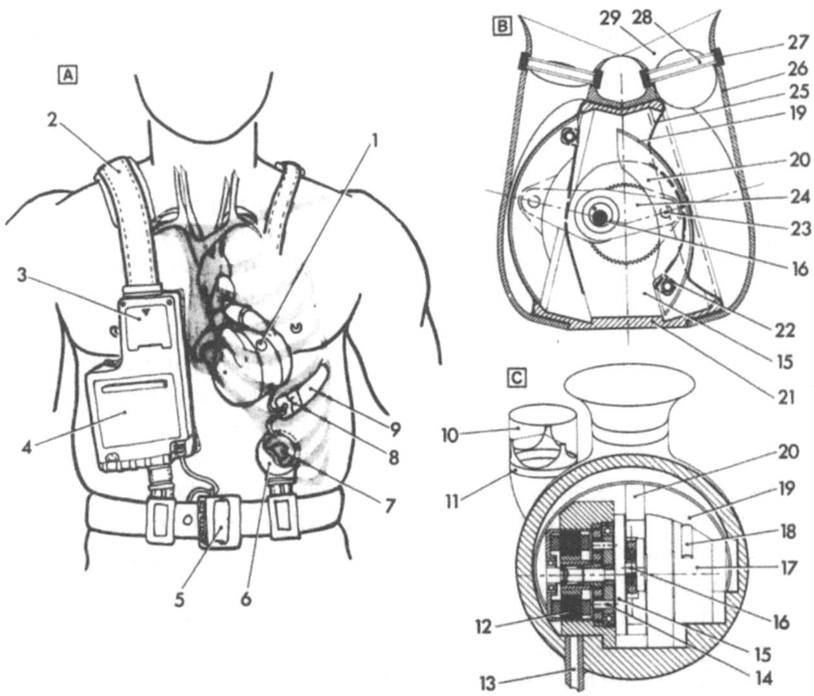


**Fig. 1A–C.** Helmholtz total electromechanical artificial heart system: **A** Overall view of the system components. *1*, Artificial heart (pump unit); *2*, holster; *3*, control display; *4*, exchangeable NiCd battery module; *5*, fastener with integrated diagnostic plugs; *6*, primary transmission coil; *7*, implanted scondary receiver coil; *8*, internal buffer battery; *9*, semi-rigid compliance system. **B** Cross-sectional view in displacement axis plane. *21*, Housing frame; *22*, flat beam spring; *23*, hinge joint pivot; *24*, pusher-plate rod; *25*, diaphragm layers; *26*, pump chamber housing; *27*, quick connector; *28*, atrial disc inlet valve; *29*, atrial sewing cuff. **C** Cross-sectional view perpendicular to *B*. *10*, Arterial sewing cuff; *11*, PUR tri-leaflet outlet valve; *12*, brushless DC motor; *13*, wire cable and compliance vent; *14*, reduction gear; *15*, hypocycloid gear; *16*, excentric crank; *17*, electronic unit; *18*, diaphragm contact sensor; *19*, pusher plate; *20*, pusher plate holder

intracorporeal buffer battery. Some research groups are working on the improvement of rechargable NiCd battery packs. To achieve lifetimes of about 5 years for implanted devices the life of an NiCd buffer battery has to exceed 2000 cycles [4, 5]. Another function of the holster is the fixation of a transcutaneous data interface which connects the external diagnostic control and the intracorporeal control unit of the TAH. For this purpose an infrared transmitter-receiver module has already been tested in vivo by Ahn et al. [6], but many alternative data link concepts are possible and currently under development.

## Orthotopic Pump Unit

Currently, the main development activities at the Helmholtz Institute concern the orthotopic pump unit (Fig. 1B,C) and the implantable compliance system (Fig. 1A), which will be described later. The overall volume of the pump unit is 550 ml. Each pusher plate displaces 65 ml by a 20-mm linear motion. The pump unit is designed for long-term orthotopic and functional replacement of the failed natural heart. This includes an automatic adaptation to changes in organ perfusion demands. The frame of the pump unit consists of a titanium ring which contains motor and gear unit, as well as power and control electronics (Fig. 1B,C). Left and right pump chambers complete the unit and close the housing ring.

Since the anatomically available space is of prime importance, the outer geometry of the artificial heart was developed without a predetermined technical solution for the motor-gear configuration. For the evaluation of available design space for an orthotopic artificial heart an anatomical thoracic model has been generated. For this purpose, data from various sources [7–9] were integrated by means of a CAD [10] system. The use of a CAD system for generating an anatomical model has many advantages. Manipulation of device orientation and collision studies, as well as changes of shape and size, can be performed easily.

The resulting artificial heart design was directly transferred to manufacturing data and CNC programs. The angled displacement axes which result from the above-mentioned anatomical studies are a typical example of this concept. Most other electromechanical devices are cylindrical. The close arrangement of the in- and outlet ports of the pump chambers support the proper fitting of all components under consideration of the anatomical constraints.

A suitable pump chamber concept for the artificial heart was the chamber of the pneumatically driven paracorporeal left ventricular assist pump (LVAP, version IV) which was previously developed at the Helmholtz Institute [11]. This pump provides the required pump characteristics, as well as good flow conditions with a uniform velocity distribution, and generates low shear rates and low hemolysis. A good washout for preventing thrombus formation and proven durability are further advantages. PUR Tri-leaflet valves 23.5 mm in diameter, which are used in the aortic and pulmonary position of the TAH, show extreme low pressure gradients (e.g., 3.8 mmHg at 30 min peak flow [12]). Disc valves 27 mm in diameter are used as inlet valves in the atrial position because of the small anatomical design space.

Recently conducted animal experiments with the further developed Helmholtz LVAD [13] allow first statements on expected TAH biocompatibility of blood-contacting surfaces and diaphragms.

Each diaphragm consists of a safety and a blood-side membrane which is manufactured by thermoforming of 0.15-mm polyurethane foil. The thermoforming mold corresponds to the diaphragm geometry in end-diastolic pusher-plate position. Because of the spherical pusher-plate surface (Fig. 1B), the diaphragm deforms in a circular rolling fold which expands in a concentric way during ejection phase. The pusher plates move the diaphragms into the end-systolic position without strain, due to their exactly adapted sphere radius. The safety membrane takes over most of the mechanical load. To provide a seamless blood-contact surface a biocompatible polyurethane solution is used for the inner coating of the pump chamber. A critical link between artificial device and natural tissue are the sewing cuffs, with their quick-connection systems (Fig. 1B). New quick connectors are currently under development. The compilation of quantitative requirements is very difficult, because these parts have to connect in a reliable way under body environmental conditions. Also, problems of thrombus formation have to be considered, since connectors are a notorious source of this type of complication.

## Energy Converter

### General Requirements

In contrast to the commonly used design of artificial heart components around a highly integrated motor-gear unit, the available space within the housing served as the main design parameter for the motor-gear unit. Besides the self-evident requirements of reliability, lifetime, and biocompatibility, some additional properties of a motor-gear configuration were established.

The displacement gear should be able to transform the unidirectional constant rotational movement of an electric motor into translatory pusher-plate movements. The active adaptation to the organ perfusion demand should be achieved by controlling the rotational speed of the motor. These properties eliminate position and switch devices which decrease reliability. The generated displacement curves should permit output curves similar to those of the natural heart. This leads to a concept with a systolic duration of 40% of the cycle time and a passive filling time of 60%. It is expected that due to venous inflow of blood the diaphragm contacts the resting pusher plate a few milliseconds before displacement begins. Thus, a full-empty mode which supports the washout behavior and a short residence time of blood can be assumed.

### Gear Unit

The requirements of design space, displacement axes, and displacement curves are realized with a combination of three different types of basic gears: First, a planetary wheel for generating a hypocycloid motion; second, two piston rods

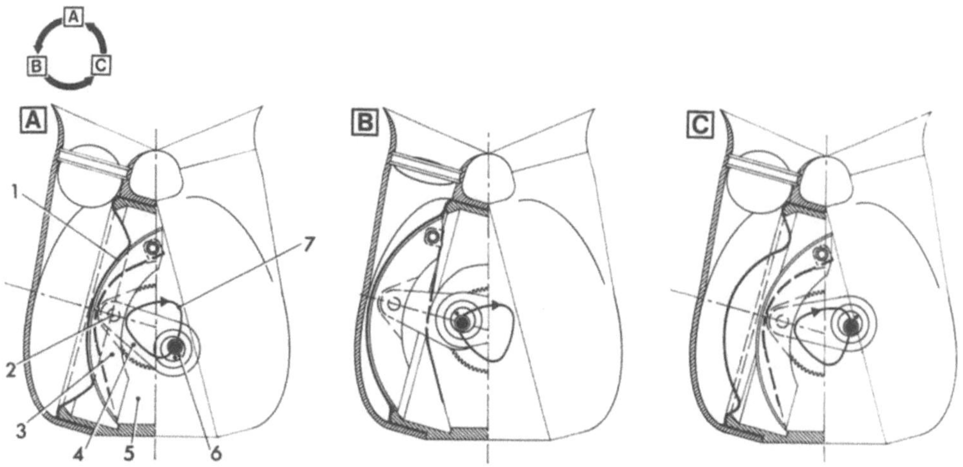


**Fig. 2A–C.** Working cycle, demonstrated for one pump chamber. **A** Transition from resting phase to beginning of ejection phase: *1*, Diaphragm; *2*, hinge joint pivot; *3*, pusher-plate holder; *4*, pusher-plate rod; *5*, motor-gear unit fixation; *6*, excentric crank; *7*, hypocycloid motion curve of the rod bearing. **B** End of ejection phase. **C** Transition from returning to resting phase

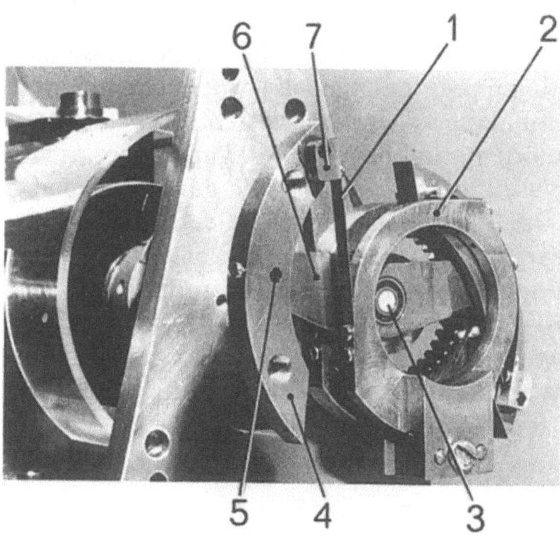


**Fig. 3.** Experimental beam spring configuration of the Helmholtz lab-type TAH. *1*, Flat beam spring; *2*, bending and fixation frame; *3*, excenter crank; *4*, pusher plate holder; *5*, hinge joint pivot; *6*, pusher-plate rod; *7*, beam spring joint

and four flat beam springs which are linked with the pusher-plate holder (Figs. 2, 3); third, a highly integrated reduction gear which increases the torque of a brushless DC mini-motor (Fig. 4).

Both pusher plates are actuated in a phase-shifted (150°), alternating way. One working cycle is schematically demonstrated for the left pump chamber (Fig. 2). The piston rod is excentrically supported within the mentioned planetary wheel and pivoted at the pusher-plate holder by a hinge joint. Additionally, the pusher-plate holder is guided by two flat beam springs on each side (Fig. 3). When the planetary wheel displaces the piston rod (or the pusher plate), the excentric

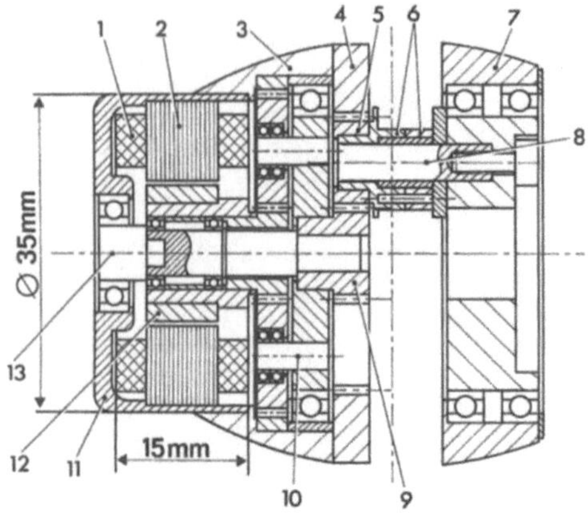


**Fig. 4.** Motor-gear unit: *1*, Stator windings; *2*, lamination stack; *3*, reduction gear frame; *4*, hypocycloid gear frame; *5*, planetary wheel; *6*, excenters; *7*, crank bearing frame; *8*, crank; *9*, central driving wheel; *10*, reduction stage; *11*, motor housing; *12*, rotor with permanent magnets; *13*, main shaft

bearing describes a three-edged hypocycloid [14]. This hypocycloid motion generator provides a special displacement behavior for both pusher plates. The pumping cycle is divided into three phases:

1. Ejection phase (Fig. 2, A–B)
2. Pusher-plate returning phase (Fig. 2, B–C)
3. Pusher-plate resting phase (Fig. 2, C–A)

The last two phases correspond to the pump filling phase which is nearly 60% of the total cycle time. During the resting phase the planetary wheel is in the rear position and the beam springs are bent along a special curve geometry (Fig. 2A). This provides a proper pusher-plate orientation until diaphragm contact occurs again. Currently, a spring metal is used as material for this guiding element. Carbonized fibers are planned for the final device. During ejection phase the beam springs provide a nearly linear motion of the pusher plate. The proper orientation of the pusher plate is supported by the mentioned rolling folds and equilibrium forces due to the hydrostatic pressure distribution within the blood-filled pump chamber. All types of linear sliding guides are eliminated. Therefore, this electromechanical drive system works like clockwork with high inherent system efficiency and low wear and friction effects.

## Motor

Motor and reduction gear were designed as final elements of the energy converter (Fig. 4). The main requirement was the available space for its structural parts. The geometry of the motor-reduction gear unit is determined by the remaining space between the end-diastolic pusher-plate position and the hypocycloid gear unit. The required rated and maximum motor torques at different beat rates were experimentally evaluated in circulatory mock loop tests (see Figs. 5, 6).

Two different types of motors and their principle functions which fulfill the requirement of very high performance per volume have been investigated for use in the TAH. The first appropriate motor type of interest is a piezoelectric ultra-

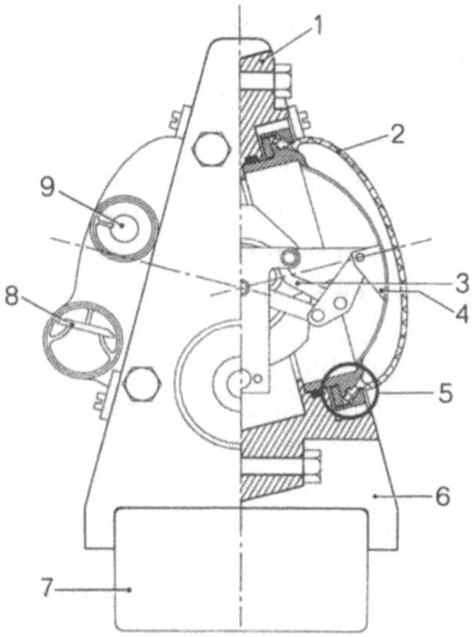


**Fig. 5.** Helmholtz lab-type TAH: *1*, Fixation frame; *2*, pump chamber housing; *3*, experimental gear unit; *4*, pusher plate; *5*, diaphragm-housing junction; *6*, rear plate; *7*, mounting base; *8*, inlet valve; *9*, outlet valve

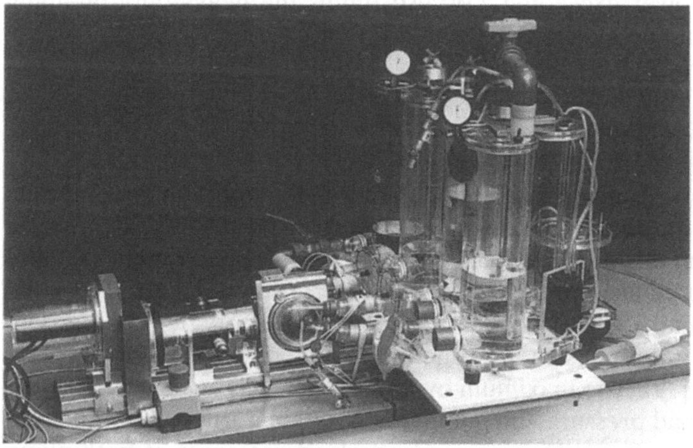

**Fig. 6.** Complete in vitro test bench

sonic traveling-wave motor [15, 16]. The rotor is in contact with the stator where traveling waves are generated by piezoelectric waves. These types of motors commonly have three times higher performance densities than conventional actuators and generate high torques at low rotational speeds, such that reducing gears can be eliminated. A further advantage is the large variety of potential design configurations. However, currently the main disadvantage is the limited lifetime, due to the unsolved problems of material properties of the lining layer between rotor and stator.

The other alternative is brushless DC motors. New developments in the field of permanent magnets and sensorless commutation [17] place this new technology in the foreground. Due to the above-mentioned problems of piezoelectric motors, a DC motor is also our alternative of choice.

In vitro experimental results with the Helmholtz lab-type TAH (see Figs. 5 and 6) accompanied by calculated requirements have been performed for the brushless DC motor design. The results allowed a reliable determination of the performance of the mentioned brushless DC motor for the first in vivo test TAH configuration. A first predesign was made in cooperation with the Laboratory of Electrodynamics and Electrical Machines at the Swiss Federal Institute of Technology, Lausanne. For this purpose a specially developed software was used [18]. The result was an eight-pole sensorless commutated brushless DC motor with an internal rotor. It was built by the ETEL Company, Switzerland. The dimensions and other features of the high-energy density motor are shown in Fig. 4. It is only 35 mm in diameter and 15 mm long, so it fits properly into the remaining space of the pump-unit frame. It produces only 4.5 W thermal losses at a mean motor output power of 13 W. A root mean square (RMS) output torque of 0.05 Nm can be generated within a rotational speed range from 1400 to 2500 rpm. Together with the highly integrated reduction gear (Fig. 4), with a reduction ratio of 18 and an estimated efficiency of 95% an RMS torque of 0.85 Nm can be achieved. The motor with a rated power exceeding 7 W also fulfills the heavy-duty pumping mode at 120 beats/min and 120 mmHg mean afterload.

## TAH Control

The task of the final artificial heart control system is the adaptation of pump rate and finally of pump output to ensure sufficient organ perfusion. The choices made in control system design and adjustment generally depend on one or more parameters which can be used to determine body perfusion demands.

Furthermore, the final TAH control has to ensure full-empty pumping at both pump chambers. A comprehensive introduction to different control concepts is given by Ruchti et al. [19]. The maximum overall efficiency is achieved when the relation between preload pressure and pump rate is within normal limits and full-empty pumping is maintained. The pre- and afterload pressures at both pump chambers can be used as input parameters. In a first approach a Fuzzy-Control system was built that uses an indirect method to detect left atrial pressure, which again controls pumping speed and output. In general, this concept follows the ideas of other groups [20–22] which try to simulate Frank-Starlings law: "High venous returns cause an increase of cardiac output." The difference in TAH control is that the increasing ventricular stroke volume of the natural heart is replaced by pump rate acceleration of the artificial heart. First in vitro test results are presented below.

## Compliance System

A compliance chamber system with a mainly rigid housing which does not traumatize surrounding tissues has been designed. It consist of two parts:

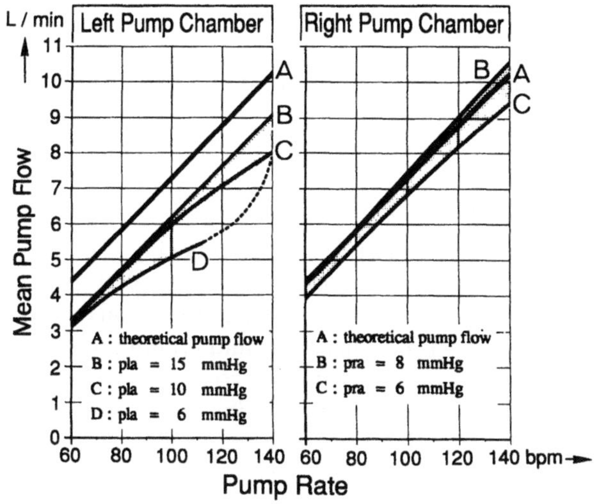


**Fig. 7.** Mean left and right output flows at different preloads

- A semi-rigid mean pressure compensator (MPC) which contains 70 ml of a hydraulic fluid (e.g., silicone oil)
- A very small compliance chamber (CC) with a volume of 25 ml

Both parts are connected via a special adjustment throttle through which fluid can pass from one compartment to the other. The MPC compensates long-term changes of internal gas pressure wich may be due to atmospheric pressure changes or other environmental pressure effects. The CC compensates short-term changes of gas volume caused by pump action. First in vitro experiments with a simple compliance system showed that the internal gas pressure oscillated between ±10 mmHg. With a lab-type TAH (see next paragraph) it was proven that the pump performance was similar to performances which are obtained with open-vented artificial hearts (Fig. 7). Compliance development is only beginning, but the first tests are of great promise.

## Experimental Results

For first in vitro testing a Helmholtz lab-type TAH was built at an early stage of development as a necessary tool for the development and design procedure. The lab type provides some of the most important features of the final artificial heart. Together with data from computer-assisted simulation, the experimental investigation will eventually lead to an iterative improvement of the quantitative synthesis of all structural parts and groups. Current in vitro testing is carried out by means of a lab-type version with a theoretical stroke volume of 73 ml [10]. The above-mentioned beam springs are replaced by a previously developed linkage gear for linear pusher-plate guiding (Fig. 5). The following functional characteristics and design elements are implemented:

- Internal pump chamber design including diaphragm and pusher-plate design
- Pusher-plate kinematics (e.g., resting phases and angled displacement axes)

- Different valve types of interest (currently, Björk-Shiley Monostrut or PUR Tri-leaflet valves)
- Totally sealed housing frame coupled with different types of compliance chambers
- Sensors and pump performance-control systems (conventional and fuzzy based)
- Other structural parts in different stages of development

The housing of this lab type essentially consists of four elements (Fig. 5):

Two semi-fixation frames for the pump chamber units, one rear plate with a sealed passage for the driving shaft of the externally located experimental electric motor, and one transparent front plate with measurement and compliance connectors. Each pump chamber unit represents a separate structural group. It consists of housing and diaphragm fixed on a mounting ring. Additionally, it contains Björk-Shiley monostrut valves 27 and 23 mm in diameter used as in- and outflow valves, respectively. Other valve types can be easily tested as well. The pump chamber unit exhibits high flexibility for the experimental investigation of different structural parts. The test setup further consists of a PC for data acquisition, motor speed control, and sensor control testing. As shown in Fig. 6, it also contains measurement equipment and energy supply, an experimental drive unit (RS-11 6001C, Harmonic Drive GmbH, Limburg, Germany), and a driving torque measurement instrument (IT 5 w-n, Staiger Mohilo & Co GmbH, Schorndorf, Germany).

Each pump chamber of the lab-type TAH is coupled with a left or right mock circulation. A 36% water-glycerol mixture is used as the test fluid. The design of the mock loops has been published previously [23]. Left and right in- and outflow curves are measured with inductive flow probes (CA 24 mm, Zepeda Instruments, Seattle, WA, USA), and pressure curves are measured with DMS probes (CDX III, Cobe Laboratories GmbH, Heimstetten, Germany). Finally, an experimental compliance chamber coupled with the sealed lab-type housing is used for compliance measurements and simulation. The main areas of current investigation are:

- Measurement of pump performance depending on pre- and afterload, pump rate, pump chamber geometry, diaphragm, and valve types
- Measurement of pulsatile pressure and flow
- Visualization of flow within the pump chamber
- Investigation of volume compensation characteristics for reducing or even omitting the implantable compliance chamber
- Testing of control sensors and control concepts
- Functional testing of all structural parts

## Measurement of Pump Performance

The primary application goal of an artificial heart is to ensure sufficient blood perfusion of all organs. Therefore, the mean pump flow performance (cardiac output) of an artificial heart is of most interest and has been tested first [24]. The mean pump flow of each pump chamber of the lab type was investigated as a function of pump rate and pre- and afterload pressures (Fig. 7). During those tests the lab type was operated with a housing frame vented to atmospheric pressure. Therefore, all compliance effects such as negative pressures behind the diaphragms are absent.

The mean flow was determined by averaging the flow curves measured by inductive flow probes behind the left and right outflow valves. The shaded areas in Fig. 7 represent mean pump flows which were generated at different preloads or filling pressures. In this study, for all pump rates the afterload conditions were kept constant at a mean pressure of 100 mmHg and 18 mmHg for the left and the right pump chamber, respectively. The "A" lines in Fig. 7 represent the theoretical mean pump flows. They are calculated by multiplying theoretical stroke volume and pump rate and are identical for both chambers. At 15 mmHg filling pressure the maximum pump flow of the left chamber is about 0.7 l/min lower than the theoretical mean pump flow. The mean pump flow decreases with a reduction of the left filling pressure. At 6 mmHg preload and pump rates above 120 beats/min, a mean pump flow above 5.3 l/min cannot be achieved due to limited filling. Despite this effect, the organ perfusion can be ensured. At 10 mmHg preload a mean pump flow of 8.3 l/min can be obtained easily at 140 beats/min. The right pump achieves significantly higher flows than the left pump. At 6 mmHg filling pressure the flow is only 0.5 l/min below the theoretical pump flow. At 8 mmHg the pump flow even exceeds the theoretical pump flow due to dynamic effects like filling during ejection phase. The left-right balance was not the aim of this first study, but the results give quantitative criteria for reducing the theoretical stroke volume of the right pump chamber to obtain a balance. Furthermore, the results show the advantages of the resting phase of the pusher plates, which provides better free filling.

From an engineering point of view, the next point of interest was the mechanical power to generate the previously described pump outputs [24]. These data were the basis for the development of a brushless DC motor. For these measurements the preloads were 10 and 6 mmHg for left and right pump, respectively. The afterload conditions were kept unchanged. The input work at the motor shaft was calculated by integration of the torque curves which were recorded by

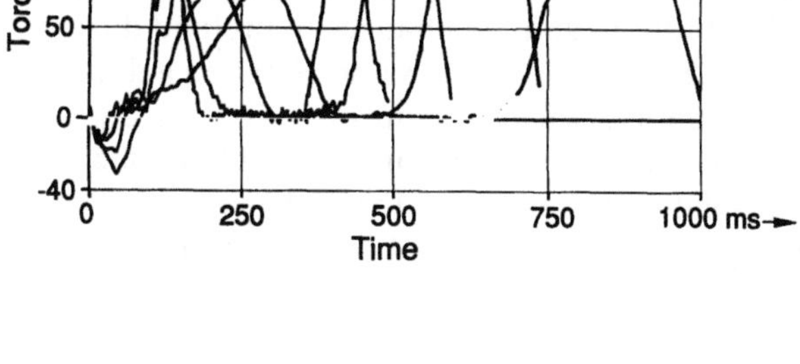


**Fig. 8.** Gear output shaft torque (validated in vitro)

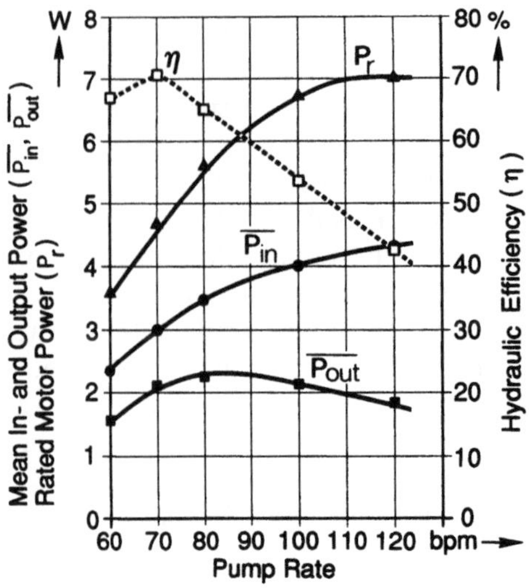


**Fig. 9.** Mean in- and output power, rated motor power, and hydraulic efficiency

a torque meter. The torque curves have two characteristic peaks (Fig. 8) for left and right ejection. Because of the phase-shifted pusher-plate kinematics, there is a certain time period with zero torque during each cycle. The zero torque period is a function of beat rate. During torque measurements left and right output flows and pressure curves downstream of the outlet valves were also measured and used for the calculation of the hydraulic efficiency of all active structural pump parts between gear unit drive shaft and outlet valves [24]. The energy for fluid acceleration was disregarded because its overall part of the whole energy output is only 1%. The hydraulic efficiency reaches its maximum of 70% at 70 beats/min pump rate. At higher pump rates it decreases due to the decrease of the mean output power and the increase of the mean input power (Fig. 9). The rated motor power, which is defined as the mean square root of the actual input power, is also depicted in Fig. 9. It was an important criteria for the brushless DC motor design. The value of 65–70% for hydraulic efficiency at 60–80 beats/min is remarkably high. It demonstrates the high efficiency of the gear system concept of the Helmholtz lab-type TAH.

## Testing of Control Sensors and Control Concepts

In a first test protocol the simulated left atrial pressure (LAP) was changed suddenly and randomly in steps, e.g., 5, 15, 10, 15, 5 mmHg (Fig. 10). The LAP alternations were generated by a displacement volume which was pushed into the open atrial fluid reservoir of the mock circulation. Figure 10 shows, in the upper panel, the fast adaptation of the beat rate to sudden changes in preload during a test cycle of 700 s. The lower panel of Fig. 10 shows the same effect on a different time scale. Adaptation to increased preload is achieved during 4–8 beats, depending on the preload level (see dots on lower curves of Fig. 10). Preload decrease may cause a slow filling and pusher-plate interference with the diaphragm. Therefore, the decrease of pump rate is generated in only 2–4 beats (Fig. 10).

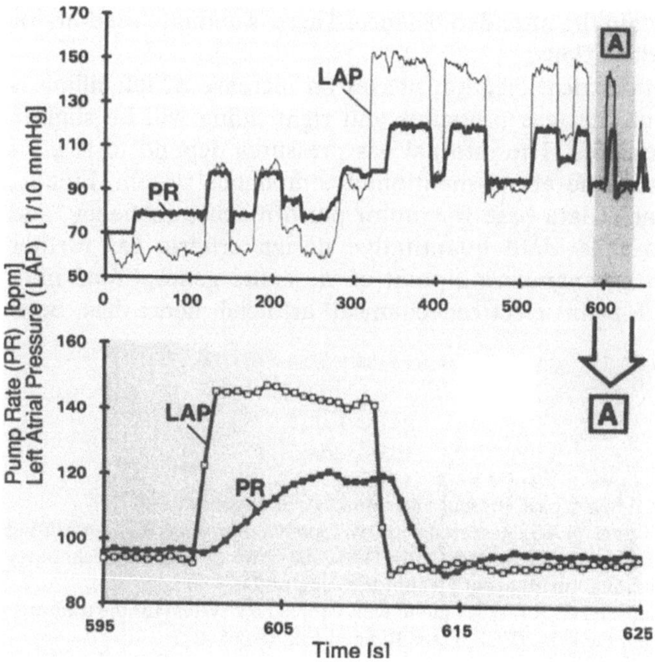


**Fig. 10.** In vitro results of automatic fuzzy-based preload output control. *A (lower panel)*, Increased time scale depiction of window *A* in upper panel; *LAP*, left atrial pressure; *PR*, pump rate

# Discussion

The tests presented and measurements obtained are examples to demonstrate the usefulnes of a lab-type TAH as a developmental tool for an advanced version of a total artificial heart and especially its energy converter. Out of the broad range of tests and studies conducted, selected results are presented which serve for the solution of specific aspects. At 10 mmHg left atrial preload and passive filling a mean pump flow of 5 l/min can be easily obtained at a pump rate of 80 beats/min (Fig. 7). If the reduced stroke volume of 65 ml of the final device is taken into account, this flow is obtained at 90 beats/min. The most surprising result is the high hydraulic efficiency values of about 70% at 60–80 beats/min (Fig. 9). This effect can be related to the resting phase of the pusher plates, which provides better free filling. The application of Fuzzy-Control and first in vitro testing results concerning automatic pump output control prove the feasibility of this control method. The novel gear unit which transforms a uniform, unidirectional rotational motor movement into translatory pusher-plate movements with resting phase in end-diastolic position is the most important feature of the Fuzzy-Control concept.

Since the geometries of left and right pump chambers are identical in the current lab-type version, a left-right-balance cannot be expected, but the results give quantitative design criteria for reducing the theoretical stroke volume of the right pump chamber to obtain the intended balance. There is enough freedom for right-chamber design modifications.

Because of the nonsymmetrical ejection phases an increase of left filling is expected with negative internal gas pressures and right filling will be slightly decreased by positive pressures. The internal gas pressures depend to a great extent on the adjustment of the above-mentioned compliance system. Finally, the results provide a reliable data base for motor performance, efficiency, and energy consumption and thus yield quantitative design criteria for further development steps. From an engineering point of view, the general feasibility of the overall concept for an electromechanical artificial heart has been demonstrated.

## References

1. Pantalos GM (1993) Artificial heart: past, present and future. Artif Organs 10:826–827
2. Sherman C, Daly B, Dasse K et al. (1983) Research and development of systems for transmitting energy through intact skin. Final technical report (N01-HV-0-2903-3) for devices and technology branch, DHVD, NHLBI. National Institutes of Health, Washington DC
3. Schuder JC, Gold JH, Stephenson HE (1971) An inductively coupled RF system for the transmission of 1 kW of power through the skin. IEEE Trans Biomed Eng 18:265–273
4. Powers RA, Wolga AE, Ochs BD, Yu LS, Kung RTV (1993) Life testing of implantable batteries for a total artificial heart. ASAIO J 39:M663–M667
5. MacLean GK, Aiken PA, Adams WA, Mussivand T (1993) Evaluation of nickel-cadmium battery packs for mechanical circulatory support devices. ASAIO J 39:M423–M426
6. Ahn JM, Kang DW, Kim HC, Min BG (1993) In vivo performance evaluation of a transcutaneous energy and information transmission system for the total artificial heart. ASAIO J 39:M208–M212
7. Fujimoto LK, Jacobs GB, Przypyz J et al. (1984) Human thoracic anatomy based on computed tomography for development of a totally implantable left ventricular assist system. Artif Organs 4:436–444
8. Fujimoto LK, Smith WA, Jacobs GB et al. (1985) Anatomical considerations in the design of a long-term implantable human left ventricle assist system. Artif Organs 4:361–374
9. Carter BL, Morehead J, Wolpert SM, Hammerschlag SB, Griffiths HJ (1977) Cross-sectional anatomy, computed tomography and ultrasound correlation. Appleton Century Croft, New York
10. Kaufmann R, Reul H, Rau G (1992) Electromechanical artificial heart with a new gear type and angled pump chambers. Int J Artif Organs 8:481–487
11. Knierbein B (1990) Konstruktion, Fertigung und Test von pneumatisch angetriebenen Membranpumpen zur Herzunterstützung. Thesis, University of Aachen, p 170
12. Eilers R, Harbott P, Reul H, Rakhorst G, Rau G (1994) Design improvements of the HIA-VAD based on animal experiments. Artif Organs 7:473–478
13. Rakhorst G, Hensens AG et al. (1992) Evaluation of a protocol for animal experiments with Helmholtz left ventricular assist devices. Cor Eur 4:155–159
14. Kaufmann R, Reul H, Rau G, Bitdinger R (1993) Pulsierend arbeitende Blutpumpe der Forschungsgesellschaft für Biomedizinsche Technik (German patent no DE 41 29 970)
15. Schadebrodt G, Salomon B (1990) The piezo travelling wave motor – a new drive element in actuation. AEG Press Release (pri 9973e/1990)
16. Tomikawa Y, Ogasawara T (1989) Ultrasonic motors – constructions/characteristics/applications. Ferroelectrics 91:163–178
17. Jufer M (1992) Smart motor technology – advantages and performance comparison. Report 92/205 of Laboratory of Electromechanics and Electrical Machines. Swiss Federal Institute of Technology

18. Perriard Y (1992) Methodologie de conception d'activateurs pour ventricule d'assistance cardiaque implantable. Thesis no 1085, Ecole Polytechnique Federale de Lausanne
19. Ruchti TL, Brown RH, Jeutter DC, Feng X (1993) Identification for systemic arterial parameters with application to total artificial heart control. Ann Biomed Eng 21:221–236
20. Rosenberg G, Landis DL, Donachy JH, Brighton JA, Stallsmith J, Pierce WS (1979) Design of the Pennsylvania State University artificial heart and electronic automatic control system. In: Unger F (ed) Assisted circulation. Springer, Berlin Heidelberg New York, pp 344–352
21. Takatani S, Harasaki H, Suwa S, Murabayashi S, Sukalac R, Jacobs G, Kiraly G, Nosé Y (1981) Pusher-plate type TAH system operated in the left and right free-running variable rate mode. Artif Organs 2:132–142
22. Kung RTV, Ochs B (1991) Self-regulation of an electrohydraulic total artificial heart In: Akutsu T, Koyanagi H (eds) Artificial heart, vol 3. Springer, Berlin Heidelberg New York, pp 173–181
23. Knierbein B, Reul H, Eilers R, Lange R, Kaufmann R, Rau G (1992) Compact mock loops of the systemic and pulmonary circulation for blood pump testing. Int J Artif Organs 1:40–48
24. Kaufmann R, Reul H, Rau G (1994) The Helmholtz total artificial heart labtype. Artif Organs 7:537–542

# Part VI
# Cardiac Transplantation

# Introduction

F. Unger

It is now nearly 30 years ago that Christian Barnard performed the first human cardiac transplantation in South Africa. Today it is indispensible in treating end-stage cardiac failure. In 1993, 2500 hearts were transplanted in Europe. The major difficulties involve harvesting donor organs and chronic rejection. There are also certain restraints concerning newborns and very old patients. In addition to all the technical activities, the ethical issues have taken on new social importance, and a serious philosophical basis for harvesting must be established. The present definitions of brain death are no longer sufficient.

The five-year survival rates for cardiac transplantation are excellent. Based on these good results, the technique was expanded to en bloc heart-lung transplantation. Nataf et al. report on heart transplantation at La Pitie in France, Haverich and Karck report on a special problem in pulmonary reperfusion, especially in clinical lung transplantation, and Cooper brings up the idea of xenotransplantation, which poses a very special challenge for overcoming the entire rejection mechanism.

# Heart Transplantation: Current Experience at La Pitié, Paris

P. Nataf, I. Gandjbakhch, A. Pavie, V. Bors, R. Dorent, M. Desruennes, P. Leger, E. Vaissier, J.P. Levasseur, A. Cabrol, J. Szefner, and C. Cabrol

## Introduction

Clinical application of heart transplantation goes beyond 25 years of experience. Advances in the detection of early rejection, improvement of organ preservation procedures, and introduction of new immunosuppressive therapy protocols have allowed dramatic progress in the results of heart transplantation. This analysis reviews the results of more than 800 heart transplantations performed in our department since 1968 and describes several particular procedures used in our transplantation program.

## Recipient Selection

Potential candidates for the procedure are patients with end-stage heart disease and limited life expectancy. Ultimately, a transplant must be considered when the patient is in stage IV or IIIb and, in the case of failure, refractory to all medical treatment, with no other therapeutic possibility.

Classical medical treatment, consisting in a low sodium diet, digitalis and diuretics, the use of vasodilatators and, more particularly, calcium inhibitors and angiotensin II inhibitors by improving in a substantial way the functional status and the survival of these patients, has delayed the necessity for surgical intervention. However, it is necessary to avoid reaching a stage of global cardiac insufficiency with anasarca and irreversible pulmonary, renal, or hepatic lesions.

The supervention of an acute irreversible cardiac failure, limiting the survival from a few hours to a few days does not often allow a compatible graft to be found in such a short time. In these cases circulatory assistance by extracorporeal artificial ventricles, or especially by a fully implantable-type Jarvik 7 artificial heart, may allow the circulation to be maintained until a graft becomes available.

Acquired experience allows us to discount other patients who would not benefit from transplantation. Although some classical contraindications are neglected, such as small infections, gastrointestinal disorders, non-insulin-dependent diabetes, and absolute age limits, a few remain absolute: severe pulmonary hypertension, uncontrolled infection, refractory gastroduodenal ulcer or severe colic diverticulosis, as well as systemic illness, recent malignancies, or diffuse amyloidosis.

The most common absolute contraindication is the existence of pulmonary hypertension due to the irreversible elevation of pulmonary vascular resistance. Pulmonary hypertension can be responsible for a severe failure of the right ventricle immediately after the transplantation in the operating room or in the intensive care unit.

The degree of acceptable pulmonary artery hypertension or vascular resistance is difficult to define [1]. Our present policy, in the presence of an elevated pulmonary vascular resistance (PVR), is to evaluate its severity as precisely as possible at the first pretransplant examination and to appreciate the importance of a spasmodic factor (a 20% fall or more in PVR after vasodilatator tests demonstrates this effect). It is important to carefully and regularly follow its evolution by echo Doppler during the period before transplantation in order to detect any progressive increase which necessitates urgent transplantation.

If the PVR is equal to or less than 6 Wood units (WU) an orthotopic transplantation is performed and usually is successful. A PVR between 6 and 8 WU indicates, rather than a heterotopic procedure, an orthotopic procedure with an oversized donor, with a vigorous heart (necessitating no drug), and preferably harvested on site in order to shorten its ischemic time. For patients with more than 8–10 WU a heart-lung transplant is preferable.

The register of the International Society for Heart and Lung Transplantation [2] in 1993 shows that the patients concerned are more often affected by idiopathic cardiomyopathies (50%) or ischemic heart disease (43%). Only 4% of heart transplant recipients have valvular disease. In our series, the main indications for cardiac transplantation remain idiopathic cardiomyopathies – 41%, and ischemic diseases – 40% [3, 4]. However, their relative incidences have varied before and after 1986 (Fig. 1). Out of indications for myocardial dysfunction after neglected valvular disease, which remain rare because of early treatment of valvulopathies, new indications have appeared such as retransplantation for early graft failure, irreversible acute rejection, or graft arteriosclerosis. These retransplantation procedures concerned 24 patients in our series.

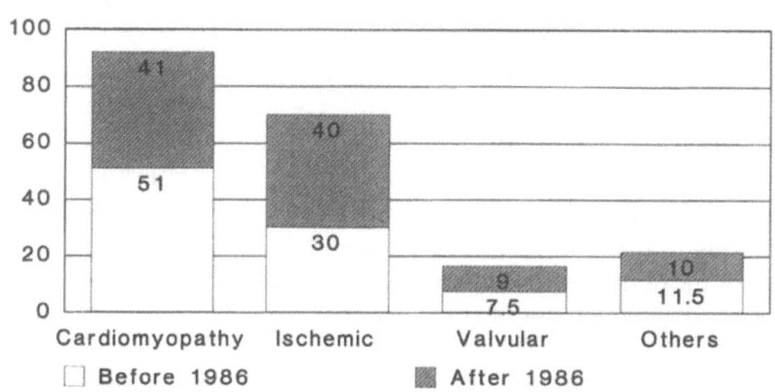


**Fig. 1.** Number of patients per indication leading to heart transplantation at La Pitié before and after 1986

Other indications were hypertrophic cardiomyopathies ($n$ = 28), congenital diseases ($n$ = 20), and restrictive cardiomyopathies ($n$ = 13) due to toxic myocarditis, amyloidosis, or systemic diseases.

## Donor Organs and Myocardial Protection

It has become more and more difficult to obtain a suitable donor due to the increase of transplantations performed and shortage of donors. Because of the donor shortage, the quality of the graft can be diminished by the necessity to accept older donors (more than 50 years). Provided that the function of the heart is carefully assessed, the use of such donors can be quite satisfactory.

Investigations to improve myocardial preservation should also be performed [5–8].

In 1989, we introduced a blood cardioplegia and warm reperfusion protocol in our heart transplantation program. More than 300 grafts were preserved with this method and cardiac recovery was significantly better with this method when compared with standard crystalloid myocardial protection [9].

Cardioplegia induction on the donor graft is performed with a perfusion of cold crystalloid solution (PLEGISOL, Abbott Laboratories). After excision, the heart is transferred in an isothermic container maintaining a constant temperature between 4° and 6°C without ice contact (TRANSPLANTHERMM, cardicorp S.A).

Perfusion of a first dose of blood for cardioplegia is immediately started on the arrival of the graft in the operating room. Cardiac reperfusion of a half dose of blood solution without potassium is performed every 20 min. Myocardial warm reperfusion is started before aortic declamping.

## Results and Postoperative Course

In our series of orthotopic heart transplantations [3], in-hospital mortality (1 month) was 26%. This rate was 14% for the 340 ambulatory patients under age 55 years who had no history of previous cardiac surgery (Fig. 2).

Multiple organ failure (49%) was the main cause of in-hospital mortality. Early graft failure occurred in 22% of patients, infection in 14%, pulmonary embolism in 7%. A technical problem was the cause of death in 8% of patients. Several variables were significantly associated with an increased operative mortality (age >55; ischemic cardiomyopathy; retransplantation; heterotopic heart transplantation; previous operation; circulatory assist device; see Table 1). For 280 patients with two or more of these risk factors, in-hospital mortality was 36%.

Rejection is rarely observed in the early days post transplantation because "hyperacute rejection" resulting from the presence of cytotoxic antibodies directed against the donor lymphocytes is avoided, either by performing a pretransplant direct cross-match (recipient serum against donor lymphocytes), or by detecting the presence and calculating the percentage of reactive antibodies in

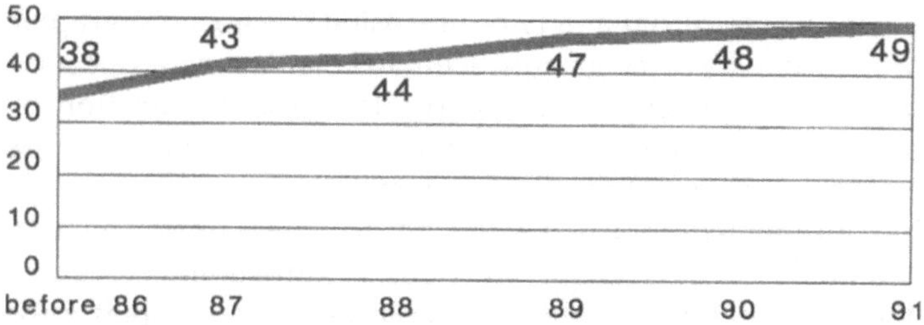


**Fig. 2.** Evolution of heart transplant recipients' mean age from prior to 1986 and up to 1991. For patients >55 years, $n = 245$; for patients >60, $n = 96$

**Table 1.** Heart transplantation at La Pitié – risk factors

| Factor | *p* |
|---|---|
| Age > 55 | <0.05 |
| Ischemia | <0.05 |
| Retransplantation | <0.001 |
| Heterotopic Tx. | <0.001 |
| Previous operation | <0.05 |
| Inotropic drugs | <0.001 |
| Mechanical circulatory assistance | <0.001 |

the recipient serum tested against a panel of potential donor lymphocytes. Recently, however, hyperacute rejection has occurred despite a compatible direct lymphocytotoxic cross-match [10]. In such cases the recipient's serum contained cytotoxic antibodies against a panel of endothelial cells. Unfortunately, the detection of such antibodies is not yet possible for clinical application, although plasmaphereses can prevent their consequences.

Acute rejection is a constant threat from the fifth postoperative day through the first year. At our center, cyclosporin A (CsA) considerably decreased the frequency and severity of rejection overall.

In most cases, CsA suppressed the usual clinical, electrical, and hemodynamic symptoms of rejection. Early diagnosis of rejection, which is so important to counteract the short- and long-term consequences of such lesions, remains a current problem in cardiac transplantation.

Presently, the only way to be certain of an ongoing rejection is a histological diagnosis (which, unfortunately, is an invasive method) by introducing a cardiac bioptome percutaneously and obtaining a small piece of right ventricular endomyocardium. Microscopic examination will reveal important lymphocyte infiltration and myocyte necrosis.

Many noninvasive methods are being evaluated, such as cytoimmunologic monitoring or urinary polyamine measurements. Simpler methods, such as the detection of changes in cardiothoracic ratio and cardiac volume on conventional chest X-rays, may be helpful [11]. Serial and two-dimensional echocardiographic findings, considered worthwhile by some groups, seem to correlate with rejection episodes [12]. Interestingly, in our experience, early detection of rejection by echo Doppler studies (isovolumic relaxation time and pressure half-time) is quite satisfactory and is now our routine technique for rejection control [13].

Secondary infections, although diminished with CsA, have remained frequent. They are bacterial pneumonia but also fungal infections. Careful donor screening is essential to avoid the frequent transmission of diseases such as toxoplasmosis and cytomegalovirus (CMV) infection.

The treatment of CMV can benefit by early detection with a CMV antigen test and by use of an antiviral agent: DHPG [14].

Whatever, the cause of pulmonary infection, its identification is often difficult and may require special tests, e.g., tracheal aspiration, fine-needle aspiration biopsy, and bronchoalveolar lavage.

Another concern in using CsA is nephrotoxicity, which can be acute during the first postoperative days. It is more common in sick patients with functional renal insufficiency due to a long-lasting cardiac failure treated with diuretics. Renal damage develops rapidly, causing oliguria, anuria, and death. This side effect prompted us as early as 1981 to follow two principles for immediate immunosuppression therapy: First, delayed use of CsA until the patient's renal function and hemodynamics improve; second, use of CsA in low doses.

However, the ideal immunosuppressive regimen is still to be determined. Our present postoperative protocol consists of azathioprine (1–2 mg/kg/day) and a 5-day course of rabbit antilymphocyte globulin (2.5 mg/kg/day), which are started after the operation. CsA therapy is gradually started to achieve a CsA serum level of 200 ng/ml–300 mg/ml. Corticosteroids are administered (1 mg/kg/day) on the fifth postoperative day. When rejection occurs, high doses of steroids and the use of antithymocyte globulin may be required.

## Late Complications

Careful early use off CsA almost suppressed the early nephrotoxic complications, but chronic nephrotoxicity is still observed. This is demonstrated by an elevated serum creatinine level, more pronounced in older patients and aggravated by the used of nephrotoxic antibiotics sometimes used to treat severe infection (Fig. 3). These lesions are characterized histologically by tubular atrophy and interstitial fibrosis without glomerular alteration and can be prevented by using low doses of CsA. Nevertheless, if they appear, they are potentially reversible by discontinuing CsA and switching to a more conventional therapy [16]. The experimental and clinical use of a new analog of CsA, cyclosporin G, was not really advantageous [17]. FK 506 is being investigated.

The systemic hypertension (Fig. 4) observed at 5 years in almost all patients treated with CsA also remains a threat; despite extensive studies by our group and others [18], we have been unable to find any alteration of the renin angiotensive system or of the aldosterone level, and the only abnormal finding

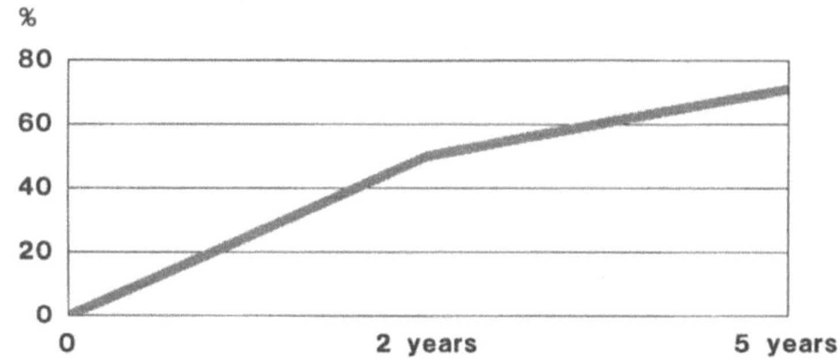


**Fig. 3.** Incidence of renal insufficiency following heart transplantation. Risk factors: age >40 years, nephrotoxic antibiotics. Postoperative dialyzed patients: 1.4%

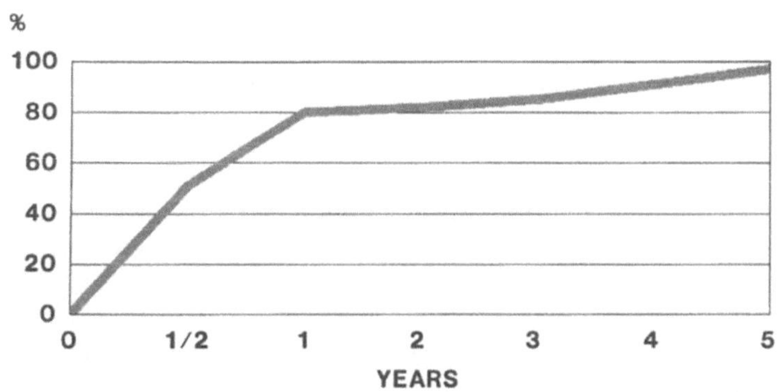


**Fig. 4.** Incidence of systemic hypertension following heart transplantation

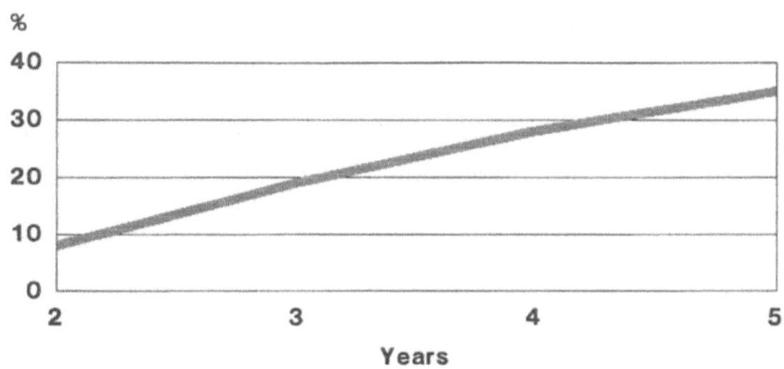


**Fig. 5.** Incidence of coronary lesions following heart transplantation among 374 coronary artery angiographies

was a persistent hypervolemia. This systemic hypertension is best treated by administration of calcium channel blockers.

Finally, one of the most intriguing and dangerous problems in cardiac transplantation is the occurrence of occlusive coronary lesions (Fig. 5). We must

**Table 2.** Rheumatic complications after heart transplantation at La Pitié

| Complication | Percent |
|---|---|
| Gout | 17 |
| Hyperuricemia | 76 |
| Hip necrosis | 3.8 |
| Vertebral osteoporosis | 4.9 |

**Table 3.** Malignancies after heart transplantation at La Pitié

| | Percent |
|---|---|
| Lymphoma | 1.2 |
| Skin cancer | 10 |
| Others | 2.9 |

distinguish between lesions already present on the donor heart (such as coronary atherosclerosis) or lesions induced during transplantation (such as coronary embolism) and three types of coronary artery lesions seen in our series after transplantation: early inflammatory arteritis, late obliterative fibrous arteritis, and late atherosclerosis.

Early inflammatory arteritis occurs on the small coronary arteries generally between 3 and 18 months after transplantation. It is characterized by lymphocyte infiltration, arteritis, and sometimes thrombosis. Its etiology is immunological and it represents a rejection lesion that is potentially reversible [19]. Late obliterative fibrous arteritis usually occurs 2 years post transplantation on large and medium-sized vessels. The lesions are essentially fibrosis of the intima with disruption of the media without lymphocyte infiltration. It possibly represents the end stage of inflammatory arteritis, and it is slowly progressive. Late atherosclerosis usually occurs 2 years after transplantation on the large coronary arteries. The lesions are essentially fibrotic, with atheromatous deposits similar to the usual coronary atheroma. They are the same lesions previously described (late obliterative fibrous arteritis) in patients with high-risk factors for atheroma, which infiltrate these lesions with lipidic plaques. The angiographic appearence is typical, with diffuse multiple distal lesions. It is rapidly progressive, silent (without angina) in the denervated heart, and detected only by routine coronary angiography. It usually cannot be treated by coronary artery bypass and requires retransplantation. The frequency are severity is a major threat to transplantation and deserve future research, in which the nutritional status of transplant patients must be considered [20].

Several other late complications are observed. Tables 2 and 3 show the frequency of rheumatic complications and malignancies after heart transplantation noted in our series.

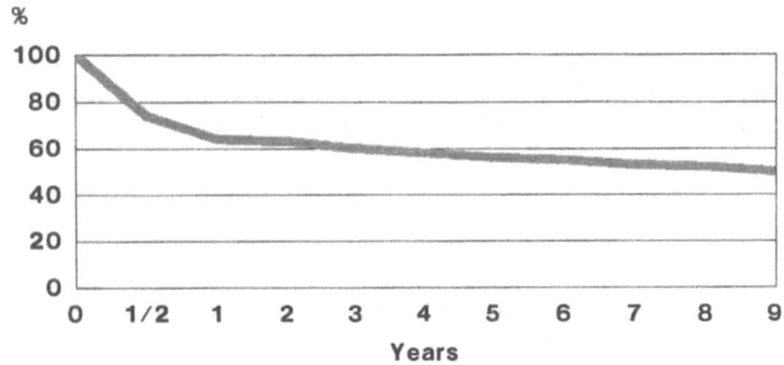


**Fig. 6.** Actuarial survival curve following heart transplantation, including in-hospital mortality

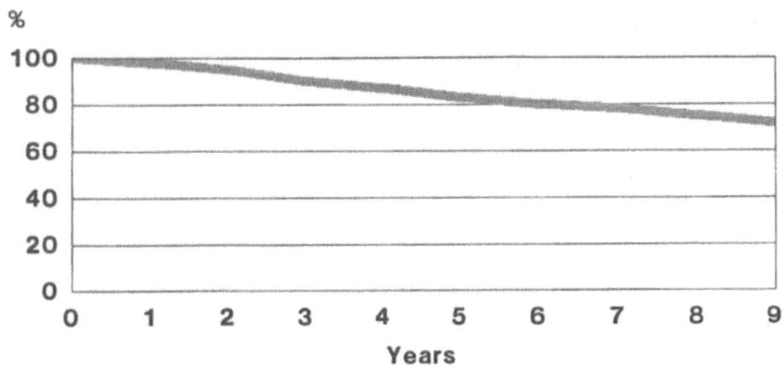


**Fig. 7.** Actuarial survival curve following heart transplantation, excluding in-hospital mortality

**Table 4.** Heart transplantation at La Pitié – causes of late mortality

| Cause | Percent mortality |
|---|---|
| Acute rejection | 37 |
| Graft arteriosclerosis or fibrosis | 32 |
| Infection | 11 |
| Malignancy | 10 |
| Others | 10 |

# Survival

The introduction of CsA in 1981 has been associated with a marked improvement in patient survival: 15% before CsA and 75% after CsA. The actuarial survival rate at 9 years is 68% in the CsA group, early mortality excluded (Figs. 6 and 7). Table 4 shows the causes of late deaths.

At Stanford, Pittsburgh, and at our center, where older and borderline suitable recipients have undergone transplantation, results have been acceptable. Similarly, the quality of the functional results is remarkable, in that survivors are leading normal familial, social, professional, and often physically active lives. This functional quality is confirmed by hemodynamic studies demonstrating normal behavior of the grafted heart in spite of persistent denervation.

## References


1. Addozissio LJ, Gersony WM, Robbins RC et al. (1987) Elevated pulmonary vascular resistance and cardiac transplantation. Circulation 76:5
2. The Registry of the International Society for Heart and Lung Transplantation (1993) Tenth official report. J Heart Lung Transplant 12:541–548
3. Cabrol C, Nataf P, Pavie A et al. (1993) Heart transplantation in 1992: the La Pitié experience. Transplant Proc 25:820–821
4. Nataf P, Gandjbakhch I, Pavie A et al. (1993) Heart transplantation: update. In: Terasaki P (ed) Clinical transplants 1992. UCLA Tissue Typing Laboratory, Los Angeles
5. Takakashi A, Chambers DJ, Braimbridge MV, Hearse DJ (1988) The effects of time, temperature and storage environment on the long-term preservation of the globally ischemic rat heart. J Mol Cell Cardiol 20:78
6. Swanson DK, Pasaoglu I, Berkoff HA, Southard JA, Hegge JO (1988) Improved heart preservation with UW preservation solution. J Heart Transplant 7:456–467
7. Darracott-Cankovic S, Carg N, Wheeldon D, Large S, Wells F, Wallwork J (1991) Myocardial preservation for transplantation: a study of 300 human donor hearts. J Heart Transplant 10:1
8. Darracott-Cankovic S, Stovin PGI, Wheeldon D, Wallwork J, Wells F, English TAH (1989) Effect of donor heart damage on survival after transplantation. Eur J Cardiothorac Surg 3:525
9. Nataf P, Pavie A, Bracamontes L, Bors V, Cabrol C, Gandjbakhch I (1992) Myocardial protection by blood cardioplegia and warm reperfusion in heart transplantation. Ann Thorac Surg 53:525–526
10. Trento A, Hardesty R, Griffith B, Zerbe T, Kormos R, Bahnson H (1988) Role of the antibody to vascular endothelial cells in hyperacute rejection in patients undergoing cardiac transplantation. J Thorac Cardiovasc Surg 95:37
11. Laczkovics A, Grabenwoger F, Teufelsbauer H, Dock W, Wollenek G, Wolner E (1988) Noninvasive assessment of acute rejection after orthotopic heart transplantation: value of changes in cardiac volume and cardiothoracic ratio. J Cardiovasc Surg 29:582
12. Hosenpud J, Norman D, Cobanoglu M, Floten H, Conner R, Starr A (1987) Serial echocardiographic findings early after heart transplantation: evidence for reversible right ventricular dysfunction and myocardial edema. J Heart Transplant 6:343
13. Desruennes M, Corcos T, Cabrol A et al. (1988) Doppler echocardiography for the diagnosis of acute cardiac allograft rejection. J Am Coll Cardiol 12:63
14. Watson FS, O'Connel JB, Ambert IJ et al. (1988) Treatment of cytomegalovirus pneumonia in heart transplant recipients with 9 (1,3 dihydroxy-2-propoxymethyl)-guanine (DHPG). J Heart Transplant 7:102
15. Grant HE, Hegberg RC, Billigham ME, Baldwin JC, Jamieson SW (1988) Analysis of the immunosuppressive and nephrotoxic effects of cyclosporin G. J Heart Transplant 7:119
16. Stevens L, Halbrook H, Berron K, Spears C, Hormuth D (1988) Conversion from cyclosporine to azathioprine in heart transplant recipients. J Heart Transplant 7:119
17. Rottemburg J, Mattei MF, Cabrol A et al. (1985) Renal function and blood pressure in heart transplant recipients treated with cyclosporine. J Heart Transplant 4:404
18. Oyer P, Stinson E, Jamieson S et al. (1983) Cyclosporin A in cardiac allografting: a preliminary experience. Transplant Proc 15:1227

19. Yowell RL, Hammond EH, Bristow MR, Watson FS, Renlund DG, O'Connel JB (1988) Acute vascular rejection involving the major coronary arteries of cardiac allograft. J Heart Transplant 7:191
20. Gredy KL, Herold LS (1988) Comparison of nutritional status in patients before and after heart transplantation. J Heart Transplant 7:123

# The Efficacy of Calcium Channel Blockers in Pulmonary Reperfusion

A. HAVERICH and M. KARCK

## Introduction

The growing number and success of lung transplantations in the treatment of end-stage pulmonary disease has led to an increased demand for safe preservation methods to prolong the ischemic tolerance of donor organs. Since many investigations indicate that the efficacy of measures of donor organ protection for transplantation is limited, when confined to the use of preservation solutions for flushing and storage alone, more recent studies have focused on reperfusion modalities and their implications for postischemic functional and metabolic recovery [17, 23]. The optimum method for reperfusion of the lung after global ischemia, however, still has to be defined. This is particularly true for lung transplantation, where the early postoperative organ function may be transiently but critically impaired [20]. Attempts to prevent this temporary functional derangement, which has been referred to as the reimplantation response, have concentrated on minimizing injury during preservation of the lung before transplantation, rather than during the initial phase of reperfusion [11].

This study focuses on the effects of the calcium antagonists nifedipine and diltiazem, administered in the early phase of postischemic reperfusion, which is known to be most susceptible for calcium influx into cells, as the capacity to sequester calcium is severely impaired [1]. We used a rabbit model, applying 2 h of normothermic ischemia of the left lung. Thereafter, oxygenation and hemodynamic aspects of pulmonary circulation, as well as extravascular fluid accumulation as an estimate of pulmonary edema formation, were investigated.

## Material and Methods

Rabbits (chinchilla gray, 3–4 kg), positioned on their back were anesthetized with ketamine (25 mg/kg i.m.) and pentobarbital (12 mg/kg i.v.), tracheotomized, and ventilated with oxygen/nitrous oxide (50:50). Lines for blood gas analysis, fluid supply, and pressure monitoring were inserted in the right carotid artery, the right jugular vein, and, after median sternotomy, in the pulmonary artery and left atrium. An electromagnetic flowprobe (Hellige, Germany) was placed around the aorta for measurements of cardiac output, and both lung hili were snared after exposure. Normothermic ischemia of the left lung was maintained for 2 h after hilus occlusion by applying a heating lamp mounted 1 m above the loosely adapted chest walls. At the end of ischemia, left lung reperfusion was started, while the right hilum was kept occluded until the experiment was terminated at 210 min.

Hemodynamic measurements included the systemic pressure, pulmonary artery pressure, left atrial pressure, and cardiac output. Pulmonary vascular resistance was calculated before, during, and after left lung ischemia until termination of the experiment 210 min after restoration of the blood flow through the left lung. Then, the left lung was harvested for determination of extravascular lung water content according to the method of Pearce, as an indicator of pulmonary edema [19]. At the time of the hemodynamic measurements arterial blood gas samples were taken. No positive inotropic agents were administered throughout the experiments.

## Experimental Groups

Group I ($n = 7$) served as a control group with occlusion of the right hilum for 210 min without previous ischemia of the left lung. In group II ($n = 7$), the left hilum was occluded for 2 h before reperfusion was started and maintained for 210 min, while the right hilum was occluded. In group III ($n = 6$) and group IV ($n = 8$) the conditions were the same as in group II, but diltiazem (62.5 μg/kg i.v., group III) or nifedipine (3 μg/kg i.v., group IV) was administered during the first 20 min of reperfusion (Fig. 1).

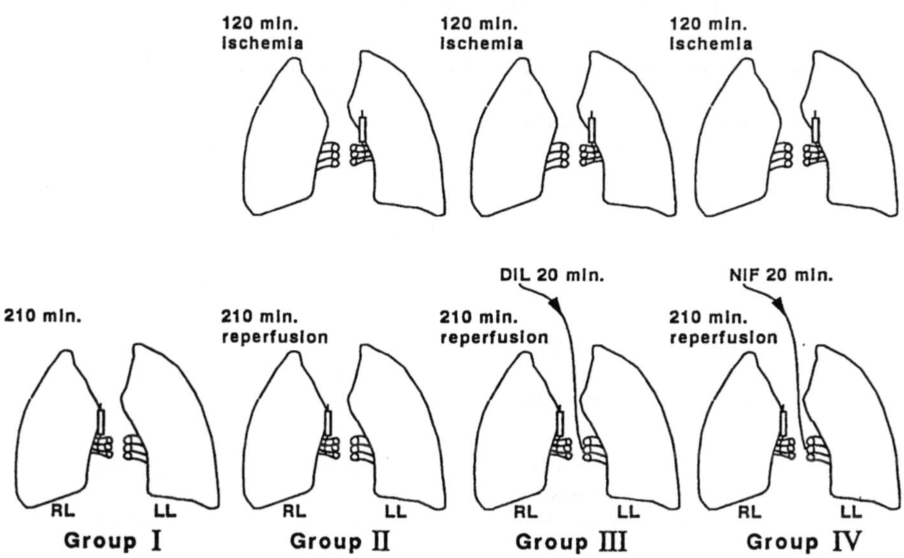


**Fig. 1.** Experimental groups: Group I – Perfusion of the left lung for 210 min without previous ischemia (control); the right hilus was kept occluded. Group II – 120 min normothermic ischemia of the left lung with subsequent reperfusion for 210 min with the right hilus kept occluded. Group III – as in group II, but diltiazem (*DIL*) as additive to the reperfusate. Group IV – as group II, but nifedipine (*NIF*) as additive to the reperfusate

**Statistical Analysis**

All data are expressed as median and Q1/Q3 quartiles. Nonparametric methods were used for data evaluation. Comparison of groups was carried out with the Kruskal-Wallis test [18]. When significant differences were found, further analysis using the Mann-Whitney Test was performed. Statistical significance was set at $p < 0.05$.

## Results

Arterial oxygenation after 210 min of reperfusion was measured at 257 mmHg (227/291) in group I, 261 mmHg (200/291) in group II, 208 mmHg (175/281) in group III, and 247 mmHg (166/307) in group IV (Fig. 2). No statistically significant differences were found among the groups.

During the preischemic period, no statistically significant hemodynamic differences were found among the groups. Hilus occlusion resulted in an increase of median pulmonary artery pressure and decrease of cardiac output; however, these were not statistically significant (Table 1). At the end of the (re)perfusion period of the left lung, median pulmonary vascular resistance was elevated in group II (5120 dynes/s $\cdot$ $cm^{-5}$), group III (5518 dynes/s $\cdot$ $cm^{-5}$), and group IV (4324 dynes/s $\cdot$ $cm^{-5}$), when compared with group I (3390 dynes/s $\cdot$ $cm^{-5}$), although not statistically significant (Fig. 3).

Measurement of the extravascular water content in the left lung revealed an increase after 210 min of reperfusion in group II (73 g/g wet weight) when

**Table 1.** Pulmonary hemodynamic parameters (median and Q1/Q3 quartiles)

| | Preischemic | Ischemia left lung (at 60 min) | (Re)perfusion left lung (at 15 min) | (Re)perfusion left lung (at 210 min) |
|---|---|---|---|---|
| Group I | | | | |
| PAP (mmHg) | 13 (10/17) | – | 15 (12/18.5) | 14 (11/18) |
| LA (mmHg) | 7 (5.5/9) | – | 4 (3.5/6) | 4 (3/7) |
| CO (ml/min) | 262 (205/306) | – | 230 (193/281) | 240 (210/291) |
| Group II | | | | |
| PAP (mmHg) | 17.5 (16/18) | 19 (15/22) | 18.5 (15/20) | 16 (13/18) |
| LA (mmHg) | 5 (4/6) | 5 (5/5) | 4.5 (3.5/6) | 5 (3/6) |
| CO (ml/min) | 232 (205/306) | 210 (180/239) | 230 (193/281) | 172 (112/210) |
| Group III | | | | |
| PAP (mmHg) | 14 (14/15) | 16.5 (16/18) | 16 (13.5/19.5) | 17 (14/19.5) |
| LA (mmHg) | 6.5 (6/7) | 6.5 (6/8) | 8 (7/9) | 6.5 (6/8) |
| CO (ml/min) | 230 (130/300) | 202 (142/320) | 123 (120/195) | 152 (100/187) |
| Group IV | | | | |
| PAP (mmHg) | 16 (13/19) | 19 (16.5/21.5) | 18 (17/22) | 16 (14/19) |
| LA (mmHg) | 5.5 (4/7.5) | 5.5 (3.5/8) | 6 (4.5/18) | 6 (4/10) |
| CO (ml/min) | 251 (220/332) | 223 (178/263) | 194 (168/231) | 185 (140/200) |

*PAP*, Pulmonary artery pressure; *LA*, left atrial pressure; *CO*, cardiac output

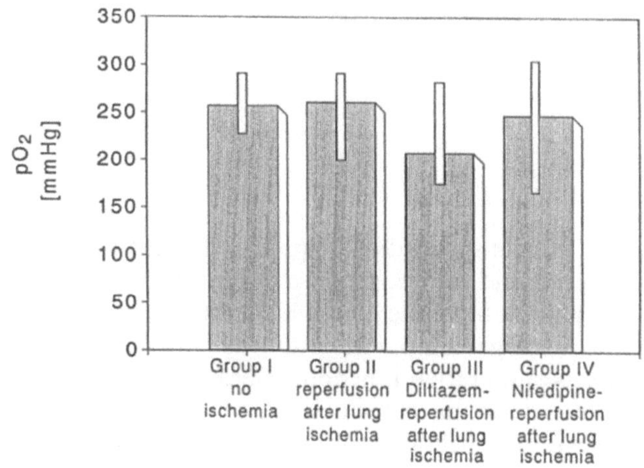


**Fig. 2.** Arterial oxygenation after 210 min reperfusion of the left lung

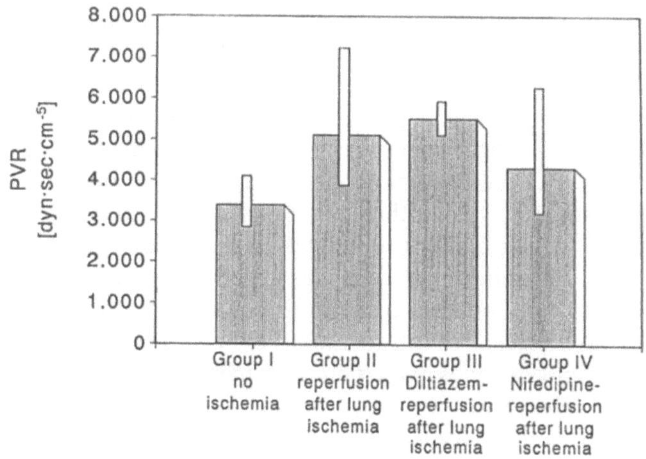


**Fig. 3.** Pulmonary vascular resistance (*PVR*) after 210 min reperfusion of the left lung

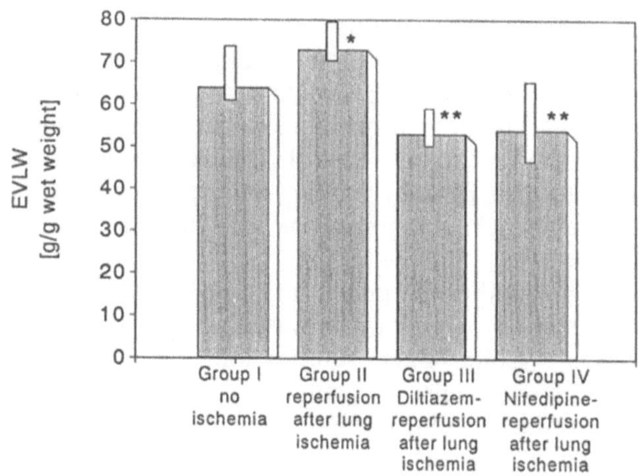


**Fig. 4.** Extravascular lung water content (*EVLW*) in the left lung after 210 min of reperfusion. *, $p < 0.0125$ versus group I; **, $p < 0.001$ versus group II

compared with group I (64 g/g wet weight; $p < 0.0125$). No such increase was measured in groups III and IV (53 g/g wet weight, 54 g/g wet weight; $p < 0.001$) (Fig. 4).

## Discussion

Distant procurement of organs for transplantation requires effective preservation to reduce injury during ischemia and the initial phase of reperfusion [5]. This is particularly important in transplantation of the lung, which not only is regarded as more susceptible to ischemic damage compared with other organs, but also may undergo severe temporary postoperative functional derangement [15, 20]. Studies on pulmonary protection as yet have focused mainly on measures to improve the initial organ preservation, such as flush perfusion or maintainance conditions during ischemia [13, 16, 21, 26–28].

Experimental studies on controlled reperfusion, however, have been the subject of a few reports only: Breda and co-workers observed improved postischemic lung performance after reperfusion with leukocyte-depleted blood. They discussed the generation of oxygen free radicals in leukocytes as a reason for the reperfusion injury [3]. This suggestion was supported by our previous observation that addition of oxygen free-radical scavengers during postischemic lung reperfusion results in a reduction of pulmonary edema formation and improved postischemic pulmonary function [6, 7]. Another trigger of reperfusion injury, besides the generation and release of oxygen free radicals, was found to reside in the calcium metabolism. $Ca^{++}$ influx into the cells has been shown to have a deleterious effect, especially during reperfusion, when the capacity to sequester $Ca^{++}$ is severely impaired [1]. An increase of intracellular $Ca^{++}$ can be followed by activation of thromboxane and leukotrienes, which on their part lead to induction of platelet activation and the release of vasoactive prostaglandins in the lung, with a subsequent increase in pulmonary vascular resistance and membrane permeability [16].

From studies on myocardial protection there is evidence that this pathophysiologic mechanism, leading to the developement of tissue edema and eventually to cell death, can be counteracted by supplementation of a calcium antagonist to the preservation solution, which prevents massive intracellular accumulation of $Ca^{++}$ ions [2]. This group of pharmacologic substances was introduced by Fleckenstein, who was the first to note that the plateau phase of the action potential could be made to disappear by treating smooth muscle tissue prior to depolarization with agents which antagonize the slow calcium channel [8].

In an experimental study of normothermic pulmonary ischemia, Hachida's group reported a significant reduction of pulmonary vascular resistance after ischemia following administration of Collins-Sachs solution for pulmoplegia supplemented with the potent calcium antagonist verapamil [11]. A possible explanation for this observation is the reduction of transmembrane cellular $Ca^{++}$ influx during ischemia, thereby minimizing release of prostaglandins which could increase pulmonary vascular resistance. The same group subsequently developed a new preservation solution for the lung (UCLA solution) containing 10.0 mg/l verapamil, in order to prevent $Ca^{++}$ influx during ischemia (rather than upon reperfusion) and observed improved pulmonary function after 6 h of global hypothermic ischemia in a canine autotransplantation model [12]. In this study, however, a second flush using UCLA solution without verapamil was found to be neccessary before the onset of reperfusion in order to avoid negative inotropic effects of this drug.

In the present study we observed an increase in the extravascular lung water content as a measure for pulmonary edema in all groups after 2 h of left lung ischemia, as measured at the end of the reperfusion period. Pulmonary edema formation is a consistent result of prolonged ischemia and represents the earliest and most frequent problem during reperfusion after ischemic damage [24]. Determination of lung water is therefore a useful marker of the quality of lung preservation and has been successfully employed previously in preservation studies [4, 25]. The increase in extravascular lung water, however, was significantly less pronounced when the calcium antagonists nifedipine also diltiazem were administered during early postischemic reperfusion. This reduction may be interpreted as a result of significant decrease of the cellular $Ca^{++}$ uptake, which is known as the final common pathway of ischemic injury and is inevitably followed by cellular water uptake [15].

The hemodynamic data acquired in this study matched the results of the lung water measurements, inasmuch as a tendency towards reduction in cardiac output and an increase in pulmonary vascular resistance were observed in all groups exposed to ischemia of the left lung.

The reduction in the lung water content afforded by administration of nifedipine or diltiazem during reperfusion was not accompanied by significant improvement of pulmonary hemodynamics in groups III and IV. However, this observation is not contradictory, since in particular the parameters pulmonary artery pressure and pulmonary vascular resistance are sensitive to disturbances in autoregulation due to hilus occlusion. Thus they were reported as less reliable parameters in the assessment of the quality of lung preservation previously [14, 15].

From our study, we therefore conclude that nifedipine and diltiazem, administered as an additive to the reperfusate after pulmonary ischemia, may be of use in pulmonary preservation as required in clinical lung transplantation by limiting early postoperative fluid accumulation in the lung parenchyma. Since nifedipine and diltiazem do not exhibit a negative inotropic effect compared with verapamil, addition of these substances during reperfusion would also decrease the cardiac risk after pulmonary ischemia.

## References

1. Allen BS, Okamoto F, Buckberg GD, Acar C, Partington M, Bugyi H, Leaf J (1986) Reperfusate composition: benefits of marked hypocalcemia and diltiazem on regional recovery. J Thorac Cardiovasc Surg 92:564–572

2. Balderman SC, Chan AK, Gage AA (1984) Verapamil cardioplegia: improved myocardial preservation during global ischemia. J Thorac Cardiovasc Surg 88:57–66
3. Breda MA, Hall TS, Scott S, Baumgartner WA, Borkon MA, Brawn LD, Hutchins, Reitz BA (1985) Twenty-four hour lung preservation by hypothermia and leucocyte depletion. Heart Transplant IV(3):325–329
4. Castagne JT, Shors E, Benfield JR (1972) The role of perfusion in lung preservation. J Thorac Cardiovasc Surg 63:521–526
5. Corris PA, Odom NJ, Jackson G, McGregor CGA (1987) Reimplantation after lung transplantation. J Heart Transplant 6:234–237
6. Cremer J, Jurmann M, Dammenhayn, Wahlers T, Haverich A, Borst HG (1989) Oxygen free radical scavengers to prevent pulmonary reperfusion injury after heart lung transplantation. J Heart Transplant 8:330–336
7. Dammenhayn L, Jurmann M, Schäfers HJ, Haverich A (1987) Effects of catalase during reperfusion of the ischemic lung. Eur Surg Res 19[S1]:14
8. Fleckenstein A (1964) Die Bedeutung der energiereichen Phosphate für Kontraktilität und Tonus des Myokards. Verh Dtsch Ges Inn Med 70:81–99
9. Gardner TJ, Stewart JR, Casale AS, Downey JM, Chambers DE (1983) Reduction of myocardial ischemic injury with oxygen-derived free radical scavengers. Surgery 94:4432
10. Gharagozloo F, Melendez FJ, Hein RA, Shemin GJ, DiSesa VJ, Cohn LJ (1988) The effect of superoxide dismutase and catalase on the extended preservation of the ex vivo heart for transplantation. J Thorac Cardiovasc Surg 95:1008–1013
11. Hachida M, Morton DL (1988) The protection of the ischemic lung with verapamil and hydralazine. J Thorac Cardiovasc Surg 95:178–183
12. Hachida M, Morton DL (1989) A new solution (UCLA formula) for lung preservation. J Thorac Cardiovasc Surg 97:513–520
13. Hall TS, Borkon M, Gurtner GC, Brawn J, Hutchins GM, Reitz BA, Baumgartner WA (1988) Improved static lung preservation with corticosteroids and hypothermia. J Heart Transplant 7(5):348–352
14. Hardy JD, Eraslan S, Dalton ML (1963) Autotransplantation and homotransplantation of the lung: further studies. J Thorac Cardiovasc Surg 46:606–615
15. Haverich A, Scott WC, Jamieson SW (1985) Twenty years of lung preservation – a review. Heart Transplant IV(2):234–240
16. Hoffner JE, McMurtry IF, Repine JE (1982) Platelet-activating factor stimulates platelets to produce pulmonary hypertension and edematous lung injury in isolated perfused rabbit lungs. Clin Res 30:430A
17. Jurmann M, Schäfers HJ, Dammenhayn L, Haverich A (1988) Oxygen-derived free radical scavengers for amelioration of reperfusion damage in heart transplantation. J Thorac Cardiovasc Surg 95:368–377
18. Kruskal WH, Wallis WA (1952) Use of ranks in one criterion variance analysis. J Am Stat Assoc 47:583–621
19. Pearce ME, Yamashita J, Beazell J (1964) Measurement of pulmonary edema. Circ Res 16:482–488
20. Prop J, Ehrie MG, Crapo JD, Niewenhuis P, Wildevuur CRH (1984) Reimplantation response in isografted rat lungs. J Thorac Cardiovasc Surg 87:702–711
21. Reichart BA, Novitzky D, Cooper DKC, Cunningham MS, Rose AG (1987) Successful orthotopic heart-lung transplantation in the baboon after five hours of cold ischemia with cardioplegia and Collins' solution. J Heart Transplant 6:15–22
22. Scholz H (1988) Pharmakologie der Calcium-entry-Blocker. In: Lawin P, Anger C (eds) Adalat pro infusione in der perioperativen Phase. Thieme, Stuttgart, pp 1–8
23. Shlafer M, Kane PF, Kirsh MM (1982) Superoxide dismutase plus catalase enhances the efficacy of hypothermic cardioplegia to protect the globally ischemic, reperfused heart. J Thorac Cardiovasc Surg 83:830–839
24. Stevens GH, Sanchez MM, Chappel GL (1973) Enhancement of lung preservation by prevention of lung collapse. J Surg Res 14:400–405

25. Taft PM, Collins GM (1976) Warm ischemic injury of the lung. J Thorac Cardiovasc Surg 72:784–787
26. Veith FJ, Crane R, Torres, M Colon I, Hagstrom JWC, Pinsker Koerner SK (1976) Effective preservation and transportation of lung transplants. J Thorac Cardiovasc Surg 72:97–105
27. Veith FJ, Montefusco C, Kamholz SL, Mollenkopf FP (1983) Lung transplantation. Heart Transplant 2:155–164
28. Wahlers T, Haverich A, Fieguth HG, Schäfers H, Takayama T, Borst HG (1986) Flush perfusion using Euro-Collins solution vs cooling by means of extracorporeal circulation in heart-lung preservation. J Heart Transplant 5:89–98

# Cardiac Xenotransplantation

D.K.C. Cooper

## Introduction

It is generally accepted that there is a shortage of suitable human organs for purposes of transplantation. In July 1993, the total number of patients on the United Network for Organ Sharing (UNOS) waiting list in the USA had risen to 31868 [1], almost double the number registered in 1988. Almost 3000 patients were awaiting a heart transplant. These data indicate that the demand for organs in the USA is increasing by about 10–15% each year and will certainly exceed 30000 per year for the foreseeable future. Worldwide, this number can be increased by at least a further 50%, and possibly 100%.

Furthermore, the median waiting period for several types of donor organs increased significantly during 1988–1991 [2] (and has continued to increase since then). In particular, patients in need of a liver or heart waited approximately twice as long in 1991 as they did 4 years earlier.

Any estimate of the current need for organs each year worldwide, however, does not take into account other important factors, the influence of which it is currently difficult to assess accurately. The first of these factors is whether the number of patients on the waiting list fully reflects the number who might benefit from an organ transplant. At our own center in Oklahoma City we have assessed more than 600 patients for possible heart transplantation during the past 7 years. Less than half, however, have been added to the waiting list for a donor organ. The remainder were declined for various reasons, generally because they had one or more contraindications.

Much of our reluctance to accept the borderline patient is based on the knowledge that the number of donors is strictly limited, and we feel obliged to utilize this scarce resource as carefully and responsibly as possible. Many consider it no longer justified to transplant an organ into a patient considered to be at high risk of not surviving the first few postoperative days.

If there were an unlimited supply of donor organs, as would be the case if xenotransplantation were successful, this ethical barrier would be largely removed. The very sick or borderline patient could be given his or her chance without jeopardizing the future of the more stable candidate. The decision regarding retransplantation of organs, which with heart or lungs is less frequently successful, would similarly prove less of an ethical dilemma.

The second factor, which is more important in our assessment of the future demands for xenografting, relates to the current status of allografting in countries where, for religious or cultural reasons, cadaveric organ donation is rare or nonexistent. Japan is the prime example of a country with advanced medical technological skills and yet where, for cultural reasons, cadaveric allotransplantation is virtually nonexistent. The impact of successful xenotransplantation in such a society would be enormous.

The advantages of xenotransplantation are obvious. Not only would the supply of donor organs be unlimited, but these organs would be available electively when required. Transplant operations could therefore be carried out on routine operating lists, and no potential recipient would need to die for lack of a suitable organ. Of equal importance would be the possibility of pretreating either the donor or the recipient to enhance acceptance of the graft, as the transplant procedure could be planned for a specific day – an advantage which is not, of course, possible with regard to cadaveric organ donation. In addition, donor organs would not be subjected to the effects of brain death, which can be damaging, particularly to the heart. Chronic infection is proving an increasing problem with human donors, particularly with regard to the transfer of hepatitis and HIV; techniques are available to breed potential donor animals that would be infection free (gnotobiosis).

## Definitions

*Xenotransplantation* refers to the transplantation of organs or tissues from an animal of one species into an animal of another species. The entire field has recently been thoroughly reviewed [3]. With regard to man, it clearly refers to the use of a donor other than man. The terms *concordant* and *discordant* xenografting [4] are used frequently to refer respectively to transplantation between closely related animal species (e.g., baboon-to-man) and between distantly related animal species (e.g., pig-to-man).

With regard to the histopathology of the rejection that takes place, we should probably confine our terms to (a) *cellular* rejection, (b) *vascular* (denoting antibody-mediated or humoral) rejection, and (c) *mixed* rejection [5]. Vascular rejection may be *hyperacute* (in that it occurs within minutes or a few hours after transplantation) but may be more delayed and can even occur some days after transplantation.

## Immunobiology

### Concordant Xenografting

When xenotransplantation is carried out between closely related species, there are usually no or very low detectable levels of anti-donor species (xenoreactive) antibody in the host at the time of transplantation. The antibody titer may rise during the first few days after transplantation. In a proportion of recipients, rejection will be cellular and will follow the normal sequence of events seen after allografting. In another proportion, however, rejection will be vascular or of a mixed nature.

The relative proportion of cases where cellular (rather than vascular) rejection will result varies, depending on the two animal species involved and possibly on the organ transplanted. For example, in chimpanzee-to-man renal transplants, rejection was mainly of a cellular nature [6]. In vervet monkey-to-baboon cardiac transplants, 80% of the hearts showed features of vascular rejection with or without cellular rejection [7].

### Discordant Xenografting

Rejection between widely differing species is uniformly vascular and generally hyperacute. There is increasing evidence that vascular rejection of discordant xenografts in man is entirely or largely a result of antibody-mediated complement activation through the classical pathway. Histopathologically, the features of vascular rejection consist of massive capillary destruction with severe interstitial hemorrhage and edema [5]. Intravascular thrombosis resulting from platelet and/or fibrin thrombi is relatively rarely observed by light microscopy but can be documented on electron microscopy. Degenerative changes are evident in the myocytes, and contraction band necrosis may be present.

## Concordant Cardiac Xenografting

Some recent progress has been made in extending heart survival utilizing either a combination of total lymphoid irradiation (TLI) and pharmacologic immunosuppression [8] or heavy immunosuppressive therapy alone [9]. It would seem, therefore, that combinations of the drugs available at the present time, or becoming available in the near future, might lead to prolongation of xenograft function utilizing a closely related donor species in man.

Several new pharmacologic immunosuppressive agents are currently under investigation that may prove more efficient in preventing not only the cellular rejection that takes place in concordant xenografting, but also the antibody-mediated rejection that can occur following the production of new antibody by B lymphocytes. Several of the drugs currently under investigation, such as brequinar sodium, mycophenolate mofetil (RS61443), and 15-deoxyspergualin, have been shown to have relatively potent anti-B-cell activity [10–25].

For example, infant baboons (age 9–19 months), splenectomized and immunosuppressed with a combination of antilymphocyte globulin, FK506, and methotrexate, with methylprednisolone being used as rescue therapy for rejection, have survived for up to 127 days with an orthotopically transplanted rhesus monkey heart [9]. Mean graft survival in four surviving animals has been 80 days, but three other animals died between 35 and 96 days of pulmonary infection or renal failure associated with drug therapy.

A combination of TLI and cyclosporine-based immunosuppression has led to survival of heterotopically placed rhesus monkey hearts in baboons for periods in excess of 1 year [8]. Whether such regimens will be well tolerated by ill patients awaiting heart transplantation remains uncertain, but, clearly, such heavy immunosuppressive programs are likely to be associated with a higher incidence of infection and de novo malignancy than is associated with allografting at the present time.

There are considerable logistic and ethical problems that need to be addressed with regard to concordant xenografting in man. In particular, there is an inadequate number of the larger nonhuman primates (e.g., chimpanzees) and the size of other nonhuman primates (e.g., baboons) would be inadequate to allow orthotopic heart transplantation in adults. Furthermore, there would likely be major public criticism of transplant teams that utilize nonhuman primates as donors on a large scale.

It seems unlikely, therefore, that concordant xenotransplantation will become a routine clinical reality. It is possible that a role for the nonhuman primate as an organ donor for man will be found in heart transplantation in neonates and infants, but, again, the controversy this will undoubtedly engender may prohibit its development.

However, there have been five clinical heart transplants using nonhuman primates as donors for man [25], the most recent being in 1984 [26] (Table 1). Survival of concordant grafts has been for a maximum of only 20 days.

## Discordant Cardiac Xenografting

For a number of reasons, the pig has been identified as a potential donor for man [27]. These reasons include (a) availability in large numbers, (b) inexpensive breeding and maintenance, (c) suitable size for the smallest or largest of humans, (d) availability of pathogen-free (gnotobiotic) animals, and (e) considerable similarities of anatomy and physiology with man.

Four heart transplants have been carried out using the pig or sheep as donors for man [25], the most recent being in 1992 [28] (Table 1). Maximum survival has been 24 h.

Hyperacute vascular rejection has, to date, proved to be an insurmountable problem. Progress is taking place in the laboratory, however, and it would seem that the most likely solution to the problem will come from one of the following approaches.

One promising approach would appear to be the depletion or inhibition of xenoreactive (anti-pig) antibodies in the host. If the xenoreactive antibody titer can be temporarily significantly or totally depleted, or in some other way "neutralized", then an organ grafted during this critical period may not undergo vascular rejection even when the antibody titer returns to its normal level. The period of time during which antibody depletion or neutralization is required remains uncertain but may be as short as 1–3 weeks. The resulting state that is achieved, termed "accommodation" [29], enables survival of an organ graft in the presence of specific antibodies directed against antigens expressed on the surface of the organ. Normal levels of complement are also present. Although this state

**Table 1.** World experience in clinical heart xenotransplantation (based on [25])

| Year | Surgeon | Institution | Donor | Type | Outcome | Reference |
|---|---|---|---|---|---|---|
| 1964 | Hardy | University of Mississippi Jackson, Mississippi, USA | Chimpanzee | OHT | Functioned 2 h (Heart too small) | [49] |
| 1968 | Cooley | Texas Heart Institute, Houston, Texas, USA | Sheep | OHT | Immediate cessation of function (? Vascular rejection) | [50] |
| 1968 | Ross | National Heart Hospital, London, UK | Pig | HHT | Cessation of function within 4 min (? Vascular rejection) } | [51] + personal communication |
| 1968 | Ross | National Heart Hospital, London, UK | Pig | Perfused with human blood but not transplanted | Immediate cessation of function (? Vascular rejection) } | |
| 1969 | Marion | Lyon, France | Chimpanzee | ?OHT | Rapid failure (? Raised pulmonary vascular resistance) | [52] |
| 1977 | Barnard | University of Cape Town, Cape Town, South Africa | Baboon | HHT | Functioned 5 h (Heart too small) | [53] |
| 1977 | Barnard | University of Cape Town, Cape Town, South Africa | Chimpanzee | HHT | Functioned 4 days (Probable vascular rejection) | [53] |
| 1984 | Bailey | Loma Linda University, Loma Linda, California, USA | Baboon | OHT | Functioned 20 days (Vascular rejection) | [26] |
| 1992 | Religa | Silesian Academy of Medicine, Sosnowiec, Poland | Pig | OHT | Functioned 24 h (Cause of failure uncertain) | [28] |

*OHT*, Orthotopic heart transplantation; *HHT*, heterotopic heart transplantation

has not been achieved after discordant xenografting, it has been clearly documented after the transplantation of ABO-incompatible organs, both experimentally [30, 31] and clinically [32], where the mechanism of antibody-mediated rejection is very similar.

Antibody depletion can be carried out by extracorporeal immunoadsorption utilizing columns of specific immunoadsorbents that are directed only against the specific antibody whose removal from the plasma is desired. These immunoadsorbents must therefore consist of either (a) the antigen itself (or a cloned or synthetic antigen) or (b) a cross-reactive antigen [33].

There is increasing evidence that the pig epitopes against which human anti-pig antibodies are directed are carbohydrate structures, most probably galactose structures in the α configuration (αGall-3Gal) [34–36]. Pretransplant extracorporeal immunoadsorption using an αGall-3Gal immunoadsorbent (or the continuous intravenous infusion of αGall-3Gal to bind the anti-pig antibodies for a period of several days) may therefore be successful in allowing accommodation to develop. When this form of therapy is combined with pharmacologic immunosuppressive therapy, prolonged xenograft function might be achieved.

The recent development of genetically engineered pigs that express certain human complement-inhibiting proteins [37] may result in their resistance to the effects of human complement on pig tissues. This may prove a significant step forward in our efforts to overcome the hyperacute rejection that destroys discordant animal grafts within minutes or hours.

For example, decay-accelerating factor (DAF, CD55), membrane co-factor protein (MCF, CD46), and CD59 (protectin, homologous restriction factor) are membrane inhibitors of complement that are present on a wide variety of cell types. These inhibitors block the activity of autologous complement but not of xenogeneic complement from a distantly related species. Lysis of human cells by human complement occurs when these regulatory proteins are deficient. Preliminary data have shown that the expression of human complement-inhibiting molecules on rodent cells protects them from human antibody/complement-mediated lysis [38].

There is some evidence, however, that even if the complement cascade is inhibited, vascular rejection might still occur within the first week after transplantation, and that this may be associated with another mechanism involving xenoreactive antibodies and cellular infiltration [39, 40]. It would therefore seem that our efforts must be directed primarily towards discovering some means of abrogating the effect of these antibodies, both to prevent activation of the complement system and also to inhibit other mechanisms dependent on the antibody-antigen interaction.

We therefore proposed an alternative approach to the development of a pig that might prove a universal donor of organs for man, namely the genetic engineering of a pig that does not express αGal on its vascular endothelium [41]. The expression of terminal α-galactose depends on the proper function of a single gene encoding for the enzyme α-galactosyltransferase [42]. If this gene were "knocked out" by homologous recombination, then there would be no target for the human anti-αGal antibodies. Although this "knock out" technique has not yet been carried out in the pig, it has been established in the mouse [43, 44] and, with the current rate of advance in the field of genetic engineering, it is likely that it will prove feasible in the pig within a few years.

If hyperacute vascular rejection could be overcome, then it remains to be seen whether the currently available drugs will prevent cellular rejection in this model. The incidence and rapidity of onset of graft atherosclerosis remains unknown in both concordant and discordant models.

## Unresolved Problems

The major unresolved immunological barrier is clearly the problem of hyperacute antibody-mediated rejection. The severity of the cellular response to a discordant organ also remains unknown and may prove to be a more significant barrier than is anticipated [45].

There is the risk that even if hyperacute rejection can be overcome, the early development of graft atherosclerosis might take place. There is some optimism, however, that this may not occur, as in long-functioning, ABO-incompatible renal allografts in patients in whom accommodation has been achieved there does not appear to be a higher incidence of graft atherosclerosis [32]. However, there is little significant experience in this field following heart transplantation [46].

One point requires more detailed experimental study. Animal hearts could be used as temporary "bridges" to allografting in patients who are developing cardiogenic shock but cannot be controlled by other means. However, it remains uncertain whether retransplantation with an allograft could then be successfully achieved, as there is conflicting evidence as to whether antibodies will develop that might cause early failure of the subsequent allograft.

Finally, questions have been raised regarding whether the metabolic "milieu interieur" of the human host will allow normal function of a pig organ [4]. Pig hearts have functioned in nonhuman primates for several days [47], and it seems likely that this will not prove to be a problem (although function of other organs, such as the liver, may prove less satisfactory).

In line with these scientific developments, there would appear to be a growing acceptance of xenotransplantation among the public. A Partnership for Organ Donation Survey in the USA recently confirmed that whereas 85% of those questioned said they would accept an organ allograft, 51% said that they would accept an organ transplant from an animal if a suitable human organ were not available [48].

Just as the early pioneers of open heart surgery from the 1950s did not envisage heart surgery on the scale it is performed today, I believe we do not envisage the role of xenotransplantation as it may be in 40–50 years' time. The ready availability of a new organ to replace a diseased one will prove too great a temptation to the average patient or physician to allow either to persevere with inadequate medical therapy that maintains the patient in a suboptimal quality of life.

# References


1. UNOS Update (1993) 9(7):46
2. UNOS Update (1993) 9(1):29
3. Cooper DKC, Kemp E, Reemtsma K, White DJG (eds) (1991) Xenotransplantation: the transplantation of organs and tissues between species. Springer, Berlin Heidelberg New York
4. Calne RY (1970) Organ transplantation between widely disparate species. Transplant Proc 2:550
5. Rose AG, Cooper DKC, Human PA, Reichenspurner H, Reichart G (1991) Histopathology of hyperacute rejection of the heart – experimental and clinical observations in allografts and xenografts. J Heart Transplant 10:223
6. Reemtsma K, McCracken BH, Schlegel JU et al. (1964) Renal heterotransplantation in man. Ann Surg 160:384
7. Cooper DKC, Human PA, Rose AG, Rees J, Keraan M, Reichart B, du Toit E, Oriol R (1989) The role of ABO blood group compatibility in heart transplantation between closely related animal species. An experimental study using the vervet monkey-to-baboon cardiac xenograft model. J Thorac Cardiovasc Surg 97:447
8. Norin AJ, Roslin MS, Panza A et al. (1992) TLI induces specific B-cell unresponsiveness and long-term monkey heart xenograft survival in cyclosporine-treated baboons. Transplant Proc 24:508
9. Kawauchi M, Gundry SR, Alonso de Begona J et al. (1993) Prolonged survival of orthotopically transplanted heart xenografts in infant baboons. J Thorac Cardiovasc Surg 106:779
10. Demasi R, Araneda D, Gross U, Daniel H, Thomas FT (1989) 15-Deoxyspergualin (DOSP) is a potent immunosuppressive agent in xenografts. Eur Surg Res 21:35
11. Valdivia LA, Monden M, Gotoh M, Nakano Y, Tono T, Mori T (1990) Evidence that deoxyspergualin prevents sensitization and first-set cardiac xenograft rejection in rats by suppression of antibody formation. Transplantation 50:132
12. Burlingham WJ, Grailer AP, Hullett DA, Sollinger HW (1991) Inhibition of both MLC and in vitro IgG memory response to tetanus toxoid by RS61443. Transplantation 51:545
13. Grailer AP, Nichols J, Hullett DA, Sollinger HW, Burlingham WJ (1991) Inhibition of human B-cell responses in vitro by RS61443, cyclosporine A and $DAB_{486}$IL-2. Transplant Proc 23:314
14. Allison AC, Almquist SJ, Muller CD, Eugui EM (1991) In vitro immunosuppressive effects of mycophenolic acid and an ester pro-drug RS61443. Transplant Proc 23[Suppl 2]:10
15. Tepper MA, Petty B, Bursuker I, Pasternak RD, Cleveland J, Spitalnik GL, Schacter B (1991) Inhibition of antibody production by the immunosuppressive agent, 15-deoxyspergualin. Transplant Proc 23:328
16. Cramer DV, Chapman FA, Jaffee BD et al. (1992) The prolongation of concordant hamster-to-rat cardiac xenografts by brequinar sodium. Transplantation 54:403
17. Morikawa K, Oseko F, Morikawa S (1992) The suppressive effect of deoxyspergualin on the differentiation of human B lymphocytes maturing into immunoglobulin-producing cells. Transplantation 54:526
18. Leventhal JR, Flores HC, Gruber SA et al. (1992) Evidence that 15-deoxyspergualin inhibits natural antibody production but fails to prevent hyperacute rejection in a discordant xenograft model. Transplantation 54:26
19. Leventhal JR, Platt JL, Flores HC, Gruber SA, Matas AJ (1992) Inhibition of natural antibody synthesis by cyclophosphamide or 15-deoxyspergualin fails to prevent xenograft rejection in the guinea pig-to-rat model. Transplant Proc 24(2):551
20. Ulrichs K, Kaitschick J, Bartlett R, Muller-Ruchholtz W (1992) Suppression of natural xenophile antibodies with the novel immunomodulating drug leflunomide. Transplant Proc 24:718
21. Gannedahl G, Karlsson-Parra A, Totterman TH, Tufveson G (1993) 15-Deoxyspergualin inhibits antibody production in mouse-to-rat heart transplantation. Transplant Proc 25:778
22. Schmidbauer G, Hancock WW, Wasowska BA, Sablinski T (1993) Rapamycin treatment prevents and/or erases sensitization and abrogates accelerated rejection of vascularized organ allografts. Transplant Proc 25:712

23. Daloze P, Chen H, Lo H, Xu D, Shan X, Wu J (1993) Rapamycin's long-term effects on humoral and cellular immune responses in the rat. Transplant Proc 25:721
24. Hasan RI, Sriwatanawongsa V, Wallwork J, White DJ (1993) Consistent prolonged "concordant" survival of hamster-to-rat cardiac xenografts by inhibition of anti-species antibodies with methotrexate. Transplant Proc 25:421
25. Cooper DKC, Ye Y (1991) Experience with clinical heart xenotransplantation. In: Cooper DKC et al. (eds) Xenotransplantation. Springer, Berlin Heidelberg New York, p 541
26. Bailey LL, Nehlsen-Cannarella SL, Concepcion W, Jolley WB (1985) Baboon-to-human cardiac xenotransplantation in a neonate. J Am Med Assoc 254:3321
27. Cooper DKC, Ye Y, Rolf LL Jr, Zuhdi N (1991) The pig as potential organ donor for man. In: Cooper DKC et al. (eds) Xenotransplantation. Springer, Berlin Heidelberg New York, p 481
28. Czaplicki J, Blonska B, Religa Z (1992) The lack of hyperacute xenogeneic heart transplant rejection in a human. J Heart Lung Transplant 11:393
29. Bach FH, Platt J, Cooper DKC (1991) Accommodation – the role of natural antibody and complement in discordant xenograft rejection. In: Cooper DKC et al. (eds) Xenotransplantation. Spring, Berlin Heidelberg New York, p 81
30. Cooper DKC, Ye Y, Kehoe M et al. (1992) A novel approach to "neutralization" of preformed antibodies: cardiac allotransplantation across the ABO-blood group barrier as a paradigm of discordant xenotransplantation. Transplant Proc 24: 566
31. Cooper DKC, Ye Y, Niekrasz M et al. (1993) Specific intravenous carbohydrate therapy – a new concept in inhibiting antibody-mediated rejection: experience with ABO-incompatible cardiac allografting in the baboon. Transplantation 56:769
32. Alexandre GPJ, Squifflet JP, De Bruyere M, Latinne D, Reding R, Gianello P, Carlier M, Pirson Y (1987) Present experience in a series of 26 ABO-incompatible living donor renal allografts. Transplant Proc 19:4538
33. Van Breda Vriesman PJC (1989) The future of plasmapheresis in host manipulation. In: Hardy MA (ed) Xenograft 25. Excerpta Medica, Amsterdam, p 267
34. Good AH, Cooper DKC, Malcolm AJ, Ippolito RM, Koren E, Neethling FA, Ye Y, Zuhdi N, Lamontagne LR (1992) Identification of carbohydrate structures that bind human anti-porcine antibodies: implications for discordant xenografting in humans. Transplant Proc 24:559
35. Oriol R, Ye Y, Koren E, Cooper DKC (1994) Carbohydrate antigens of pig tissues reacting with human natural antibodies as potential targets for hyperacute vascular rejection in pig-to-man organ xenotransplantation. Transplantation 56:1433
36. Cooper DKC, Good AH, Koren E, Oriol R, Malcolm AJ, Ippolito RM, Neethling FA, Ye Y, Romano E, Zuhdi N (1993) Identification of α-galactosyl and other carbohydrate epitopes that are bound by human anti-pig antibodies: relevance to discordant xenografting in man. Transplant Immunol 1:198
37. Langford GA, Yannoutsos N, Cozzi E, Lancaster R, Elsome K, Chen P, Richards A, White DJG (1994) Production of pigs transgenic for human decay accelerating factor. Transplant Proc 26:1400
38. White DJG, Oglesby T, Kiszewski MK, Tedja I, Hourcade D, Wang MW, Wright L, Wallwork J, Atkinson JP (1992) Expression of human decay accelerating factor or membrane cofactor protein genes on mouse cells inhibits lysis by human complement. Transplant Proc 24:474
39. Inverardi L, Samaja M, Marelli F, Bender JR, Pardi R (1992) Cellular immune recognition of xenogeneic vascular endothelium. Transplant Proc 24:459–461
40. Leventhal JR, Dalmasso AP, Cromwell JW, Platt JL, Manivel CJ, Bolman RM, Matas AJ (1993) Prolongation of cardiac xenograft survival by depletion of complement. Transplantation 55:857–866
41. Cooper DKC, Koren E, Oriol R (1993) Genetically engineered pigs. Lancet 342:682
42. Galili U, Shohet SB, Kobrin E, Stults CLM, Macher BA (1988) Man, apes and Old World monkeys differ from other mammals in the expression of α-galactosyl epitopes on nucleated cells. J Biol Chem 263:17755–17762
43. Capecchi MR (1989) Altering the genome by homologous recombination. Science 244:1288–1292
44. Condorcet JP (1992) Knock-out a la pelle! Med Sci 8:1091–1096

45. Moses RD, Auchincloss H (1991) Mechanism of cellular xenograft rejection. In: Cooper DKC et al. (eds) Xenotransplantation. Springer, Berlin Heidelberg New York, p 101
46. Cooper DKC (1990) A clinical survey of cardiac transplantation between ABO-blood group-incompatible recipients and donors. J Heart Transplant 9:376
47. Cooper DKC, Lexer G, Rose AG, Keraan M, Rees J, du Toit E (1988) Effects of cyclosporine and antibody adsorption on pig cardiac xenograft survival in the baboon. J Heart Transplant 7:238
48. The Gallup Organization (1993) The American public's attitudes toward organ donation and transplantation, conducted for the Partnership for Organ Donation, Boston
49. Hardy JD, Kurrus FE, Chavez CM, Neely WA, Webb WR, Eraslan S, Turner MD, Fabian LW, Labecki JD (1964) Heart transplantation in man: developmental studies and report of a case. J Am Med Assoc 188:1132
50. Cooley DA, Hallman GL, Bloodwell RD, Nora JJ, Leachman RD (1968) Human heart transplantation: experience with 12 cases. Am J Cardiol 22:804
51. Ross DN (1969) In: Shapiro H (ed) Experience with human heart transplantation. Butterworths, Durban, p 227
52. Marion P (1969) Les transplantations cardiaques et les transplantations hepatiques. Lyon Med 222:585
53. Barnard CN, Wolpowitz A, Losman JG (1977) Heterotopic cardiac transplantation with a xenograft for assistance of the left heart in cardiogenic shock after cardiopulmonary bypass. S Afr Med J 52:1035

# Part VII
# Extracorporeal Respiratory Support

# Introduction

F. Unger

New emphasis is given in these chapters to extracorporeal membrane oxygenation, a routine clinical method in patients with respiratory failure. Gattinoni, a pioneer in this area, reports on his experience in adults, as do Pearson and Firmin in children. Zwischenberger focusses on the implantable IVOX pump, an approach which can very easily be realized in the clinical process.

# Extracorporeal Respiratory Support in Acute Respiratory Failure

L. Gattinoni, L. Brazzi, P. Pelosi, and A. Pesenti

## Introduction

Mechanical ventilation with high minute ventilation, high levels of peak inspiratory pressures, high levels of positive end-expiratory pressure (PEEP), and high inspiratory fractions of oxygen represents the most common ventilatory management of patients with severe adult respiratory distress syndrome (ARDS). However, mechanical ventilation does not offer the proper environment for the healing of the lungs, since both pulmonary [1, 2] and systemic complications [3, 4] have been attributed to positive-pressure breathing.

Several ventilatory techniques have been proposed to decrease the mechanical lung damage due to high lung ventilatory volumes and pressures, such as high-frequency jet ventilation [5], inverse-ratio ventilation [6, 7], and controlled hypoventilation [8]. However, all the conventional attempts to compensate for impaired pulmonary function simply exploit the residual capacity for gas exchange of the diseased lung. In fact, due to the high inhomogeneity of the ARDS lung lesions, as evidenced by recent computer tomographic (CT) studies [9–12], very little can be done to improve the efficiency of the ventilatory support, and further improvement in the outcome of ARDS possibly requires the substitution of the alveolar-capillary function to limit lung damage.

The rationale for extracorporeal support rests in the assumption that mechanical ventilation is disadvantageous per se in the ARDS lung, and that lung rest provides a better environment for healing.

In this chapter we will discuss: (a) the structural-functional characteristics of the ARDS lung; (b) the rationale for extracorporeal support; (c) the main technical aspects of and recent improvements in the extracorporeal technique; and (d) the clinical results obtained in our institute during the past 20 years.

## Structural-Functional Characteristics of the ARDS Lung

Since its original description, ARDS has been considered a syndrome diffusely affecting the lung parenchima, as usually shown on antero-posterior chest radiographs. However, computer tomographic studies have shown that the lung lesions (densities on the CT scan) are primarily located in the dependent part of the lung [9–11], the nondependent regions apparently being saved. This suggests a nonhomogeneous distribution of the lung alterations. Some regions of the lung have an apparently normal inflation, while others appear poorly aerated or consolidated [12]. Therefore, only one third to one half of the lung tissue participates in tidal gas exchange, an amount similar to that present in a normal lung of a baby ("baby lung") [13]. This concept has further evolved with subsequent studies in which the analysis of the CT section of the entire lung has been shifted to a regional analysis, which allows a more detailed comprehension of regional distibution of edema and ventilation. Regional analysis of the ARDS lung showed that the edema is distributed throughout the lung parenchima and, consequently, that the residual ventilated part of the lung ("baby lung") is also diseased. The ARDS lung structure may therefore be modeled as follows: the primary disease causes a diffuse endothelial alteration, leading to diffuse lung edema; the increase in lung weight, produced by edema, causes a progressive deflation of the pulmonary units along the ventral-dorsal axis in the supine position (atelectasis areas) [14–16]. As a consequence, at 0 cm $H_2O$ PEEP, the ARDS lung is nearly collapsed from halfway down [16], and the ventilation is preferentially distributed to the nondependent lung regions since the dependent regions are collapsed and/or consolidated [12]. The ventilation/perfusion ($V_A/Q$) studies are consistent with the described model [17]. In fact the gasexchange in ARDS is characterized by true shunt (pulmonary flow perfusing the noninflated regions) and normal $V_A/Q$ (gasexchange in the "baby lung") [18]. The $CO_2$ clearance occurs only into the "baby lung", according to its ventilation and perfusion. Despite a near normal $PaCO_2$ usually observed in early ARDS, the specific ventilation, i.e., the ratio of ventilation to the lung gas volume, may be 10–20 times higher than normal. In fact, due to the reduced size of the "baby lung" (in severe cases 1/5 of the size of a normal lung), ventilation levels of 8–10 l/min are correspondingly lower than those of a normal lung with minute ventilation of 40–50 l/min. Since tidal volumes usually applied in normal lungs are approximately triple the actual capacity of the acutely injured lung, they really overdistend and overventilate the functional lung tissues (specific hyperventilation). Furthermore, the ventilated tissues are, as described above, not only reduced in size but also affected by the disease process. Such a continued stress may produce interstitial emphysema, cyst formation [19], and systemic gas embolism [20] which may further damage the functional residual part of the lung, thereby prolonging the need for mechanical ventilation and increasing the risk of lung tissue injury.

With time, the anatomical structure of the lung changes: edema is partially readsorbed, fibrous processes occur, and phenomena termed emphysema-like lesions progressively develop.

Total static lung compliance (TSLC), which reflects the mechanical properties of the aerated and potentially recruitable lung regions [12], in early ARDS shows a biphasic contour, characterized by the presence of an inflection point in the ascending limb of the pressure-volume curve. Later in ARDS, this biphasic contour is lost as a more uniform and reduced compliance characterizes the entire spirometric range .

In early-stage ARDS patients gas exchange improves and shunt is reduced when PEEP is set above the inflection point [21]. In fact, PEEP acts as a counterforce which prevents the compression atelectasis induced by increased superimposed pressure, due to edema, on the dependent lung regions [15]. In contrast, in late-stage ARDS patients, in whom intra-alveolar fibroproliferation has replaced edema, air spaces are unrecruitable by the action of PEEP [22]. In fact, the transmission of hydrostatic forces throughout the lung parenchima is likely prevented by the presence of fibrous structure. Furthermore, it is possible that $V_A/Q$ maldistribution and oxygen diffusion impairment may play a role in determing hypoxemia in the late stages. The anatomical basis of the $CO_2$ retention in late ARDS is most likely the emphysema-like lesions: the alveolar dead space increases and the alveolar ventilation decreases unavoidably [23, 24].

In conclusion, the treatment of ARDS lung is characterized by increased ventilation related to the dimension of the residual ventilatable lung to obtain adequate $CO_2$ removal. PEEP is required to recruit collapsed regions, while a high oxygen inspiratory concentration is needed to reduce the hypoxemia induced by shunt. Specific hyperventilation [25], high peak pressures [26, 27], and increased inspiratory oxygen concentration [28] are all known determinants of pulmonary damage. Therefore, the "best" treatment for the diseased lung should be to keep the lung at rest, avoiding all the reported disadvantages of conventional ventilatory management.

Although it has not been proven directly that lung rest provides a better environment for healing, it has been reported that this treatment approach could prevent hyaline membrane formation [29, 30], with an improvement of renal function and hemodynamics [31].

## Development of the Lung Rest Hypothesis

The hypothesis that lung rest can be obtained using an artificial lung with extracorporeal circulation was originally derived from several animal experiments designed to test a spiral-coil membrane lung especially designed for $CO_2$ removal in chronic lung disease [32].

Testing these carbon dioxide membrane lungs (CDML) in spontaneous breathing animals in 1977, Kolobow et al. found that by removing $CO_2$ through the CDML the spontaneous ventilation decreased proportionally to $CO_2$ removal artificially [33]. By removing 100% of the $CO_2$ metabolically produced, the animals could be kept completely apneic while an amount of oxygen equal to that consumed (apneic oxygenation) was provided without ventilation [34]. In other words, the normal physiological reaction to a reduced need for $CO_2$ removal was a reduction in tidal volume and in the minute ventilation rate, resulting in a reduced elimination of $CO_2$ through the natural lung while maintaining blood $PCO_2$ at the normal level. This control was such that any increase or decrease in extracorporeal $CO_2$ removal within a few seconds was reflected by the animals in an increase/decrease in breathing and, more specifically, in an increase/decrease in alveolar ventilation [33].

The reduced need for mechanical ventilation for $CO_2$ removal (since $CO_2$ was partially removed by the artificial lung) could be useful in reducing the negative effects of mechanical ventilation. Thereby, using the extracorporeal support, the two main respiratory functions, i.e., oxygenation and $CO_2$ removal, were dissociated: 70–80% of oxygenation occurred through the natural lungs, while these were kept inflated with pressure sufficient to keep open the recruitable regions; clearance of total $CO_2$ minute production occurred mainly through the artificial lung being kept apneic, while three to five sighs were provided each minute to preserve the functional residual capacity (low frequency positive pressure ventilation – extracorporeal $CO_2$ removal, LFPPV-ECCO$_2$R) [35]. Here we will discuss this technique, which is the most familiar to us, describing its evolution during the past 20 years.

## Technique

LFPPV-ECCO$_2$R is performed by a veno-venous bypass [35, 36]; catheters are usually inserted after a bolus of intravenous heparin (100 U/kg) using a femoro-femoral cannulation even if a jugulo-femoral approach is possible. Spring-wire reinforced catheters up to 34 F are positioned percutaneously, using a modified Seldinger technique [37]. The patients are paralyzed and receive a light intravenous anesthesia throughout the procedure.

The extracorporeal apparatus consists of a blood section (artificial lung, blood pump, blood circuit), a gas section (flow meter, gas lines, humidifiers), a monitoring setup (blood flow meter, differential pressures across the membrane lung, temperature), and feedback safety controls for venous return and differential pressures. The system is regulated by a thermostat.

The extracorporeal circuit is assembled and primed with Ringer's lactate, following $CO_2$ flushing to prevent bubble formation. Immediately before the connection the priming solution is substituted with heparinized whole blood at 37°C.

As regards the artificial lung, we routinely use the Medtronic-Carmeda (Medtronic, Anaheim, CA; Carmeda BioActive Surface, Stockolm, Sweden) microporus heparinized lungs [38], which allow a decrease of systemic anticoagulation but tend to plasma leakage after a few days of use. The hydrophobic pores, in fact, after a variable time of contact with blood, become hydrophilic, with consequent leakage of plasma [39]. This leads to frequent changes of the artificial lungs. The problem, however, now seems close to being solved, as a new model of the Medtronic-Carmeda heparinized artificial lung (ECLA III) did not show any plasma leakage in the last patients we treated (up to 3 weeks).

For blood pumping, a centrifugal pump (Biomedicus Medtronic) with a heparinized pump head is actually used. The main advantage of this device is that it may be used without a reservoir. The reservoir, in fact, which is mandatory with roller pumps, may be considered a weak point of the circuit, especially when heparinized circuits are used due to the low blood flow speed with consequent formation of clotting and thrombi and possible formation of emboli. In contrast, the major disadvantage of the heparinized centrifugal pump is the tendency for deposition of small clots near the shaft of the rotor, which may cause hemolysis. To prevent this problem we change the pump head every 5 days.

When the patient has been connected to the extracorporeal circuit, blood flow is slowly started, with close attention paid to the body temperature and hemodynamic parameters. After 20–30 min, it is usually possible to set the extracorporeal blood flow at the maintenance rate. Clearance of the total $CO_2$ minute production (200–400 ml/min) occurs mainly through an artificial lung and requires a blood flow of 1.5–2.5 l/min with a ventilation in the artificial lung of 10–20 l/min. While oxygen transfer by the artificial lung is strictly dependent on extracorporeal blood flow (ECBF), the $CO_2$ clearance is less dependent on ECBF ($ECCO_2R$ increases linearly only with the logarithm of ECBF) [32]. Consequently, the amount of $ECCO_2R$ depends on the surface area of the artificial lung and its level of ventilation.

PEEP is set in order to maintain mean airway pressure at the same level as during the previous mechanical ventilation period, while the ventilation of the natural lung is decreased to 2–4 breaths/min. A small catheter positioned into the carina delivers 100% oxygen to provide for the oxygen consumption during the long expiratory pause (apneic oxygenation).

Bleeding is the main complication during long-term bypass, even though heparin-coated circuits with heparinized artificial lungs have reduced the need for systemic anticoagulation. Nevertheless, relatively low heparin doses by continuous intravenous infusion (15 000–30 000 U/day) to maintain an activate clotting time (Hemocron, Int. Technidine, NJ) between 180 and 210 s have been chosen to minimize the consequences of systemic anticoagulation. Systemic heparin is discontinued only if major bleeding occurs or when surgical maneuvers are required.

The weaning process starts immediately: first from $FiO_2$, second from pressures. When oxygenation increases, the $FiO_2$ of the ventilators is decreased first, using a target $PaO_2$ of 80–100 mmHg. When the target $PaO_2$ is maintained with a ventilatory setting at an $FiO_2$ of 40%, the $FiO_2$ of the gas mixture ventilating the artificial membrane lung is decreased stepwise to an $FiO_2$ of 21%. If oxygenation is still maintained at the target value we start decreasing the PEEP level.

When $PaO_2$ remains stable between 80 and 100 mmHg, with an $FiO_2$ in the ventilator of 40% and in the membrane lung of 21% and a PEEP level between 5 and 10 cm $H_2O$, the patient ventilatory setting is shifted to spontaneous/assisted ventilation.

The disconnection from bypass is considered when the patient is able to tolerate spontaneous/assisted ventilation for 6–12 h, with the same level of $FiO_2$ and PEEP either in the ventilator or in the membrane lung. Fist of all, the gas flow through the artificial lungs is stopped, and second, if the patient is able to maintain a viable gas exchange without any extracorporeal support, the catheters are removed. Percutaneous cannulation does not require any surgical repair.

## Clinical Experience

At our center, we now select patients for $ECCO_2R$ according to three entry criteria: (a) severe hypoxemia [40, 41]; (b) low respiratory compliance; and (c) lack of positive response to PEEP. Severe hypoxemia is defined according to the criteria originally devised in 1974 by the National Heart, Lung and Blood Institute, which funded a prospective multicenter, randomized trial to compare extracorporeal membrane oxygenation (ECMO) and continuous positive-pressure ventilation with continuous positive-pressure ventilation alone in ARDS (ECMO study) [42]. Patients admitted to the study were selected according to fast and slow entry criteria (ECMO criteria). Fast entry criteria selected patients with an arterial oxygen pressure ($PaO_2$) of less than 50 mmHg for more than 2 h when measured at an inspiratory oxygen fraction of 100%, and a PEEP 5 cm $H_2O$ or greater. Slow entry criteria selected patients with a $PaO_2$ of less than 50 mmHg for more than 20 h when measured at an $FiO_2$ of 60% or greater, a PEEP 5 cm $H_2O$ or greater, and a right-to-left shunt greater than 30% after 48 h of maximal medical therapy [43].

The second criterion we apply for selection of patients is the total static lung compliance (TSLC). In fact, we reported that patients with a TSLC lower than 25 ml/cm $H_2O$ could not be maintained on pressure control – inverse ratio ventilation (PC-IRV) or continuous positive airway pressure (CPAP), while all the patients with a TSLC higher than 30 ml/cm $H_2O$ were successfully treated with CPAP [44]. The borderline patients, with TSLC between 25 and 30 ml/cm $H_2O$, had to be treated with prolonged PC-IRV or with LFPPV-$ECCO_2R$ if PC-IRV resulted in a significant rise in $PaCO_2$. Therefore, a TSLC lower than 30 ml/cm $H_2O$ measured at 10 ml/kg during anesthesia and paralysis was added as an entry criteria for extracorporeal support [45].

Recently, we added a third entry criterion for starting extracorporeal support, trying to discriminate patients with early ARDS, in whom recruitment of the tissue poorly or noninflated into the inflated compartment could be expected, from those with late ARDS, characterized by diffuse fibrosis, emphysema-like lesions, and lack of improvement in gas exchange by application of PEEP. Actually, no patient with a reasonable increase in oxygenation and a consistent clearing of the densities to the CT scan when PEEP is increased from 5 to 15 cm $H_2O$ undergoes extracorporeal support [46].

The only exclusion criteria, in our center, are the contraindications to systemic anticoagulation; neither the patients's age nor the length of previous mechanical ventilation are considered criteria of exclusion.

Since 1979, we have treated 94 patients with LFPPV-$ECCO_2R$ (mean age 31.2 years ± 11.1); 89 had ARDS of varying etiology (pneumonia 63%, post-traumatic 21%, embolism and sepsis 16%), while the others had acute respiratory failure due to alveolar proteinosis (three patients), chronic obstructive pulmonary disease (one patient), and recurrent pneumothorax due to bullous emphysema (one patient), All the non-ARDS patients survived. Survival rate in ARDS patients was 43% for pneumonia, 42% for post-traumatic respiratory failure, and 57% for embolism and sepsis. These data are similar to those reported in the European experience, which involves more than 300 patients with a mortality of 47% (personal communications).

As regards the causes of death, it is worth nothing that 27 of the 49 patients who died in our series became hypoxemic despite $ECCO_2R$, and in some of them the intrapulmonary shunt approached 100%. These observations suggest that when life is sustained with extracorporeal support, the lung may deteriorate and completely lose the ability to perform gas exchange even during ARDS, a syndrome in which only a few deaths are usually attributed to hypoxemia, multiple-organ failure always being claimed as the major cause of death [47, 48].

A number of prognostic factors have been proposed in the literature as predictors of mortality in ARDS [44, 45]. We reported in 1986 that the only discriminant, in our $ECCO_2R$ population, between survivors and nonsurvivors was the level of $PaCO_2$ before bypass, which was significantly higher in nonsurvivors than in survivors [45]. This parameter has lost some of its significance in the past few years due to the increasing use of permissive hypercapnia before $ECCO_2R$. Important factors now appear to be: the presence of barotrauma [44 of 89 (49%) had a chest tube positioned for pneumothorax drainage and 29 (66%) died], the level of peak inspiratory pressure (peak inspiratory pressure before bypass was significantly more elevated in nonsurvivors) and the number of failed organs (nine patients had failure of more than three organs besides the lung and none of them survived) before $ECCO_2R$.

As regards the response to $ECCO_2R$, it was reported in 1986 [45] that an improvement in lung function was always seen within 48 h after the beginning of bypass, this group of patients (responder group) being the only group in which survivors were observed. During the past several years, an increased frequency in survivors in the nonresponder group has been obtained (oxygenation improved only after 1 or 2 weeks of bypass). Two main reasons might explain the "late responders": first of all, the changes in entry criteria, with a selection of patients with an underlying lung pathology unexpected to show rapid improvement in oxygenation (PEEP unresponsive); second, the possibility of longer and safer bypass due to percutaneous cannulation and heparinized artificial lungs, which has drastically decreased the incidence of bleeding. In fact, if we compare the population treated between 1979 and 1988 with that treated between 1988 and 1992, we find that blood transfusions are now 1/3 of what they were before ($360 \pm 363$ vs. $976 \pm 830$ ml/day, $p = 0.05$), while the time on bypass of survivors is actually more than double what it was before ($153 \pm 128$ vs. $467 \pm 321$ h; $p = 0.001$) with no change in duration was regards nonsurvivors ($237 \pm 152$ vs. $243 \pm 299$; $p =$ n.s.).

Based on all these observations, we believe that in the future $ECCO_2R$ will become less invasive, safer, and simpler in management. If this target is reached, it will be possible to perform this nonconventional respiratory treatment not only as a last resort in a selected group of patients with high expected mortality (ECMO criteria), but also in early ARDS, avoiding the lung damage produced by long periods of mechanical ventilation. To date, however, since extracorporeal support is considered an experimental technique, its application should be limited to particularly selected patients at a few referral centers with sufficient motivation, technical skills, and manpower.

## References


1. Kumar A, Pontoppidan H, Falke KJ et al. (1973) Pulmonary barotrauma during mechanical ventilation. Crit Care Med 1:181–186
2. Baeza OR, Wagner RB, Lowery BD et al. (1975) Pulmonary hyperinflation: a form of barotrauma during mechanical ventilation. J Thorac Cardiovasc Surg 80:790–803
3. Qvist J, Pontoppidan H, Wilson RS et al. (1975) Hemodynamic responses to mechanical ventilation with PEEP: the effect of hypervolemia. Anesthesiology 42:45–55
4. Hall SV, Johnson EE, Hedley-White J (1974) Renal hemodynamics and function with continuous positive pressure ventilation in dog. Anesthesiology 41:452–461
5. Rouby JJ (1986) Jet ventilation a haute fréquence. Aspects techniques, physiopathologie, principales indications. In: Lemaire F (ed) La ventilation artificielle. Collection d'Anesthésiologie et de Réanimation. Masson, Paris, pp 141–168
6. Gattinoni L, Marcolin R, Caspani ML (1985) Constant mean airway pressure with different patterns of positive pressure breathing during the adult respiratory distress syndrome. Bull Eur Physiopathol Respir 21:275–279
7. Pesenti A, Marcolin R, Prato P et al. (1985) Mean airway pressure vs positive end-expiratory pressure during mechanical ventilation. Crit Care Med 13:34–37
8. Hickling KG, Henderson SJ, Jackson R (1990) Low mortality associated with low volume pressure limited ventilation with permissive hypercapnia in severe adult respiratory distress syndrome. Intensive Care Med 16:372–377
9. Gattinoni L, Mascheroni D, Torresin A et al. (1986) Morphological response to positive end-expiratory pressure in acute respiratory failure. Computerized tomography study. Intensive Care Med 12:137–142
10. Maunder RJ, Schuman WP, McHugh et al. (1986) Preservation of normal lung regions in adult respiratory distress syndrome: analysis by computed tomography. J Am Med Assoc 255:2563–2565
11. Gattinoni L, Pesenti A, Avalli L et al. (1987) Pressure volume curve of the total respiratory system in acute respiratory failure. Am Rev Respir Dis 136:730–736
12. Gattinoni L, Pesenti A, Torresin A et al. (1986) Adult respiratory distress syndrome profiles by computed tomography. J Thorac Imag 1986; 1:25–30
13. Gattinoni L, Pesenti A, Baglioni S et al. (1988) Inflammatory pulmonary edema and positive end-expiratory pressure: correlations between imaging and physiologic studies. J Thorac Imaging 3:59–64
14. Gattinoni L, Pelosi P, Vitale G et al. (1991) Body position changes redistribute lung computed tomographic densities in patients with acute respiratory failure. Anesthesiology 74:15–23
15. Gattinoni L, D'Andrea L, Pelosi P et al. (1993) Regional effects and mechanism of positive end-expiratory pressure in early adult respiratory distress syndrome. J Am Med Assoc 269:2122–2127
16. Pelosi P, D'Andrea L, Vitale G et al. (1994) Vertical gradient of regional lung inflation in adult respiratory distress syndrome. Am Rev Respir Dis Am J Respir Crit Care Med 149:8–13
17. Dantzker DR, Brook JC, Dehart P et al. (1979) Ventilation-perfusion distributions in the adult respiratory distress syndrome. Am Rev Respir Dis 120:1039–1042
18. Gattinoni L, Pesenti A, Bombino M et al. (1988) Relationship between lung computed tomographic density, gas exchange and PEEP in acute respiratory failure. Anesthesiology 69:824–832
19. Albelda SM, Gefter WB, Kelley MA et al. (1982) Ventilatory-induced subpleural air cysts: clinical, radiographic and pathologic significance. Am Rev Respir Dis 127:360–365
20. Marini JJ, Culver BH (1989) Systemic air embolism consequent to mechanical ventilation in ARDS. Ann Intern Med 110:699–703

21. Suter PM, Fairlay HB, Isenberg MD (1975) Optimum end-expiratory airway pressure in patients with acute pulmonary failure. N Engl J Med 292:284–289
22. Lamy M, Fallat RL, Koeninger E et al. (1976) Pathologic features and mechanisms of hypoxemia in adult respiratory distress syndrome. Am Rev Respir Dis 114:267–284
23. Pontoppidan H, Geffen B, Lowenstain E (1972) Acute respiratory failure in the adult. N Engl J Med 287:690
24. Slavin G, Nunn JF, Crow J, Pore' CJ (1982) Bronchiolectasis: a complication of artificial ventilation. Br Med J 28:931–934
25. Mascheroni D, Kolobow T, Fumagalli R et al. (1985) Respiratory failure following induced hyperventilation. An experimental study. Crit Care Med 13:330
26. Dreyfuss D, Basset G, Soler P et al. (1985) Intermittent positive pressure hyperventilation with high inflation pressures produces pulmonary microvascular injury in rats. Am Rev Respir Dis 132:880–884
27. Webb H, Tierney DF (1974) Experimental pulmonary oedema due to intermittent positive pressure ventilation with high inflation pressures. Protection by positive end-expiratory pressure. Am Rev Respir Dis 110:556–565
28. Deneke SM, Fanburg BL (1982) Oxygen toxicity of the lung: an update. Br J Anaesthesiol 54:737–749
29. Pesenti A, Kolobow T, Buckhold DK (1982) Prevention of hyaline membrane disease in premature lambs by apneic oxygenation and extracorporeal carbon dioxide removal. Crit Care Med 8:11
30. Dorrington KL, McRae KM, Gardaz JP et al. (1989) A randomized comparison of total extracorporeal $CO_2$ removal with conventional mechanical ventilation in experimental hyaline membrane disease. Intensive Care Med 15:184–191
31. Gattinoni L, Agostoni A, Damia G et al. (1980) Hemodynamics and renal function during low-frequency positive pressure ventilation with extracorporeal $CO_2$ removal. Intensive Care Med 6:155–161
32. Kolobow T, Gattinoni L, Tomlinson T et al. (1977) The carbon dioxide membrane lung (CDML): a new concept. Trans Am Soc Artif Intern Organs 23:17–21
33. Kolobow T, Gattinoni L, Tomlinson T, Pierce J (1977) Control of breathing using an extracorporeal membrane lung. Anesthesiology 46:138–141
34. Kolobow T, Gattinoni L, Tomlinson T, Pierce J (1978) An alternative to breathing. J Thorac Cardiovasc Surg 75:261–266
35. Gattinoni L, Kolobow T, Tomlinson T et al. (1978) Low-frequency positive pressure ventilation with extracorporeal carbon dioxide removal (LFPPV-ECCO2R): an experimental study. Anesth Analg 55:470–477
36. Gattinoni L, Pesenti A, Kolobow T et al. (1983) A new look at therapy of the adult respiratory distress syndrome: motionless lung. Int Anesthesiol Clin 21:97–117
37. Bombino M, Marcolin R, Pesenti A et al. (1992) Percutaneous cannulation for long-term bypass. 2nd European Congress on Extracorporeal Lung Support, Marburg, p 26
38. Bindslev L, Eklund J, Worlander W et al. (1987) Treatment of acute respiratory failure by extracorporeal carbon dioxide elimination performed with a surface heparinized artificial lung. Anesthesiology 67:117–120
39. Mottaghy K, Oedekoven B, Starmans H et al. (1989) Technical aspects of plasma leakage prevention in microporous capillary membrane oxygenators. Trans Am Soc Artif Intern Organs 35:640–645
40. Gattinoni L, Kolobow T, Damia G et al. (1979) Extracorporeal carbon dioxide removal ($ECCO_2R$): a new form of respiratory assistance. Int J Artif Organs 2:183–185
41. Gattinoni L, Agostoni A, Pesenti A et al. (1980) Treatment of acute respiratory failure with low-frequency positive pressure ventilation and extracorporeal removal of $CO_2$. Lancet 2: 292–295
42. Protocol for extracorporeal support for respiratory insufficiency collaborative program. National Heart, Lung and Blood Institute, Division of Lung Disease, Bethesda, May 1974
43. Zapol W, Snider MT, Hill JD et al. (1979) Extracorporeal membrane oxygenation in severe acute respiratory failure. A randomized prospective study. J Am Med Assoc 242:2193–2196

44. Gattinoni L, Pesenti A, Caspani ML et al. (1984) The role of total static lung compliance in the management of severe ARDS unresponsive to conventional treatment. Intensive Care Med 10:121–126
45. Gattinoni L, Pesenti A, Mascheroni D et al. (1986) Low-frequency positive-pressure ventilation with extracorporeal $CO_2$ removal in severe acute respiratory failure. J Am Med Assoc 256:881–886
46. Pesenti A, Gattinoni L, Bombino M (1993) Long-term extracorporeal respiratory support: 20 years of progress. Intensive Crit Care Dig 12:15–18
47. Artigas A, Carlet J, Le Gall JR et al. (1991) Clinical presentation, prognostic factors and outcome of ARDS in the European collaborative study (1985–1987): a preliminary report. In: Zapol WM, Lemaire F (eds) Adult respiratory distress syndrome. Dekker, New York, pp 37–63
48. Montgomery AB, Stager MA, Carrico CJ et al. (1985) Causes of mortality in patients with the adult respiratory distress syndrome. Am Rev Respir Dis 132:485–489

# Extracorporeal Membrane Oxygenation in Children

G.A. Pearson and R.K. Firmin

## Introduction

The introduction of modern methods of prolonged extracorporeal life support to the United Kingdom (UK) commenced in Leicester in 1989 [1]. Up to that time, many cardiothoracic centres had had prior experience of its use, usually in the treatment of adults, dating from the late 1970s [2, 3]. The universally poor outlook for such patients, documented by the National Institutes of Health (NIH) trial in 1979 [4], caused most to abandon its use. However, extracorporeal membrane oxygenation (ECMO) had become so successful in the treatment of neonates during the 1980s, in the United States of America [5], as to become considered a standard therapy. This was the stimulus for us to start our service. In the light of more recent experience in older patients [6], we did not confine the facility to neonates, but considered any patient with a potentially reversible pulmonary or cardiopulmonary problem.

Protracted cardiopulmonary life support, provided by the creation and maintenance of an extracorporeal circulation incorporating a gas-exchange device, has been possible since the 1960s [7]. The ability to sustain such an extracorporeal circulation for prolonged periods without prohibitive degrees of haemolysis was achieved by refinements of oxygenator design [8, 9]. The bubble oxygenators that had been used for early peroperative bypass surgery were replaced, first with disc oxygenators and later with the membrane oxygenators in common use today. The term "ECMO" [10, 11] has been adopted as a generic description of the system – whether or not a membrane oxygenator is employed. By virtue of its direct approach to the maintenance of adequate gas exchange and the optional independence of the subject's cardiac function, ECMO has been widely applied with varying levels of success to situations where conventional life support is felt to be inadequate or to have failed [10, 11].

Encouraged by reports of high survival rates in patients otherwise expected to have a significant risk of mortality [12, 13], a total of 123 patients were treated at our institution, 109 of whom were infants or children. This chapter presents this consecutive paediatric series which was accumulated over 3.5 years. The neonatal data presented throughout apply to the time period up to the 1st of January, 1993, at which time the extracorporeal support of neonates within the UK became the subject of a collaborative multicentre prospective randomised trial. The data for older children are not so restricted.

## Patient Selection

### General Principles

The literature suggests that the clearest refinement in the application of ECMO, since its first inception, has been the evolution of meticulous patient selection [11]. We therefore made extensive efforts to distinguish and exclude those patients whose outcome was likely to be inevitably hopeless. The remaining population were refined by a screening process intended to ensure both that they were sick enough to justify the procedure and that they were not likely to be at prohibitive risk from it. Thus the same generic considerations were applied to all patients:

1. Does the patient have a potentially reversible pulmonary, cardiac or cardiopulmonary problem?
2. Are the neurological status and the function of other organs consistent with a reasonable outcome?
3. Is even limited heparinisation contraindicated?
4. Is there anything to be gained by further pursuit of conventional treatment, and is the patient sufficiently sick to warrant more interventional support?

### Neonates

The application of such questions to neonates involved several specific issues, the answers to which had become relatively standardised in the USA.

The potential predisposition of excessively preterm infants towards intraventricular haemorrhage [5] led to the treatment only of patients >34 weeks' completed gestation at birth. Patients with established or significant haemorrhage were excluded for fear of extension of the haemorrhage. Additionally, infants were required to be of sufficient size to allow cervical cannulation – the vascular access of choice – which becomes progressively more difficult below a birth weight of 2 kg [11].

The exclusion of patients with irreversible disease precluded the treatment of patients with severe chromosomal abnormalities and other congenital malformations that are incompatible with a reasonable quality of life (e.g. hypoplastic left heart). Similarly, babies who had suffered a severe hypoxic injury and who had associated hypoxic-ischaemic encephalopathy or established brain damage were excluded.

A history of prolonged high-pressure mechanical ventilation (>10 days) led to exclusion on the expectation that the degree of pressure-related lung damage would have reached a level that would delay lung recovery beyond the realistic time limits of ECMO perfusion [14].

Patients with severe coagulopathy prior to ECMO were avoided. We employed a somewhat arbitrary cutoff (in all age-groups) of an INR value persistently greater than 2 despite appropriate treatment.

Hence, the clinical evaluation of the neonatal ECMO candidate involved a series of clinical and laboratory investigations, during the course of which attempts were made to further optimise conventional treatment and preparations were made for cannulation. Specifically, cranial ultrasound was performed, looking for lesions involving the brain parenchyma which could have been associated with a poor neurological outcome. It was also intended to detect significant haemorrhage in the lateral ventricles, i.e. extending beyond the subependymal or choroidal regions. Echocardiography was performed in order to provide an evaluation of pulmonary haemodynamics and to detect covert presentations of cyanotic heart disease such as total anomalous pulmonary venous connection [15–17].

Disease severity amongst the neonates was judged with the assistance of numerical criteria as an adjunct to clinical decision-making [18]. Of the available options, the oxygenation index (OI) [19] was most commonly applied. This descriptive index was calculated as a fraction according to the formula:

$$\frac{\text{Mean airway pressure} \times FiO_2(\%)}{\text{Post-ductal } P_AO_2}$$

The numerator was thus a numerical expression of the level of ventilatory support being provided and the denominator a measure of how much oxygenation was being achieved. Values of 40 or more had been reputed to predict an 80% mortality without ECMO and so were applied prospectively in the selection of this treatment group.

Neonates (particularly those with congenital diaphragmatic hernia) also presented on occasion with intractable carbon dioxide retention, rather than hypoxia. In preference to the ventilatory indices described by Bohn et al. [20], we chose to adopt a policy of accepting patients whose partial pressure of carbon dioxide remained above 12 kpa for 3 h or more despite optimal ventilator management.

## Paediatrics

Selection of older patients was also based upon the generic questions outlined above. Unlike the neonates, there was a lack of any single uniform measure of disease severity/predictor of mortality that could confidently be applied prospectively to the population [21, 22]. Patients did, however, fall clearly into two groups: firstly, patients with mainly pulmonary failure, and secondly, patients in whom ECMO was indicated primarily for cardiac support.

In assessing those patients with respiratory failure for ECMO, information from lung biopsy, when available, carried the greatest weight [23]. Careful consideration was also given to the underlying diagnosis and its natural history to avoid placing a patient on ECMO who had a progressive or irreversible disease. The severity of secondary barotrauma due to positive-pressure mechanical ventilation was assessed clinically, with close attention paid to the duration and pressure of ventilation, the inspired oxygen concentration ($FiO_2$) and the presence or absence of bullae or air leaks. In general, ventilation at high pressures and $FiO_2$ for more than 7 days was considered a contraindication to ECMO in anticipation of progressive (fibrotic) lung damage [23]. In some rare disease processes ECMO was, almost electively, considered the only viable option, for example, in the case of a patient who had severe but relatively stable respiratory failure and required a lung wash for alveolar lipoproteinosis. ECMO was used to provide life support and suitable conditions for this to be performed (see below).

Echocardiography also formed part of the pre-ECMO evaluation in these patients. The intention was not so much to detect cases of covert cyanotic heart disease as to make an objective assessment of cardiac function and pulmonary haemodynamics [24].

The decision to employ ECMO as mechanical circulatory support was most likely when patients presented with acute severe right heart failure as a consequence of pulmonary hypertension. However, failure to wean from cardiopulmonary bypass, intractable low cardiac output and unresponsive pulmonary hypertensive crisis were all considered valid indications for intervention. Despite having the facility to perform ECMO available in the cardiac surgical unit, extensive efforts were made to establish the reason for deterioration prior to cannulation in the postoperative patients. Such a careful appraisal of cardiac status involved echocardiography and pressure and saturation measurements, looking specifically for unrelieved outflow tract obstructions and/or residual shunts.

# Method

## Cannulation and Circuit

Extracorporeal circulations were established using peripheral cannulation, and cannulae were selected according to their flow characteristics [25], as well as ease of placement. Different techniques of cannulation were used, according to the weight of the patient and the degree of cardiac dysfunction. In patients less than 15 kg, cannulae were, by preference, inserted after surgical cutdown under general anaesthesia. In some older patients cannulae were inserted percutaneously or using a combined technique of percutaneous insertion into a surgically exposed vessel. Only in the rare instance of failure to wean from preoperative bypass was transthoracic cannulation contemplated. Peripheral cannulation was even preferred for post-operative patients on the cardiac intensive care unit [26].

Cervical cannulation permits vascular access with optimal blood flow characteristics and was preferred exclusively in the neonates. For the larger patients, again, the right internal jugular vein was the favoured site for the venous drainage cannula. The provision of mechanical circulatory assistance was possible through a venoarterial cannulation (involving the right common carotid artery); however, the venovenous route was preferred in all age-groups where possible. This cannulation was perceived as advantageous in terms of myocardial oxygenation [27] and pulmonary blood flow [28]. It was also suspected that, for a variety of reasons, it would be associated with a greater speed of pulmonary recovery even in the absence of pulmonary hypertension.

The ECMO circuits were constructed from super Tygon tubing according to the conventional Bartlett design with the addition of "Galveston" diamonds (see Fig. 1). Using this design, the various components were assembled in such a way as to avoid areas of stasis and maintain normothermia. Bypass circuits all used Scimed spirally wound silicone membrane oxygenators (0.8–2.4 $m^2$ of membrane surface area). In the patients less than 8 kg, 1/4-inch super Tygon tubing was used. In the larger patients 3/8-inch tubing was preferred. A roller pump was used in virtually all cases since our early experience of a centrifugal impeller system had been unfavourable.

The patients were heparinised (40 units/kg i.v. bolus) during the cannulation and 100–200 units of heparin were added to the circuit during priming, depending upon its priming volume. During the perfusion a continuous infusion of heparin was used to prevent thrombosis in the circuit. Recognising the risk of haemorrhagic complications during ECMO, we adopted a policy of minimal

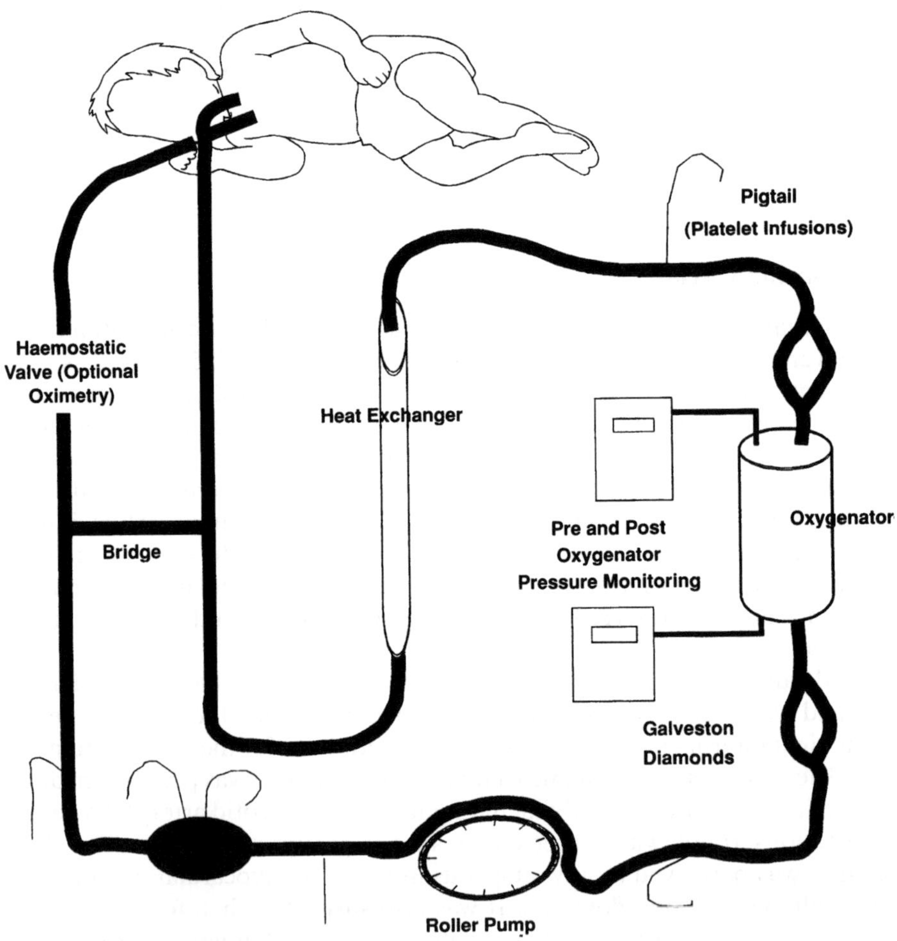


**Fig. 1.** Standard ECMO circuit constructed from ¼-inch super Tygon

heparinisation, with the degree of anticoagulation maintained as close as practicable to the perceived limits of safety. Hourly measurement of a whole-blood activated clotting time (ACT) was used as an indicator of the risk of circuit thrombosis, and a target elevation to 160–200 s was used (from the normal of 110–120 s). This normally required heparin infusion rates of 30–60 units/kg/h.

Thus, in most instances, routine operation involved blood draining from the right atrium via a cervical venous cannulation. This flow was driven by the central venous pressure and facilitated by the syphonage of a 1-m drop between the patient and the "bladder" (a small 30- to 50-ml reservoir of ovoid design to promote laminar internal flow without areas of stasis). Therefore, without untoward suction being imparted to the venous drainage line, the bladder was nonetheless distended by the spontaneous venous drainage. Any imbalance of flows depleting the bladder caused it to collapse and this feature was used to servoregulate the circuit. The bladder was housed in a box where its distension depressed a plunger that operated a tripswitch, electrically linked to the pump power supply. Hence, inadequate venous drainage or excessive pump flow caused collapse of the bladder and cessation of pump flow before suction was applied to the venous line (which could cause cavitation in the blood column or excessive haemolysis).

The pump perfused the oxygenator and then, after gas exchange, a heat exchange column where the blood was warmed to body temperature before reinfusion. The pressures within the circuit both pre and post oxygenator were monitored continuously, and changes in their relative and absolute values were used to infer the degree and position of potential occlusions in the circuit (whether mechanical or thrombotic). When using tubing of appropriate calibre the flow characteristics of the venous drainage cannula were then the rate-limiting step in terms of venous drainage, and those of the return cannula were the critical determinant of the operating pressure within the circuit between the pump and the patient.

## Principles of Gas Exchange

Carbon dioxide transfer across respiratory surfaces is, by virtue of its high solubility coefficient in water, largely a function of its diffusion gradient and the permeability characteristics of the membrane. In the native lung the diffusion gradient is maximised by replacing equilibrated (alveolar) gas with fresh gas containing little or no carbon dioxide. This process is achieved by ventilation. Arterial partial pressures of carbon dioxide therefore bear an inverse relationship to minute ventilation. By contrast, oxygen is poorly soluble in water, and the vast majority of oxygen in blood is transported using haemoglobin as a carrier molecule. This effectively imparts an upper limit on the amount of oxygen that can be carried by a given volume of blood. This limit (100% saturation of haemoglobin) is achieved at physiological partial pressures of oxygen. Once the limit is reached, further oxygen uptake necessitates more desaturated haemoglobin replacing that at the respiratory surface.

These principles [29] are independent of the gas-exchange device and therefore hold true for membrane oxygenators as well as for native lungs. Increased uptake of oxygen requires an increased exposure of blood to the respiratory surface, and carbon dioxide removal requires improved ventilation of the membrane. A variety of membrane oxygenators are available with differing internal membrane surface areas. Larger membrane surface areas with relatively narrow blood films create a greater potential for oxygenation, and this capacity is described by the "rated flow" of the membrane (defined as the point after which increases in blood flow across the membrane are not associated with increased oxygenation). Hence, the choice of oxygenator for the circuit was dictated by the requirements of the patient, size of patient, and whether the emphasis was upon oxygenation or carbon dioxide removal. Both blood flow and gas flow to the oxygenator could be adjusted during ECMO.

$CO_2$ removal was maximised by the use of a countercurrent in blood and gas flow directions. The composition of the delivered "sweep gas" was kept constant (100% oxygen) and was not used to affect the diffusion gradient for $CO_2$. Such an arrangement ran the risk of allowing the membrane surface to become wet. The additional barrier to gaseous diffusion would then deleteriously affect oxygenation. In our experience this was not problematic, providing a membrane oxygenator was used that exceeded the anticipated blood flow requirements.

Assuming adequate oxygenator function, the oxygen uptake of blood traversing the circuit (in millilitres per minute) was predetermined by the haemoglobin concentration and the level of desaturation in the blood draining to the circuit (cf. the Fick principle). Additionally, the oxygen content of this blood was used, during venoarterial circulation, as an indicator of the adequacy of tissue oxygen delivery. This could be inferred from continuous oximetry of blood traversing the afferent limb of the circuit [29]. During venovenous perfusion the phenomena of recirculation and venous admixture meant that the oxygen content of the venous drainage to the circuit was artificially elevated (by recirculation of blood recently infused into the venous circulation from the circuit) and the patient's arterial oxygen content was reduced (by mixture of blood from the circuit with venous blood that had not traversed the circuit). Hence, patients with a venovenous cannulation had effectively a physiological right-to-left shunt which, in the absence of native lung function, left them mildly desaturated. This perfusion technique was therefore reserved for patients with adequate or remediable cardiac function. Peripheral oxygen saturations of 82+% were considered acceptable provided the haematocrit was maintained around 0.4. Adequate oxygen delivery could then be expected through modest increases in native cardiac output.

In situations where the primary emphasis of extracorporeal gas exchange was upon $CO_2$ removal (extracorporeal $CO_2$ removal – ECCOR) [30], circuits were constructed to run low blood flows across a large membrane surface area, and the native lung was then required to contribute only to oxygenation. This required the assistance of low-frequency, low-pressure ventilation or (rarely) apnoeic oxygenation. Such circuits in the larger patients (>40 kg) frequently comprised two oxygenators in parallel if some contribution to oxygenation was required (higher blood flows) and in series if it was not.

## Haemodynamic Considerations

A venoarterial cannulation imparted a degree of cardiopulmonary bypass that was proportional to the relative volume of ECMO blood flow compared with the patient's cardiac output. At blood flow rates sufficient to achieve adequate oxygenation (in the absence of native pulmonary function – 100 ml/kg/min) a reduction in pulsatility of the patient's arterial circulation was common. Nonpulsatile circulation was very rare, however. Since most patients' cardiac output exceeded this basal flow rate, nonpulsatile circulation was generally limited to patients with profound myocardial compromise. A venovenous cannulation had no direct effects in the form of circulatory assistance; however, improved oxygen delivery frequently resulted in reversal of inotropic dependence and improved haemodynamic stability.

The cardiac implications of systemic circulatory assistance provided by venoarterial cannulation were considerable. Left and right ventricular preload were reduced in proportion to the extracorporeal flow and pulmonary blood flow was reduced (in the absence of a ductus arteriosus). In contrast, left ventricular afterload was increased by the current of blood returning from the circuit [31, 32]. In situations of myocardial compromise the increase in afterload could be sufficient to exceed the left ventricle's capacity for ejection [33]. Indeed, myocardial compromise could be defined if this occurred at extracorporeal blood flow rates below the expected resting cardiac output.

In the neonatal patients great emphasis was placed upon the dangers of uncontrolled left-to-right shunting through a persistent ductus arteriosus [34]. In the majority of cases spontaneous, although somewhat asynchronous, ductal closure was observed as the high pulmonary vascular resistance responded to treatment. However, this was not a reliable phenomenon, especially in patients with congenital diaphragmatic hernia. Echocardiographic evidence of left ventricular dilatation and mitral regurgitation in such patients was interpreted as reflecting high pulmonary blood flow and an increased risk of haemorrhagic pulmonary oedema (or even pulmonary haemorrhage). Such appearances were usually distinguishable from myocardial dysfunction by the preservation of the left ventricular ejection fraction and prompted a policy of early ductal ligation on ECMO. In the event of ECMO treatment prior to surgical repair of diaphragmatic hernia, the operative ductal ligation was combined with a transthoracic reduction and repair of the diaphragmatic defect. This usually involved the positioning of a generous Gore-Tex patch to prevent tense abdominal distension.

## Ventilation

Once a patient had been established upon extracorporeal life support, the requirement for gas exchange to occur across the native lung was significantly reduced. In our cases of neonatal and paediatric ECMO, the circuit was frequently designed so that it would be obviated completely. This enabled a drastic reduction of ventilator settings from the extremes of pressure, volume and $FiO_2$ that had been required prior to ECMO. Almost all patients had severely noncompliant lung disease, although some were obstructed and some had mixed ventilatory defects. The tendency, therefore, was for reduced airway pressures to drop below a "closing pressure" and for the lung at least initially to become less compliant and the chest radiograph to "whiteout". This appearance was common in all age-groups but not universal. The radiographic appearances presumably represented the combined effects of atelectasis and capillary fluid leakage/pulmonary oedema. The aetiology of this response was probably mixed and may have included a contribution from an "inflammatory response" to extracorporeal circulation [35]. However, the appearances were temporary and resolved as lung recovery ensued during continued extracorporeal circulation.

Aside from the considerations outlined below, our practice was to use conventional ventilators in an admittedly unconventional manner. Techniques such as negative-pressure ventilation were not employed during ECMO, although this particular technique did prove useful in weaning neonates with pulmonary hypoplasia from ventilation after successful ECMO. The principle aim of ventilator management during perfusion, particularly with neonates, was to minimise the components of atelectasis and pulmonary oedema by maintaining a significant, although reduced, mean airway pressure. However, priority was also given to the issue of barotrauma. The perceived need was to minimise peak airway pressure and the gap between peak and end-expiratory pressures that, combined with the inspiratory time and gas-flow rate, would have a direct effect on the generation of shearing forces within the airways. The result was the use of long inspiration times with low peak-inspiratory pressures (PIP) and high end-expiratory pressures (PEEP) [36, 37]. A typical neonate would be ventilated therefore at pressures of 18–20/12 cm water, at a rate of 10 breaths and with an inspired time of 1 s. Such settings were at marked variance from those customary to ventilate the lung; however, ventilation was no longer necessary for gas exchange. Patients with extremes of barotrauma (multiple air leaks, bronchopleural fistulae, etc.) were extubated or left on low-pressure continuous positive airway pressure, often for several days.

Outside of the neonatal age-group, there was a marked paucity of information which could have been used to help determine the correct approach towards pulmonary care in these patients. Strict attention to fluid balance and more general issues were treated with the same priority as in other intensive care patients. The presence of the cannulation reduced the ability for extremes of postural variation. With regard to ventilator settings, airway pressure was felt to be a key issue, both in the aetiology of the trauma associated with all types of artificial ventilation and in the prevention of atelectasis and pulmonary oedema. This meant that frequently, once on ECMO, pressure ventilation was adopted for larger patients who would otherwise customarily have received volume regulated ventilation. This arrangement persisted for the duration of the perfusion.

In situations where the circuits were being used primarily for $CO_2$ removal some contribution to gas exchange (oxygenation) was required of the native lung. Again, ventilation strategies were adopted that were intended to minimise ventilator-induced lung injury, for example apnoeic oxygenation, very low frequency pressure ventilation or CPAP.

The independence of gas exchange from native lung function produced considerable advantages in terms of endotracheal toilet and the ability to perform protracted and intensive physiotherapy. The advantages are highlighted by the following examples:

1. A 17-month-old child was treated for peanut inhalation. Repeated attempts at bronchoscopy in the light of a clear history had been unsuccessful because they were associated with profound hypoxia. He was referred after 4 days on astronomical ventilator settings with multiple air leaks into pleura, mediastinum, and peritoneum. Bronchoscopy on ECMO was problem free and the foreign body was removed. Of more significance, however, was the fact that sufficient resolution of the barotrauma to allow decannulation took 284 h.

2. A 2-year-old child with biopsy-proven alveolar lipoproteinosis was referred with respiratory failure. Clinical and radiographic appearances were too severe to contemplate selective segmental bronchial lavage (the treatment of choice). Under venoarterial ECMO total pulmonary lavage was performed. After a "nitrogen washout" her functional residual capacity was replaced with pH-buffered normal saline, and tidal volumes of the same were continuously instilled and drained until the effluent was clear (6 h later). At the end of the procedure a dose of exogenous surfactant was administered. Decannulation was possible within 12 h after resolution of the radiographic abnormalities.

In a third case, ECMO was used to allow complex tracheal surgery without compromising gas exchange.

## Fluids and Nutrition

Patients of all ages tended to present for ECMO with widespread oedema. This reflected the fact that, as a rule, they had received large volumes of colloid infusion as part of their resuscitation. However, isolated acute renal failure and capillary leak phenomena were also observed. There was, in fact, a comparatively high incidence of varying degrees of pre-existent multiorgan-system failure. Tissue oedema and the continued "third space" distribution of any administered fluids were considered issues of paramount importance in their general intensive care and in the specific requirements for recovery of organ systems (particularly cardiopulmonary and hepatorenal dysfunction). Any "inflammatory response" to extracorporeal circulation could be anticipated to aggravate this problem. As a consequence, in general terms, virtually all patients were fluid restricted to some extent in the early stages of perfusion. We also adopted a very low threshold for haemofiltration and added a haemofiltration loop to the ECMO circuit:

1. If the improved perfusion associated with the instigation of ECMO did not promote a spontaneous diuresis
2. If the urine output was considered inadequate (<2 ml/kg/min in the early stages of perfusion)
3. If bypass appeared to aggravate tissue oedema in the early stages of perfusion
4. If the requirement for diuretic administration (by the above standards) was excessive or associated with unwanted side effects (such as intravascular haemoconcentration or normokalaemic metabolic alkalosis)

Enteral feeding during neonatal ECMO was very rare. In the early phases of the perfusion a reluctance to feed was due to the possibility of covert reperfusion gut injury. ECMO perfusions were frequently over in this age-group before this possibility was reliably excluded. In older patients and longer term neonatal perfusions enteral feeding was possible, but most patients received total parenteral nutrition instead. The potential detrimental effects of a catabolic state accompanying the illness led us to commence such nutrition early, although the presence of acidosis and/or jaundice or pulmonary hypertension was likely to lead to reduced doses of protein and lipid administration, respectively. Another advantage of the low threshold for ultrafiltration was that it allowed the continued administration of some form of parenteral nutrition to patients with fluid balance problems without these being exacerbated.

## Results

### Neonates

When compared with the traditional neonatal intensive care population, the ECMO selection criteria generated a group of relatively large, mature infants (63 babies, mean birthweight 3.3 kg, SD 0.54 kg, mean gestation 38 weeks, range 35–42 weeks). Predictably, in such a population severe cardiopulmonary failure stemmed from a small number of diagnoses; meconium aspiration syndrome, sepsis (including congenital pneumonia), respiratory distress syndrome (more rarely than in more preterm infants) and congenital diaphragmatic hernia. These were united by the complication of high pulmonary vascular resistance, manifest as persistent pulmonary hypertension of the newborn. This maladaptation of the transitional circulation also occurred in apparent isolation, usually after a perinatal hypoxic insult. Such pathophysiology was almost universal in our neonatal series, although the extent of its contribution to the presentation varied between cases.

The neonatal results are summarised in Table 1, alongside statistics from the extracorporeal life-support organisation (ELSO), whose series now comprises 8000 neonatal ECMO perfusions. Six patients have been separated because ECMO was used after cardiac surgery, and these are included in Table 3.

Strictly speaking, these neonatal data should not be directly compared, since the series presented comprises a different population from the predominantly American ELSO statistics. These data also include the effects of whatever learning curve was experienced, both by our ECMO centre and by those neonatologists who referred patients to us. An anticipated reduction in the threshold for referral in response to high survival rates was not observed, and the mean oxygenation index at the point of referral was 73 (range 35–357). The blood gases of the neonates prior to ECMO demonstrated mean arterial pH 7.26 (SD 0.24) and the mean $P_AO_2$ was 6.52 (SD 4.82). It can be seen from the table that patients with congenital diaphragmatic hernia fare less well and justify separate consideration (see below).

**Table 1.** Neonatal results

| Diagnosis | No. of patients | No. survived[a] n (%) | ELSO no. | Survival[a] (%) |
|---|---|---|---|---|
| PPHN/PFC | 16 | 11 (69) | 1008 | 83 |
| MAS | 21 | 20 (95) | 2997 | 93 |
| CDH | 12 | 6 (50) | 1543 | 58 |
| RDS | 4 | 2 (50) | 982 | 84 |
| Sepsis | 6 | 2 (33) | 1197 | 76 |
| Other | 4 | 1 (25) | 293 | 76 |
| Total | 63 | 42 (67) | 8020 | 81 |

*PPHN/PFC*, Persistent pulmonary hypertension of the newborn/persistent foetal circulation; *MAS*, meconium aspiration syndrome; *CDH*, congenital diaphragmatic hernia; *RDS*, respiratory distress syndrome

[a] Survival data refer to survival to discharge from hospital; ELSO data as of July 1993; Leicester data up to December 31, 1992

Of the total of 63 neonates presented here, 31 received a venovenous cannulation and 31 a venoarterial. One additional patient had a venovenous cannulation revised to venoarterial because of subsequent deterioration with septicaemic shock (nonsurvivor). Perfusions lasted for a mean of 123 h (range 36–405 h).

## Congenital Diaphragmatic Hernia

Patients with congenital diaphragmatic hernia did not constitute a homogeneous group. Clinical assessment prior to ECMO revealed a variety of different interactions of three components in the aetiology of their cardiopulmonary failure:

1. Pulmonary hypoplasia secondary to lung compression in utero
2. Pulmonary hypertension and persistent fetal circulation
3. The compression of existing lung tissue by hernial contents, particularly if they had been allowed to become distended with air

Such patients were referred both pre- and postoperatively and had been accepted even in the absence of a recognised honeymoon period [38] or, in some cases, without ever having had a normal blood gas (including preductal) at any stage of the illness [39]. This was because it was felt that in the face of a multifactorial problem, there were nonetheless no sound criteria for reliably distinguishing patients with an inevitably fatal degree of pulmonary hypoplasia.

A total of 13 perfusions in 12 patients with congenital diaphragmatic hernia contributed to the neonatal series. Of these, all but two were venoarterial cannulations. In the analysis these complex cases significantly affect the data for neonatal perfusions. Although the survival to coming off ECMO was high (75%), three of the 12 did not survive to eventual discharge from their referral hospitals. Deaths were due to either chronic pulmonary hypoplasia or its attendant sequelae. The average duration of a perfusion for one of these patients was 180h, compared with 123 for the group as a whole. When their data are excluded from the neonatal series, the mean duration of perfusion for the rest of the group falls to 110h and the difference between the two groups is significant ($p = 0.0013$).

## Paediatrics

The older paediatric patients presented with a wide diversity of conditions and, generally speaking, without a unifying oxygen-responsive haemodynamic pathophysiology. Notwithstanding this, in one notable case pre-ECMO evaluation revealed haemodynamic consequences of secondary pulmonary hypertension akin to those almost universally manifested by the neonates. In this case, of a 4-year-old boy with severe pneumonia, it was determined that a significant proportion of his hypoxia was due to a right-to-left shunt across a patent foramen ovale. This component of the shunt would have been aggravated by high-pressure ventilation (essential in his conventional support). The success of his ECMO treatment was presumably due in part to the fact that extracorporeal gas exchange avoided this particular problem. As a patent foramen ovale is present in up to 27% of the population [40], this may be an underdiagnosed phenomenon.

The 34 paediatric respiratory patients were comparatively young (mean age 32 months, range 3–100), with a significant proportion of graduates from the neonatal intensive care unit (with or without bronchopulmonary dysplasia) representing, usually with viral pneumonia. At presentation these children had a mean pH of 7.32 (SD 0.2), $P_ACO_2$ 7.47 (SD 4.61) and $P_AO_2$ 7.13 (SD 1.85). Conventional ventilation strategies varied widely across this age range and between institutions, and so contrived oxygenation or ventilation indices are, generally speaking, not useful for comparison within the group. However, all were receiving high pressures with high fractional inspired oxygen concentrations (usually 1). The results are presented by diagnosis in Table 2; again, ELSO data are included.

Of the 36 perfusions performed in this population 20 were via venovenous cannulation throughout and 15 were via a venoarterial cannulation. One additional patient had a venovenous cannulation revised to venoarterial during the perfusion because of subsequent deterioration (survivor). The mean duration of

**Table 2.** Paediatric respiratory support

| Diagnosis | No. of patients | No. survived *n* (%) | ELSO no.[a] | Survival (%) |
|---|---|---|---|---|
| Viral pneumonia | 14 | 12 (86) | 156 | 50 |
| Bacterial pneumonia | 4 | 3 (75) | 38 | 47 |
| ARDS | 7 | 5 (71) | 152 | 45 |
| Aspiration | 4 | 2 (50) | 53 | 58 |
| Other | 5 | 3 (6) | 168 | 47 |
| Total | 34 | 25 (74) | 567 | 48 |

[a] ELSO data as of July 1993

**Table 3.** Paediatric cardiac support

| Diagnosis | Number | Survived |
|---|---|---|
| Functional pulmonary atresia | 1 | 1 |
| TAPVD | 1 | 1 |
| Ventricular septal defect | 1 | 0 |
| Transposition of great arteries | 2 | 0 |
| Truncus arteriosus | 2 | 2 |
| Tetralogy of Fallot | 2 | 1 |
| Interrupted aortic arch | 1 | 1 |
| Fontan procedure | 1 | 1 |
| Atrioventricular septal defect | 1 | 0 |
| Total | 12 | 7 |

perfusions was significantly longer than in the neonates as a whole (mean 202 h, range 4–652 h, $p = 0.0005$), reflecting the relative decreased contribution of oxygen-responsive pulmonary vascular pathophysiology and an increased proportion of patients with interstitial lung damage. In our series this difference in the duration of perfusion required retains significance, despite the inclusion of some very short perfusions in which asystolic, hypothermic drowned patients where resuscitated using ECMO.

The 12 patients (six neonates and six older children) who required cardiac support presented primarily after cardiac surgery, usually for congenital heart disease (as our centre does not provide a transplant service). These small numbers reflect the fact that low cardiac output states which do not respond to inotropic support, or appropriate pulmonary vasodilatation, are not common in paediatric cardiac surgery. When they do occur they are often due to inadequate surgical repair. Hence, extensive pre-ECMO investigation of potential candidates further reduces the numbers of patients who require this treatment. The results are shown in Table 3. In common with other centres, the best results were achieved in situations where reversible pulmonary hypertension was likely to be making a significant contribution to the presentation. All of these patients received a venoarterial cannulation of mean duration 104 h (SD 53 h, range 48–244 h). These comparatively short perfusions presumably reflect the fact that myocardial recovery takes place comparatively quickly or not at all.

## Outcome/Complications

In total, this series represents over 18 000 h of prolonged bedside perfusion on the intensive care unit. During much of this time the patients were critically dependent upon the circuit for gas exchange and/or cardiac assistance. Technical complications that in any way affected the function of the circuit therefore had an immediate effect upon the patients' vital signs and required emergency treatment. The comparatively low incidence of such complications could be used to debate the necessity for continual specialist supervision of the circuit. However, as the ECMO programme developed it became clear that such complications could in some instances be anticipated or detected early, enabling prophylactic repairs using methods practised in the water lab (on isolated clear primed circuits). Mechanical complications in this series were limited to:

- Oxygenator failure ($n = 4$)
- Pump raceway rupture ($n = 2$)
- Bladder box fault ($n = 1$)
- Hospital power failure ($n = 1$),
- Cannula occlusion (VA) ($n = 1$)
- Cannula occlusion (VV) ($n = 4$), although the 14 fg Kendal double-lumen cannula for neonates is notorious for repeated minor occlusions from kinking
- Blood leak from pigtail ($n = 1$)

In all but the last case, prompt repair of the circuit was possible before the patient was unduly compromised.

The quality of the outcome of the survivors in this series is the subject of a long-term follow-up project. Not surprisingly, in a population selected by the severity of presentation and attempts to predict mortality, neurological sequelae have been identified. The incidence of some degree of developmental delay in neonatal ECMO graduates runs at around 10% of survivors. Comparative data for similarly sick conventionally treated patients will be provided by the UK Collaborative Trial. However, a review of the published literature would suggest (a) that this rate is representative of the collective experience [41–43], and (b) that similar incidences can be expected in survivors of conventional treatment for illnesses of equal severity [44].

Other anticipated demonstrations of morbidity after ECMO have also been rare. Persistent respiratory compromise has been very unusual, except in situations of pulmonary hypoplasia.

In the older children, survivors who were neurologically normal prior to the illness that caused referral have been, thus far, neurologically normal at follow-up. Additionally, we have observed a number of older patients with a short-lived choreiform movement disorder after decannulation and removal of sedation. In each case dystonic movements were apparent immediately after ECMO and resolved over days to weeks. Despite giving rise to concern, in each case the signs have resolved without obvious residual sequelae. The aetiology probably relates to the prolonged administration of multiple sedatives and muscle relaxants in a changing metabolic environment; perhaps it is a variant of the central anticholinergic syndrome [45, 46].

## Discussion

The style of ECMO support and the manner in which it is handled now differ considerably from those employed in the era of the NIH trial. Although modern treatment of older children (and adults) is not as successful as that of neonates, it is associated with much greater survival than was reported in the past and represents a significant improvement over the predicted outcome (by whatever measure) without ECMO. By contrast, ad hoc attempts to perform the procedure de novo, without these refinements, are still almost invariably associated with the survival rates that were ascribed to the technique in the 1970s. The duration of perfusion that is required for older children and specific subgroups of the neonatal population (like those with congenital diaphragmatic hernia) may vary but is generally longer than that of the "typical" neonate. Expansion of a neonatal programme to incorporate these patients needs to take into account the additional investment of time and bed occupancy that results.

Twenty years since the first successful application of ECMO in its "modern form", the evidence that the method works is impressive. The international registry, which is an almost complete record of neonatal and paediatric ECMO, reveals that in application to neonatal cardiorespiratory failure in over 8000 cases (selected by a high probability of mortality) the mean survival is over 80% and exceeds 90% in some centres. Similarly, in older children with pulmonary failure, survival rates ranging from 50 to 80% have been reported in a cumulative total of over 500 children. Nonetheless, it is apparent in all age-groups that ECMO is not a universal panacea for refractory cardiopulmonary failure.

The population of patients treated with ECMO is highly selected, both by severity of illness and by exclusion of those who would be placed at intolerable risk from the procedure or who are felt to be beyond help for reason of irreversible organ damage. However, the basis upon which such decisions are made is not uniform. The numerical indices used in an attempt to introduce uniformity to such decisions in neonates rely upon values derived from historical control studies. Similar retrospective studies do not usually support the use of such indices in the older child or produce data that is not necessarily transferable between institutions [21, 22]. Case selection in the paediatric population as a whole therefore remains somewhat empiric.

The consequence is that, despite a comprehensive and diligent record of the ECMO-treated population, there is a paucity of comparable data for non-ECMO-treated patients. Without such information a truly objective evaluation of ECMO is difficult. Over the same time period during which modern ECMO has evolved, a similar parallel refinement has occurred in "conventional" intensive care (particularly that of neonates). Thus, the validity of historical controls in patient selection and in the evaluation of ECMO statistics is questionable [47], although some degree of standardisation is useful in order to compare the outcome of patients either referred for ECMO at different points in their illness or not referred at all. It is, however, possible to argue that many fundamental issues relating to the application of ECMO remain unanswered [48, 49]. In this respect ECMO is not alone and can be ranked alongside, for example, positive-pressure ventilation of neonates or renal dialysis.

The evolution of ECMO has been punctuated by determined attempts to establish scientifically its place in intensive care by unbiased prospective comparison with more "conventional" treatment modalities, some of which – we have pointed out – would not themselves stand the same scrutiny. Profound ethical difficulties surround the design of trials involving patients who have been selected by the extreme severity of their illness and in whom a likely end point after treatment allocation is death [50]. The history of attempts to resolve such issues is intertwined inextricably with the evolution of ECMO.

The first attempt to address this problem in neonates was a trial which adopted a "play the winner" technique of randomisation [51]. This design biased future allocations proportionately according to the relative degree of success ascribed to each treatment up to that point within the trial. The results did not gain widespread acceptance because of the marked disparity in the size of the resultant two treatment populations (11 ECMO patients surviving against one conventional patient who died). This prompted a second trial which again had to address the issues generated by the perception that ECMO was a better treatment. O'Rourke et al. [52] adopted a design in which standard, unbiased, prospective allocation proceeded until there had been four deaths in each treatment group. Subsequent allocation was exclusively to the more successful technique until the differences between the two groups achieved significance. Again, the results failed to gain universal acceptance because of lack of confidence in the validity of the trial design.

At that time, however, neonatal ECMO was being extensively adopted in the USA, and in 1985, in acknowledgement of its apparent success, it was accepted as "standard" treatment. The practical necessity for further attempts at randomised study therefore became less obvious, and the ethical constraints upon trial design in the USA increased.

The initial success of Hill and co-workers in the prolonged extracorporeal support of a young adult was a somewhat atypical experience, as the results of a later multicentre randomised trial showed. Published in 1979, the trial sponsored by the NIH in the USA randomised 92 patients with adult respiratory distress syndrome to ECMO with ventilation or ventilation alone. The survival rates were less than 10 in both groups. This trial was at best difficult to interpret for various reasons. Some of the centres involved were contributing their first experiences with ECMO and reported rates and degress of complications, such as blood loss, that were excessive. Many centres continued to employ high-pressure/high-volume ventilation during ECMO. Also, a concurrent pandemic of influenza pneumonia meant that these patients dominated the trial population. For these and other reasons the results of this trial are now widely considered inapplicable to non-neonatal ECMO as practised today. The likelihood of survival in modern series is much greater than was reported then [53], and these differences are due to both patient selection and ECMO technique [54]. There is conflicting evidence as to whether a similar improvement has or has not occurred in the results of conventional treatment in this population [55, 56]. A recent attempt to objectively reassess a new method for decision-making in ventilator management by comparison in a single institution has reported unexpectedly high survival rates for "conventional" treatment [57, 58].

Reports of experience such as that outlined in this chapter and the availability of cumulative worldwide results through the ELSO registry have encouraged other centres in the UK to develop ECMO facilities. They have also stimulated a recurrence of debate as to the quality of objective proof of the efficacy of ECMO. Proponents of ECMO maintain that its widespread use can be justified without the need for further trials. Critics of the technique cite the lack of conclusive evidence from randomised controlled studies and, for neonates in the UK, possible, but unproven, differences between the UK and American perinatal populations [59]. The result has been the joint development of a protocol for a further prospective randomised controlled trial of neonatal ECMO (see below).

Similar arguments apply to the other patients who may require ECMO. As a result, there are currently plans to conduct a prospective trial of paediatric ECMO through the collaboration of centres in ELSO. This trial must be of sufficient magnitude to avoid being confounded by the errors that predictably result from the extreme diversity of respiratory failure aetiology in this population. Difficulty persists in defining suitable entry points for such a trial in terms of disease severity. The lack of any universally acceptable prognostic indicator in this population remains problematic [22]. Recently, further attempts to determine appropriately sensitive predictive indices by retrospective study have been undertaken, and results are awaited (O.D. Timmons, 1993, personal communication). Nevertheless, the situation is further complicated by the diversification of "alternative" technologies and ventilation techniques suggested for these patients that are themselves awaiting objective ratification by randomised trial.

In the cardiac population the apparent failure of conventional treatment often presents as a clear end point, making the decision whether or not to embark upon extracorporeal life support one in which there are few alternatives, and the issue to be addressed is whether there is any possibility of survival with ECMO, in the certain knowledge that there is none without. The use of ECMO in such a population therefore requires justification, which is restricted to a consideration of its yield. The difficulties in selecting potentially successful cases from the inevitably hopeless mean that the returns may be small despite heavy investment of time and expertise. Most would not contemplate the provision of an ECMO programme purely for this population, although it remains appropriate to offer this service to potential candidates when they present in a situation where the technology is routinely available [24].

## Future Developments

### Trials

The "Collaborative ECMO Trial" based in the UK has been running since January 1, 1993 and is due to present its findings in 1997. It is conventionally designed, prospective, randomised trial of neonates who satisfy established criteria for ECMO treatment. During the trial neonatal ECMO is available within the UK only through informed consent and random allocation. Appropriate patients are presented by designated collaborating centres and are then randomly assigned either to (a) transport to recognised ECMO centre and possible ECMO, or to (b) remain at the referring centre to continue more conventional treatment.

The trial thus intends to compare all aspects of an anticipated UK national ECMO service (including the effects of mortality and morbidity arising during the transfer of patients) against the alternative – conventional care in a designated neonatal centre. The results will allow comparison of differences in short-term outcome (mortality) and longer term outcome (impairment associated with disability at 1 year of age). In contrast to the earlier trials of ECMO, it can be seen that the emphasis of this trial is not just to resolve an abstracted debate about the comparative efficacy of ECMO/non-ECMO treatment. The intention is also to clarify its appropriate place in modern neonatal intensive care as practised in the UK. It is not yet clear how applicable the results of this trial will be to other health care systems.

## Technology

Technically, ECMO is continually being refined, although each change has to prove itself as an improvement in the laboratory and clinical sphere before being widely adopted. Recent advances include the refinement of venovenous techniques, the development of percutaneous cannulae and the evolution of tidal flow systems such as that used in AREC (*assistance respiratoire extracorporeal*). Here we will consider two technical advances from a large selection, both of which can be anticipated to exert major change in the near future. These are heparin-bonding chemistry and the latest developments in pump design.

The interest in heparin bonding stems from the fact that, despite the use of albumin and blood during priming to, at least in theory, coat and "pacify" the artificial surfaces of the circuit [60], the use of extracorporeal circulation is still associated with a "whole-body inflammatory response" [35], part of which includes impaired haemostasis [61]. Despite improved oxygenator design, during perfusion, platelet sequestration persists, and clotting factors and other blood proteins still tend to adhere to the circuit roughly in proportion to their concentration in plasma. Extracorporeal circulation creates a haemostatic defect which involves platelet dysfunction as well as activation of closely interrelated humoral systems such as the complement [62], coagulation, fibrinolytic [63] and kallikrein/kinin [64] systems. The effect of these factors is further complicated by the persistent necessity of anticoagulation, routinely achieved through heparin administration, in order to prevent thrombus formation within the circuit. Much research has been devoted to the possibility of reducing these problems by improving the biocompatability of the artificial surfaces which comprise the circuit [65]. A variety of potential mechanisms of heparin bonding have been explored [60]. Currently, the widely preferred option appears to be that of covalently bonding the heparin to the surface using a spacer molecule so that the active heparin molecules protrude into the lumen, making them more accessible to circulating antithrombin III (necessary in its mechanism of action) [66]. Alternatives exist, however.

Heparin-bonded tubing and hollow-fibre oxygenators have been commercially available for some time [66]. Heparin-bonded membrane oxygenators have also been developed [67]. The clinical impact of these devices remains to be assessed.

Currently, they have enabled a reduction in the requirement, but have not yet negated the need, for the systemic administration of heparin, particularly when circuits are being used at low blood flow rates.

The interest in new pump designs for ECMO use reflects the attention that is paid to the incidence of technical complications during ECMO. Orthodox roller pumps rely heavily on the integrity of a "raceway" of tubing which is continually exposed to the rollers in the pump head. The original silastic tubing, which was prone to rupture, has now been substituted with super-Tygon, which is inherently more robust, but raceway ruptures still occur. Although they are mercifully rare, this still encourages the search for other options in pump design. An example of the enthusiasm thus generated by alternative pumps was seen after the introduction of the constrained vortex system. Time and experience with the system have led in most cases to a more balanced view. The most promising development yet in this field is that of the peristaltic style of pump derived from that originally marketed by "Rhone Poulenc". With this pump a bladder/reservoir may prove to be unnecessary, since it is almost impossible to impart excessive suction to the venous line or to pump air even if the raceway is cut. Also, both inflow and outflow can be occluded without raceway rupture. The widespread introduction of a device superior to roller, centrifugal impeller, and constrained vortex pumps is likely in the near future.

## Alternative Therapies

Intensive care is currently witnessing a profusion of new developments applicable to the field of cardiopulmonary failure. This has already reached the point where it is no longer possible to refer to mechanical ventilation as a "conventional" technique. Indeed, in ECMO parlance the term "conventional" has long been corrupted to mean "non-ECMO". Novel ventilation strategies such as high-frequency jet ventilation, high-frequency oscillation, synchronised expiratory oscillation, intratracheal pressure ventilation and revised approaches to older ideas such as negative-pressure ventilation, including high-frequency negative pressure oscillation, are all available. New treatment groups are being found for more accepted techniques (such as the application of pressure-controlled inverse-ratio ventilation). Although the relative merits of these techniques are beyond the scope of this chapter, most still require extensive evaluation or reevaluation before the choice between them (and between these modalities and ECMO) can be made clearly.

Three other developments – nitric oxide (NO), liquid ventilation, and the intravenous oxygenator (IVOX) – are worthy of mention although, unlike ECMO, they offer support only to gas exchange and not circulatory support.

## Nitric Oxide

Nitric oxide is an apparently ubiquitous molecule that has multiple roles in cellular defence and communication. It has identified roles in a multitude of physiological processes including neurotransmission, gastrointestinal motility, penile erection, uterine contraction, haematopoiesis, skin growth, wound healing and inflammation. However, in the context of cardiopulmonary intensive therapy the most relevant effect is that upon smooth muscle tone, particularly that of blood vessels. Nitric oxide (endothelium-derived relaxing factor) is a lipophilic molecule that rapidly diffuses across biological membranes. Its intracellular formation from L-arginine is catalysed by the action of NO synthase enzymes. The release of NO from vascular endothelial cells is increased in response to stimuli such as shear stress and in response to platelet products, coagulation factors and hormones. The effects are to inhibit vasospasm and platelet aggregation [68]. Therapeutic nitrates exert their action through the production of NO and inhaled NO may, amongst other things, exert a selective pulmonary vasodilator effect. As NO is a toxic gas, however, dose monitoring is essential to avoid toxic effects such as methaemoglobinaemia. Nitric oxide is also a known mutagen and reacts with oxygen to form nitrogen dioxide, which is both highly caustic and toxic. Additionally, NO has been implicated in the mechanism of free-radical injury. The superoxide radical reacts with NO to generate peroxynitrite species, the decomposition of which generates a powerful oxidative stress [69]. Initial clinical experience with the gaseous administration of this molecule to intensive care patients has produced reports of improvements in oxygenation [70, 71], but its therapeutic advantages remain to be proven.

### Perfluorocarbon-Assisted Gas Exchange (PAGE)

The ability of perfluorocarbons to dissolve large quantities of oxygen and carbon dioxide leads to potential applications as blood substitutes [72] for internal gas transport and gas substitutes for ventilation. Total liquid ventilation improves gas exchange and lung compliance but requires specialised apparatus for ventilation and a method for extracorporeal $CO_2$ removal and re-oxygenation before the liquid is recycled. However, the potential advantages of partial liquid ventilation stem mainly from its low surface tension. In a surfactant-deficient animal lung, replacing the functional residual capacity with perfluorocarbon reduces the surface tension of the intrapulmonary gas-liquid interface and prevents atelectasis by bulk distension of the alveoli with a noncompressible medium. The result is improved gas exchange through a more compliant gas-ventilated lung. Laboratory studies of this technique are promising [73], and clinical trials are awaited.

### Intravenous Oxygenator

The intravenous oxygenator (IVOX) [74] comprises an elongated arrangement of a series of thin-walled, microporous, silicone-coated hollow fibres. It is inserted furled, into the inferior vena cava via the right common femoral vein, using a hollow introducer. It then opens into a configuration that produces a turbulent flow across each fibre. Oxygen is drawn through the fibres by negative pressure (to reduce the risk of gas embolism) and gas exchange occurs. Maximum gas-transfer characteristics currently approximate to an ability to oxygenate just up to 25% of the resting cardiac output. Systemic heparinisation is necessary during its use, and bleeding complications (usually during insertion) are reported. Clinical experience is currently restricted to small series of mainly adults from single institutions [75–77]. These series usually document poor survival after its application to patients who require gas-exchange assistance beyond its capabilities, or who also may have required circulatory support. There might yet exist a role for this device in an earlier application to patients at risk for ventilator-related lung damage, perhaps alongside a policy of permissive hypercapnia.

## Conclusions

Detailed record-keeping of the ECMO treatment and outcome of thousands of patients, selected by the severity of their presentation, has generated an enormous body of detailed evidence about the efficacy of ECMO. This pattern has been reflected by the microcosm of our own experience, in part presented here. However, the place of neonatal, paediatric and adult ECMO in intensive care is still debated and the issues involved in this deliberation persist, despite most attempts to resolve them.

Objective analysis requires controlled comparative information of the sort generated by conventional prospective randomised trials. However, clinical trials of life-support techniques that differ fundamentally from each other do not lend themselves to "cross-over" or "placebo-controlled" designs. Hence, because of the nature of the patients population, they may necessarily involve death as an end point. If the onus is upon the protagonists of a treatment to conceive and perform such trials, it is inevitable that they will face ethical dilemmas in the design and planning of the protocol. The result, in the case of neonatal ECMO, has been the performance of trials of adaptive and resourceful design that have, unfortunately, been difficult to interpret as a consequence. Our own response to this problem has been to design yet another trial which, if nothing else, will contribute to the debate. Notwithstanding this, the likelihood is that even the issues that this aims to fundamentally address will endure to some extent. When this is conceded in advance of the third in a series of prospective trials, it becomes germane to recall that absolute certainty is not a universal feature of the natural world [78, 79]. Expectations of the quality of proof from clinical trials must therefore be realistic [50].

In the meantime, further new treatments, of varying prospects and merits, inevitably appear. Each of these has its own group of protagonists, anxious to prove its worth. Recent trends are for this phenomenon to manifest itself in a reduction of referrals for ECMO within individual institutions and a poorer performance of ECMO than was previously experienced in that institution. This reflects the fact that ECMO referral has then been delayed and that ECMO patients have been further selected by their failure to respond to another innovative therapy. The deleterious effects of such situations are compounded if one has to contemplate transport of the patient between institutions for ECMO referral. Each new technology (including ECMO) has to be assessed in terms of its overall impact on the treatment of specific conditions. The invasive nature of ECMO may justify its use as a last resort; however, delay in referral has a profound effect upon outcome, irrespective of which pre-ECMO treatment is employed.

The correct approach remains to objectively establish the niche for each new technology by prospective randomised assessment. Wherever possible, this should occur without delaying ECMO referral for rescue therapy. The use of ECMO in such a manner can be justified, while ECMO itself continues in a concurrent evaluation, since ECMO is uniquely capable of providing cardiac and pulmonary support independent of the magnitude of native organ compromise. The merits of this approach should not only find favour amongst ECMO, protagonists, but should also appeal to the investigators of the new life-support technology, as this technology could, and should, then be instituted at an earlier stage, or less severe degress of illness, when a positive outcome is perhaps more accessible. The intravenous oxygenator, inhaled nitric oxide and perfluorocarbon-assisted gas exchange would all lend themselves to such an approach toward prospective evaluation. This could then proceed without having a detrimental effect upon ECMO statistics (and therefore patient survival). The introduction of potential future improvements in "conventional" life-support techniques should not allow any neonate or paediatric patient to die of cardiopulmonary failure without the appropriate use of ECMO being judiciously considered.

## References


1. Sosnowski AW, Bonser SJ, Field DJ, Graham TR, Firmin RK (1990) Extracorporeal membrane oxygenation. Br Med J 301:303–304
2. Hill JD, O'Brien TG, Murray JJ, Dontigny L, Bramson ML, Osborn JJ, Gerbode F (1972) Prolonged extracorporeal oxygenation for acute post-traumatic respiratory failure (shock-lung syndrome). Use of the Bramson membrane lung. N Eng J Med 286:629–634
3. Hill JD, DeLeval M, Fallat RJ, Bramson ML, Eberhart RC, Schulte HD, Osborn JJ, Barber R, Gerbode F (1972) Acute respiratory insufficiency. Treatment with prolonged extracorporeal oxygenation. J Thorac Cardiovasc Surg 64:551–562
4. Zapol WM, Snider MT, Hill JD, Fallat RJ, Bartlett RH, Edmunds LH, Morris AH, Peirce E. 2nd, Thomas AN, Proctor HJ, Drinker PA, Pratt PC, Bagniewski A, Miller RJ (1979) Extracorporeal membrane oxygenation in severe acute respiratory failure. A randomized prospective study. J Am Med Assoc 242:2193–2196
5. Bartlett RH, Gazzaniga AB, Toomasian J, Coran AG, Roloff D, Rucker R, Corwin AG (1986) Extracorporeal membrane oxygenation (ECMO) in neonatal respiratory failure. 100 cases [published erratum appears in Ann Surg 1987 205:11A]; Ann Surg 204:236–245
6. Pesenti A, Gattinoni L, Kolobow T, Damia G (1988) Extracorporeal circulation in adult respiratory failure. ASAIO Trans 34:43–47
7. Yoshinaga N et al. (1966) Application of assisting extracorporeal circulation to a patient with severe carbon dioxide intoxication. Masui 15:1041–1043
8. Kolobow T, Hayano F, Weathersby PK (1975) Dispersion-casting thin and ultrathin fabric-reinforced silicone rubber membrane for use in the membrane lung. Med Instrum (Baltimore) 9:124–128
9. Lande AJ, Dos SJ, Carlson RG, Perschau RA, Lange RP, Sonstegard LJ, Lillehei CW (1967) A new membrane oxygenator-dialyzer. Surg Clin North Am 47:1461–1470
10. Ed: Arensman RM, Devn-Cornish J (1993) Extracorporeal life support. Blackwell Scientific, Boston
11. Bartlett RH (1990) Extracorporeal life support for cardiopulmonary failure. Curr Probl Surg 27:621–705

12. Toomasian JM, Snedecor SM, Cornell RG, Cilley RE, Bartlett RH (1988) National experience with extracorporeal membrane oxygenation for newborn respiratory failure. Data from 715 cases. ASAIO Trans 34:140–147
13. Data Supplied by the Registry of the Extracorporeal Life Support Organisation
14. Kolobow T (1988) Acute respiratory failure: on how to injure healthy lungs (and prevent sick lungs from recovering. ASAIO Trans 34:31–34
15. Kimball TR, Weiss RG, Meyer RA, Daniels SR, Ryckman FC, Schwartz DC (1989) Color flow mapping to document normal pulmonary venous return in neonates with persistent pulmonary hypertension being considered for extracorporeal membrane oxygenation. J Pediatr 114:433–437
16. Zylberberg R, Cook L, Roberts J, Edmonds D, Reese A, Groff D (1987) Total anomalous pulmonary venous return: report of a case diagnosed on ECMO. J Perinatol 7:185–185
17. Pearson GA, Sosnowski A, Firmin RK, Leanage R (1992) Extracorporeal membrane oxygenation and cyanotic heart disease. Cardiology in the Young 2:359–360
18. Wetmore N, McEwen D, O'Connor M, Bartlett RH (1979) Defining indications for artificial organ support in respiratory failure. ASAIO Trans 25:459–461
19. Hallman M, Merritt TA, Jarvenpaa AL, Boynton B, Mannino F, Gluck L, Moore T, Edwards D (1985) Exogenous human surfactant for treatment of severe respiratory distress syndrome: a randomised prospective clinical trial. J Pediatr 106:963–969
20. Bohn DJ, James I, Filler RM, Ein SH, Wesson DE, Shandling B, Stephens C, Barker GA (1984) The relationship between $PaCO_2$ and ventilation parameters in predicting survival in congenital diaphragmatic hernia. J Pediatr Surg 19:666–671
21. Rivera RA, Butt W, Shann F (1990) Predictors of mortality in children with respiratory failure: possible indications for ECMO Anaesth Intensive Care 18:385–389
22. Timmons OD, Dean JM, Vernon DD (1991) Mortality rates and prognostic variables in children with adult respiratory distress syndrome. J Pediatr 119:896–899
23. Pratt PC, Vollmer RT, Shelburne JD, Crapo JD (1979) Pulmonary morphology in a multihospital collaborative extracorporeal membrane oxygenation project. I. Light microscopy. Am J Pathol 95:191–214
24. Pearson GA, Underwood MJ, Chan KC, Firmin RK (1993) Extracorporeal membrane oxygenation and paediatric cardiology. Cardiology in the Young 3:197–201
25. Montoya JP, Merz SI, Bartlett RH (1991) A standardized system for describing flow/pressure relationships in vascular access devices. ASAIO Trans 37:4–8
26. Pearson GA, Sosnowski A, Chan KC, Firmin RK (1993) Salvage of postoperative pulmonary hypertensive crists using ECMO via cervical cannulation. Eur J Cardiothorac Surg 7:390–391
27. Kinsella JP, Gerstmann DR, Rosenberg AA (1992) The effect of extracorporeal membrane oxygenation on coronary perfusion and regional blood flow distribution. Pediatr Res 31:80–84
28. Morigami K, Yamada C, Shiokawa C, Ohno K, Maekawa Y, Kinoshita H (1990) Experimental studies on extracorporeal membrane oxygenation (ECMO) perfusion for respiratory insufficiency associated with pulmonary hypertension (in Japanese). Nippon Geka Gakkai Zasshi 91:272–282
29. Bartlett RH, Cilley RE (1993) Physiology of extracorporeal life support. In: Arensman RM Cornish JD (eds) Extracorporeal lief support. Blackwell Scientific, Boston, pp 89–104
30. Gattinoni L, Pesenti A, Mascheroni D, Marcolin R, Fumagalli R, Rossi F, Lapichino G, Romagnoli G, Uziel L, Agostoni A et al. (1986) Low-frequency positive-pressure ventilation with extracorporeal $CO_2$ removal in severe acute respiratory failure. J Am Med Assoc 256:881–886
31. Berdjis F, Takahashi M, Lewis AB (1992) Left ventricular performance in neonates on extracorporeal membrane oxygenation. Pediatr Cardiol 13:141–145
32. Axelrod HI, Baumann FG, Galloway AC (1989) Left ventricular stress during extracorporeal membrane oxygenation. Ann Thorac Surg 47:330 (letter)
33. Bavaria JE, Furukawa S, Kreiner G, Gupta KB, Streicher J, Edmunds LJ (1990) Effect of circulatory assist devices on stunned myocardium. Ann Thorac Surg 49:123–128
34. Burch KD, Covitz W, Lovett EJ, Howell C, Kanto WJ (1989) The significance of ductal shunting during extracorporeal membrane oxygenation. J Pediatr Surg 24:855–859
35. Westaby S (1987) Organ dysfunction after cardiopulmonary bypass. A systemic influammatory reaction initiated by the extracorporeal circuit. Intensive Care Med 13:89–95

36. Keszler M, Subramanian KN, Smith YA, Dhanireddy R, Mehta N, Molina B, Cox CB, Moront MG (1989) Pulmonary management during extracorporeal membrane oxygenation. Crit Care Med 17:495–500
37. Keszler M, Ryckman FC, McDonald JJ, Sweet LD, Moront MG, Boegli MJ, Cox C, Leftridge CA (1992) A prospective, multicenter, randomized study of high versus low positive end-expiratory pressure during extracorporeal membrane oxygenation. J Pediatr 120:107–113
38. Johnston PW, Liberman R, Gangitano E, Vogt J (1990) Ventilation parameters and arterial blood gases as a prediction of hypoplasia in congenital diaphragmatic hernia. J Pediatr Surg 25:496–499
39. Stolar C, Dillon P, Reyes C (1988) Selective use of extracorporeal membrane oxygenation in the management of congential diaphragmatic hernia. J Pediatr Surg 23:207–211
40. Hagen PT, Scholz DG, Edwards WD (1984) Incidence and size of patent foramen ovale during the first ten decades of life: an autopsy study of 965 normal hearts. Mayo Clin Proc 59:17–20
41. Adolph V, Ekelund C, Smith C, Starrett A, Falterman K, Arensman R (1990) Developmental outcome of neonates treated with extracorporeal membrane oxygenation. J Pediatr Surg 25:43–46
42. Glass P, Miller M, Short B (1989) Morbidity for survivors of extracorpreal membrane oxygenation: neurodevelopmental outcome at 1 year of age. Pediatrics 83:72–78
43. Hofkosh D, Thompson AE, Nozza RJ, Kemp SS, Bowen A, Feldman HM (1991) Ten years of extracorporeal membrane oxygenation: neurodevelopmental outcome. Pediatrics 87:549–555
44. Brett C, Dekl M, Leonard PD et al. (1981) Developmental outcome of hyperventilated neonates: preliminary observations. Pediatrics 65:588–591
45. Rupreht J, Dworacek B (1990) Central anticholinergic syndrome during postoperative period. Ann Fr Anesth Reanim 9:295–304
46. Schneck HJ, Rupreht J (1989) Central anticholinergic syndrome (CAS) in anesthesia and intensive care. Acta Anaesth Belg 40:219–228
47. Elliott SJ (1991) Neonatal extracorporeal membrane oxygenation: how not to assess novel technologies (see comments). Lancet 337:476–478
48. Greenough A, Emery E (1990) ECMO and outcome of mechanical ventilation in infants of birthweight over 2 kg. Lancet 336:760 [letter]
49. Anonymous (1988) Persistent fetal circulation and extracorporeal membrane oxygenation (editorial) (see comments). Lancet 2:1289–1291
50. Lantos JD, Frader J (1990) Extracorporeal membrane oxygenation and the ethics of clinical research in pediatrics (see comments). N Engl J Med 323:409–413
51. Bartlett RH, Roloff DW, Cornell RG, Andrews AF, Dillon PW, Zwischenberger JB (1985) Extracorporeal circulation in neonatal respiratory failure: a prospective randomized study. Pediatrics 76:479–487
52. O'Rourke P, Crone RK, Vacanti JP, Ware JH, Lillehei CW, Parad RB, Epstein MF (1989) Extracorporeal membrane oxygenation and conventional medical therapy in neonates with persistent pulmonary hypertension of the newborn: a prospective randomized study. Pediatrics 84:957–963
53. Pesenti A, Kolobow T, Gattinoni L (1988) Extracorporeal respiratory support in the adult. ASAIO Trans 34:1006–1008
54. Anderson H III, Delius RE, Sinard JM, McCurry KR, Shanley CJ, Chapman RA, Shapiro MB, Rodriguez JL, Bartlett RH (1992) Early experience with adult extracorporeal membrane oxygenation in the modern era (see comments). Ann Thorac Surg 53:553–563
55. Suchyta MR, Clemmer TP, Orme JJ, Morris AH, Elliott CG (1991) Increased survival of ARDS patients with severe hypoxemia (ECMO criteria). Chest 99:951–955
56. Vasilyev S, McMillan S, Schaap R, Mortenson JD (1992) Survival rates for patients with acute respiratory failure in 1991–1992, utilizing mechanical ventilator augmentation of blood gas transfer. A multicenter prospective survey. Proc ledings of the 2nd Congress of the European Extracorporeal Support Organisation, Marburg, 1992, L30
57. Sittig DF, Gardner RM, Pace NL, Morris AH, Beck E (1989) Computerized management of patient care in a complex, controlled clinical trial in the intensive care unit. Compute Methods Programs Biomed 30:77–84

58. Sittig DF, Gardner RM, Morris AH, Wallace CJ (1990) Clinical evaluation of computer-based respiratory care algorithms. Int J Clin Monit Comput 7:177–185
59. Rose SJ (1990) Extracorporeal membrane oxygenation (letter; comment). Br Med J 301:1163
60. Eberhart RC (1993) Interactions of blood and artificial surfaces: in search of "heparin-free" cardiopulmonary bypass. In: Arensman RM, Cornish JD (eds) Extracorporeal life support. Blackwell Scientific, Boston, pp 105–125
61. Mammen EF, Koets MH, Washington BC et al. (1985) Haemostasis changes during cardiopulmonary bypass surgery. Semin Thromb Hemost 11:281–292
62. Chenoweth DE, Cooper SW, Hugli TE (1981) Complement activation during cardiopulmonary bypass. N Engl J Med 304:497–503
63. Stibbe J, Kluft C, Brommer EJ (1984) Enhanced fibrinolytic activity after cardiopulmonary bypass surgery in man is caused by extrinsic (tissue type) plasminogen activator. Eur J Clin Invest 14:375
64. Fuhrer G, Gallimore MJ, Heller W (1984) Studies on the components of the plasma kallikrein-kinin system in patients undergoing cardiopulmonary bypass. In: Greenbaum LW, Margolis HS (eds) Kinins IV: advances in experimental medicine and biology. Plenum, New York, pp 53–61
65. Westaby S (1987) Aspects of biocompatability in cardiopulmonary bypass. CRC Crit Rev Biocompat 3:193–234
66. Bindslev L (1988) Adult ECMO performed with surface-heparinized equipment. ASAIO Trans 34:1009–1013
67. Toomasian JM, Hsu LC, Hirschl RB, Heiss KF, Hultquist KA, Bartlett RH (1988) Evaluation of Duraflo II heparin coating in prolonged extracorporeal membrane oxygenation. ASAIO Trans 34:410–414
68. Luscher TF (1991) Endothelium-derived nitric oxide: the endogenous nitrovasodilator in the human cardiovascular system. Eur Heart J 12:2–11
69. Beckman JS, Beckman TW, Chen J, Marshall PA, Freeman BA (1990) Apparent hydroxyl radical production by peroxynitrite: implications for endothelial injury from nitric oxide and superoxide. Proc Natl Acad Sci USA 87:1620–1624
70. Kinsella JP, Neish SR, Shaffer E, Abman SH (1992) Low-dose inhalation nitric oxide in persistent pulmonary hypertension of the newborn (see comments). Lancet 340:819–820
71. Roberts JD, Polaner DM, Lang P, Zapol WM (1992) Inhaled nitric oxide in persistent pulmonary hypertension of the newborn (see comments). Lancet 340:818–819
72. Urbaniak SJ (1991) Artificial blood. Br Med J 303:1348–1350
73. Leach CL, Fuhrmann BP, Morin FC, Rath MG (1993) Perfluorocarbon-associated gas exchange (partial liquid ventilation) in respiratory distress syndrome: a prospective randomized controlled study. Crit Care Med 21:1270–1278
74. Mortenson JD, Berry G (1989) Conceptual and design features of a practical, clinically effective intravenous mechanical oxygen/carbon dioxide exchange device (IVOX). Int J Artif Organs 12:384–389
75. High KM, Snider MT, Richard R, Russell GB, Stene JK, Campbell DB (1992) Clinical trials of an intravenous oxygenator in patients with adult respiratory distress syndrome. Anesthesiology 77:856–863
76. Conrad SA, Eggerstedt JM, Morris VF, Romero MD (1993) Prolonged intracorporeal support of gas-exchange with an intravenacaval oxygenator. Chest 103:158–161
77. Kallis P, al-Saady, NM, Bennett ED, Treasure T (1993) Early results of intravascular oxygenation. Eur J Cardiothorac Surg 7:206–210
78. Hawking S (1988) The uncertainty principle. In: A brief history of time from the big bang to black holes. Transworld, London, pp 53–62
79. Gleick J (1987) A geometry of nature. In: Chaos. Sphere, London, pp 81–118

# Intravascular Membrane Oxygenation and Carbon Dioxide Removal with Permissive Hypercapnia – New Concepts in the Management of Respiratory Failure

J.B. Zwischenberger, W. Tao, V.J. Cardenas, Jr., and A. Bidani

## Introduction

Despite advances in ventilatory support, antibiotic therapy and critical care, mortality from adult respiratory distress syndrome (ARDS) remains between 50 and 77% [1–3]. Treatment of ARDS is mainly supportive, with mechanical ventilation being the mainstay of therapy. However, current techniques of ventilator management are associated with high inspiratory airway pressures (barotrauma), overdistension of normal lung regions (volutrauma), and toxic levels of inspired oxygen (oxygen toxicity), leading to exacerbated lung injury as manifested by progressive deterioration in total lung compliance, functional residual capacity, and arterial blood gas [4–6]. High positive airway pressure also contributes to cardiovascular instability [7]. Disappointing results with conventional management of ARDS patients have resulted in an increased urgency for developing alternative strategies that provide sufficient oxygenation, carbon dioxide removal, and "lung rest". Over the past 5 years, many have recognized that the primary goal of respiratory support should focus on $CO_2$ removal and $O_2$ exchange with avoidance of high tidal volumes and airway pressures. We and others have shown that a modified form of cardiopulmonary bypass, known as venovenous extracorporeal membrane oxygenation (VV ECMO), has been successful in supporting total gas exchange during severe respiratory failure [8–10], but application of this technology involves blood-surface interactions that may exacerbate lung injury [8, 11, 12]. In addition, ECMO is labor-intensive and requires expensive equipment and a highly sophisticated team.

## Functional Performance and Limitations of IVOX

A new concept in respiratory support was the development of an intravascular gas-exchange device (IVOX) by Mortensen with CardioPulmonics (Salt Lake City, UT) [13, 14] (Fig. 1). IVOX is a miniature membrane lung that consists of multiple long, crimped hollow fibers within the vena cava that provide $CO_2$ removal and blood oxygenation without the need for extracorporeal circulation or blood transfusion. The hollow fibers are joined together in a potted manifold that communicates with the dual lumen gas conduit at both its proximal and distal ends. The fibers are crimped to produce turbulent blood flow in the vena cava, thus increasing the blood/membrane contact time and blood mixing. The fibers are spiralled, allowing the device to be compressed by furling while being inserted into the vena cava through right femoral or jugular venotomy and unfurled after insertion to perform gas exchange. The membrane is coated with thromboresistance silicone to which heparin is bonded covalently.

IVOX devices are manufactured in sizes 7, 8, 9, and 10 (millimeters in transverse diameters) (Table 1). The largest device permissible is inserted into a patient for two reasons: first, a larger membrane surface area results in greater gas exchange; second, if the unfurled device does not fill the vena cava, the venous return will stream around it, minimizing the blood/membrane contact time and area.

Our group initially tested the IVOX for safety and efficacy and described experimental and clinical use of the IVOX [15–18]. Patients selected for IVOX implantation undergo evaluation of vascular access sites for size and patency with Doppler ultrasound. The IVOX is passed into the vena cava over a guide wire under fluoroscopy to ensure proper position. At the time of venotomy, the patient is given 400 U/kg of heparin as a bolus, followed by a continuous heparin infusion to maintain the activated clotting time at 200–250 s or partial thromboplastin time at 80–90 s. The patient is maintained on prophylactic antibiotics. A vacuum pump draws 100% oxgen into the multiple hollow fibers from an oxygen source via the gas inlet, and gas flow is regulated by an in-line flowmeter. The exhaust gas is analyzed for carbon dioxide concentration by a capnometer. The estimation of $O_2$ transfer can be obtained by measuring the changes in mixed venous $O_2$ saturation with the IVOX on versus a brief period with the IVOX off:

$$O_2 \text{ transfer (ml/min)} = 0.134 \times \text{Hgb} \times \text{CO} \times \text{SvO}_2 \text{ (IVOX on-IVOX off)} \times 10$$

where Hgb is the hemoglobin concentration (g/dl), CO is cardiac output (l/min), and $SvO_2$ is mixed venous $O_2$ saturation (%).

$CO_2$ removal by IVOX is the product of gas flow and $CO_2$ content:

$$CO_2 \text{ removal (ml/min)} = Q \times [CO_2]$$

where Q is the gas flow through the IVOX (ml/min) and $[CO_2]$ is the $CO_2$ concentration of the exhaust gas (%).

**Table 1.** Device properties and performance of IVOX

| Size (mm)[a] | Surface area ($m^2$) | No. of fibers | $O_2$ transfer[b] | $CO_2$ removal[b] |
|---|---|---|---|---|
| 7 | 0.21 | 589 | 40.3 | 43.8 |
| 8 | 0.32 | 703 | 45.6 | 60.2 |
| 9 | 0.41 | 894 | 54.2 | 60.1 |
| 10 | 0.52 | 1107 | 72.5 | 71.0 |

[a] Size in diameter at the site of potting of fibers. The overall size of IVOX is slightly greater.
[b] Unit in ml/min. Data based on summarized clinical trials [19].

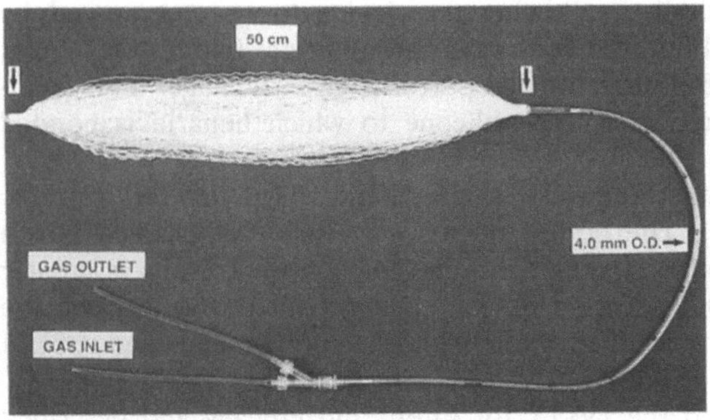


a

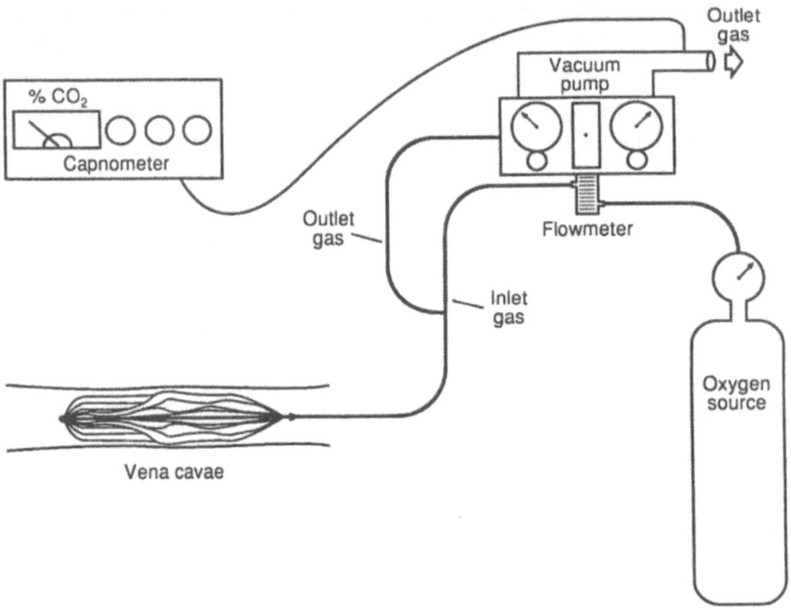


b

Implantation of IVOX in sheep or human patients did not adversely affect hemodynamic function. Due to the absence of a large foreign surface, there were fewer blood-surface interactions and less pulmonary leukosequestration or compliment activation than with ECMO [15]. However, the performance of the current design of IVOX is limited compared with the natural lungs (Table 2) [18]. Experience with IVOX in animal and human studies demonstrated an average of 40 ml/min of $CO_2$ and $O_2$ exchange, about 25–30% of the metabolic demand adults [15, 16]. Therefore, IVOX is not a device meant to substitute for ECMO or to provide total support for patients with acute respiratory failure.

An international multicenter clinical trial of IVOX was conducted for a phase-I and phase-II Food and Drug Administration (FDA) study in major critical care

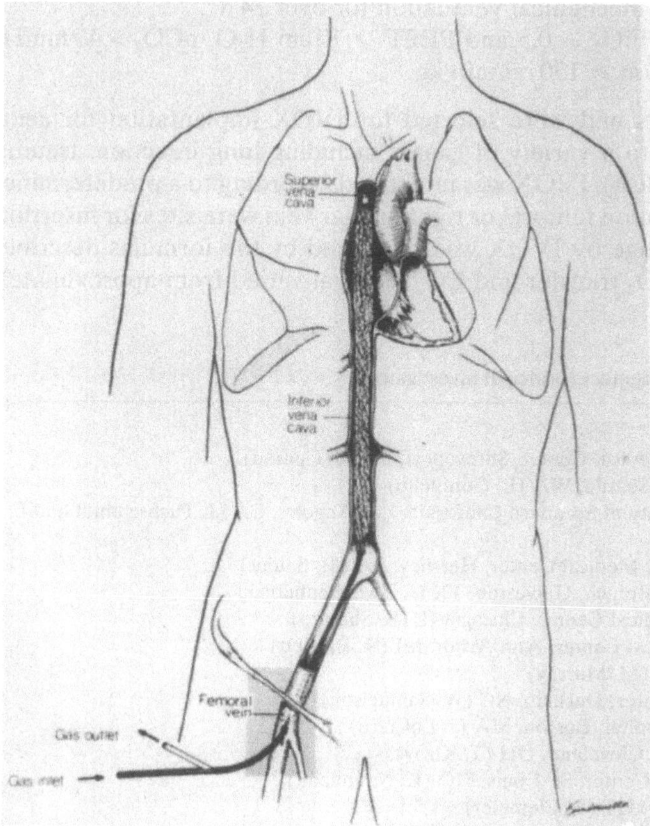


c

**Fig. 1a–c.** The intravenacaval oxygenator and carbon dioxide removal device (IVOX) (**a**), its working setup (**b**), and placement in the human body (**c**)

**Table 2.** Comparison of the natural lungs and IVOX

| | Lungs | IVOX (Size 7) |
|---|---|---|
| Surface area ($m^2$) | 70 | 0.21 |
| Barrier thickness (μm) | 0.6 | 20 |
| Gas flow (l/min) | 5–100 | <3 |
| Max $O_2$ transfer (ml/min) | 2000 | 42 |
| Max $CO_2$ removal (ml/min)[a] | 1500 | 42 |

[a] During normocapnia

centers in the United States and Europe (Table 3). From February 1990 to May 1993, a total of 164 IVOX devices were utilized in 160 clinical trial patients as a means for temporary augmentation of gas exchange in patients with severe, but potentially reversible, acute respiratory failure [19]. Basic entry criteria for the study in the United States and Europe were similar:

1. The requirement for mechanical ventilation for over 24 h
2. $pO_2 \leqslant 60$ mmHg on $FiO_2 \geqslant 0.5$ and PEEP $\geqslant 10$ cm $H_2O$, $pCO_2 > 40$ mmHg with minute ventilation $\geqslant 150$ ml/min/kg

All patients were adults and were selected for IVOX implantation for acute respiratory failure due to a variety of causes including lung infection, trauma, sepsis, and ARDS (Table 4). IVOX was implanted according to a predetermined protocol. The right common femoral or right jugular vein were sites for insertion. The $O_2$ and $CO_2$ exchange by IVOX was calculated by the formulas described above. The amount of $O_2$ transfer and $CO_2$ removal varied from approximately

**Table 3.** IVOX Clinical trial centers (principal investigators)

| |
|---|
| In the USA: |
| Louisiana State University Medical Center, Shreveport, LA (S. Conrad) |
| Harborview Medical Center, Seattle, WA (L. Gentilello) |
| Los Angeles County/University of Southern California, Los Angeles, CA (J. Tuchschmidt and F. Weaver) |
| Pennsylvania State University Medical Center, Hershey, PA (M. Snider) |
| University of Texas Medical Branch, Galveston, TX (J. Zwischenberger) |
| Northwestern University Medical Center, Chicago, IL (B. Shapiro) |
| University of Michigan Medical Center, Ann Arbor, MI (R. Bartlett) |
| Mayo Clinic, Rochester, MN (M. Murray) |
| Duke University Medical Center, Durham, NC (W. Samuelson) |
| New England Deaconess Hospital, Boston, MA (J. LoCiero) |
| Cleveland Clinic Foundation, Cleveland, OH (T. Kirby) |
| St. Louis University Medical Center, St. Louis, MO (K. Naunheim) |
| LDS Hospital, Salt Lake City, UT (T. Clemmer) |
| In Europe: |
| St. George's Hospital, London, England (E.D. Bennett) |
| Berlin Heart Institute, Berlin, Germany (N. Friedel) |
| Cochin University Hospital, Paris, France (F. Brunet) |
| University Hospital, Augsburg, Germany (S. Binder) |
| Royal London Hospital, London, England (A. Wood) |
| St. James Hospital, Leeds, England (N. Webster) |
| Freeman Hospital, Newcastle-upon-Tyne, England (L. Paes) |
| University Hospital, Linkoping, Sweden (C. Aren) |
| Santa Cruz y San Pablo Hospital, Barcelona, Spain (S. Benito) |
| University Hospital, Zurich, Switzerland (L. von Segesser) |
| Puerto de Hiero Hospital, Madrid, Spain (D. Figuera) |
| Academic Hospital, Utrecht, Holland (E.W.L. Jansen) |
| Hannover Medical School, Hannover, Germany (A. Haverich) |
| Royal Brompton National Heart and Lung Hospital, London, England (T. Evans) |
| Rudolf-Virchow University Hospital, Berlin, Germany (R. Rossaint) |
| Leicester Royal Infirmary, Leicester, London (M. Pepperman) |
| Heidelberg University Hospital, Heidelberg, Germany (A. Tanzeem) |
| University Hospital, Hamburg, Germany (G. Kreymann) |
| Papworth Hospital, London, England (D. Bethune) |
| Henri Mondor Hospital, Paris, France (H. Mentec) |
| Gutenberg Hospital, Mainz, Germany (S. Iversen) |
| Uppsala University Hospital, Uppsala, Sweden (U. Hedstrand) |

**Table 4.** Primary causes of acute respiratory failure in patients with IVOX trial [19]

| Etiology | Number of cases | Incidence (%) |
|---|---|---|
| Pneumonia/pneumonitis | 66 | 42 |
| ARDS | 40 | 27 |
| Post-shock lung injury (trauma, surgery, hemorrhage, etc.) | 39 | 26 |
| Sepsis | 25 | 17 |
| Pulmonary embolism | 6 | 4 |
| Other | 25 | 17 |

40 to 70 ml/min, depending on the size of the implanted device (Table 1). Use of IVOX was associated with immediate blood gas improvement in a majority of patients, which allowed a reduction in ventilator settings: $FiO_2$, PEEP, mean or peak airway pressure, and minute ventilation were decreased by >10% in over 60% of patients and by >25% in over 40% of patients. Overall survival of reported patients receiving IVOX is 30%; however, survival is directly related to the severity of lung injury and patient selection – patients with an increasing severity of lung injury or pulmonary malfunction, as indicated by the Murray score, oxygenation index, or intrapulmonary shunt, have a decreasing rate of survival. Unfortunately, there was no control arm to this study to evaluate improvement of survival with IVOX. Complications or adverse events associated with the use of IVOX included mechanical and/or performance problems (29%) and patient complications such as bleeding, thrombosis, infection, venous occlusion, and arrhythmia, as well as user errors which reflected the learning curve with a new device. Seven clinically recognized adverse events were probably contributory to patients' death.

In reporting individual experiences with functional performance of IVOX, Gentilello et al. [20] treated nine adult patients with acute respiratory failure with IVOX for a mean duration of 5.6 days. Mean $CO_2$ removal by IVOX (sizes 7–10) was 40–51 ml/min, and although application of IVOX was associated with an increase in $PaO_2$ and decrease in $PaCO_2$, the quantity of gas transfer was not sufficient to allow a reduction in PEEP, $FiO_2$, or minute ventilation. High et al. [21], by comparing the gas exchange of IVOX and lungs using mass spectrometry in five patients with ARDS, showed IVOX (sizes 7–9) transferred 13–84 ml/min of $O_2$ and 14–82 ml/min of $CO_2$, an amount not exceeding 29% of the total gas exchange, and only small changes in ventilator support were achieved in two patients. Jurmann et al. [22] implanted IVOX in three patients with severe respiratory failure and, in their best experience with a size-9 IVOX, only partial gas exchange support (55–74 ml/min $CO_2$ removal) and moderate reductions in ventilator settings were achieved. In their experience with eight patients, Kallis et al. [23] achieved an average of 58 (40–106) ml/min of $CO_2$ removal and 85 (68–140) ml/min of $O_2$ transfer in eight patients. Conrad et al. [24] treated two patients with size-9 and -10 IVOX, which transferred 43–92 ml/min of $O_2$ and 33–86 ml/min of $CO_2$, and achieved a significant reduction in $FiO_2$ in both patients and minute ventilation in one. In an adult patient with extended use of IVOX, von Segesser et al. showed increased $PaO_2$ that allowed a reduction in PEEP and $FiO_2$, together with improved hemodynamic function [25].

Based on the experience with IVOX worldwide to date, IVOX is useful as a "booster" lung in patients with acute respiratory failure. Measurable amounts of gas exchange (usually 30% of the metabolic demands of an adult) can be achieved to allow a measurable reduction in ventilator settings. Improvements in design and engineering will be necessary for IVOX to improve gas exchange efficiency and ease of insertion and make it a more clinically applicable device.

To allow more precise measurements on gas exchange characteristics, better definition of the contributing factors affecting the performance of IVOX, and evaluation of engineering improvements in IVOX design, an ex vivo veno-venous bypass circuit modeling the adult vena cava was used by Tönz et al. [26] and later modified by us [27]. The bypass circuit was flow controlled and temperature maintained, allowing accurate quantification of the gas exchange by IVOX at different blood flows, different hemoglobin concentrations, and different blood $pCO_2$ levels. Results with size-7 IVOX (589 fibers with 0.21 $m^2$ surface area) showed that total $O_2$ transfer increased in proportion to the blood flow up to 41 ml/min. $CO_2$ removal gradually increased from 17 to 42 ml/min as blood flow increased from 1.0 to 3.0 l/min, but higher blood flow did not further increase $CO_2$ removal. Hemoglobin concentration higher than 8.0 g/dl did not cause a proportional increase in $O_2$ transfer. However, increase of blood $pCO_2$ from 45 to 90 linearly increased the mean pressure gradient across the membrane of IVOX, doubling $CO_2$ removal from 41 to 81 ml/min (Fig. 2). Therefore, IVOX is a diffusion-limited, perfusion-dependent device whose gas exchange performance needs further improvement. In clinical applications of the current design, a normal cardiac output and hemoglobin level should be maintained for the device to perform at maximum capacity.

## Mathematical Model of IVOX

To further analyze the factors limiting $O_2$ and $CO_2$ exchange by IVOX and to explore possible ways to enhance performance, a detailed mathematical model was developed considering IVOX as multiple hollow capillary fibers which separate gas from blood by a gas-permeable membrane [28]. All fibers are assumed to behave identically with respect to gas transfer and no interfiber interaction is included. A coaxial cylinder of moving blood is assumed to surround each fiber, which is considered representative of all fibers. A surface of symmetry lying midway between adjacent fibers is assumed, across which there is no net species transfer. Thus the IVOX device is modeled, as a first approximation, in terms of a repeating unit of a single cylindrical IVOX fiber surrounded by a cylindrical sleeve of blood with closed boundaries and no net interaction between adjacent

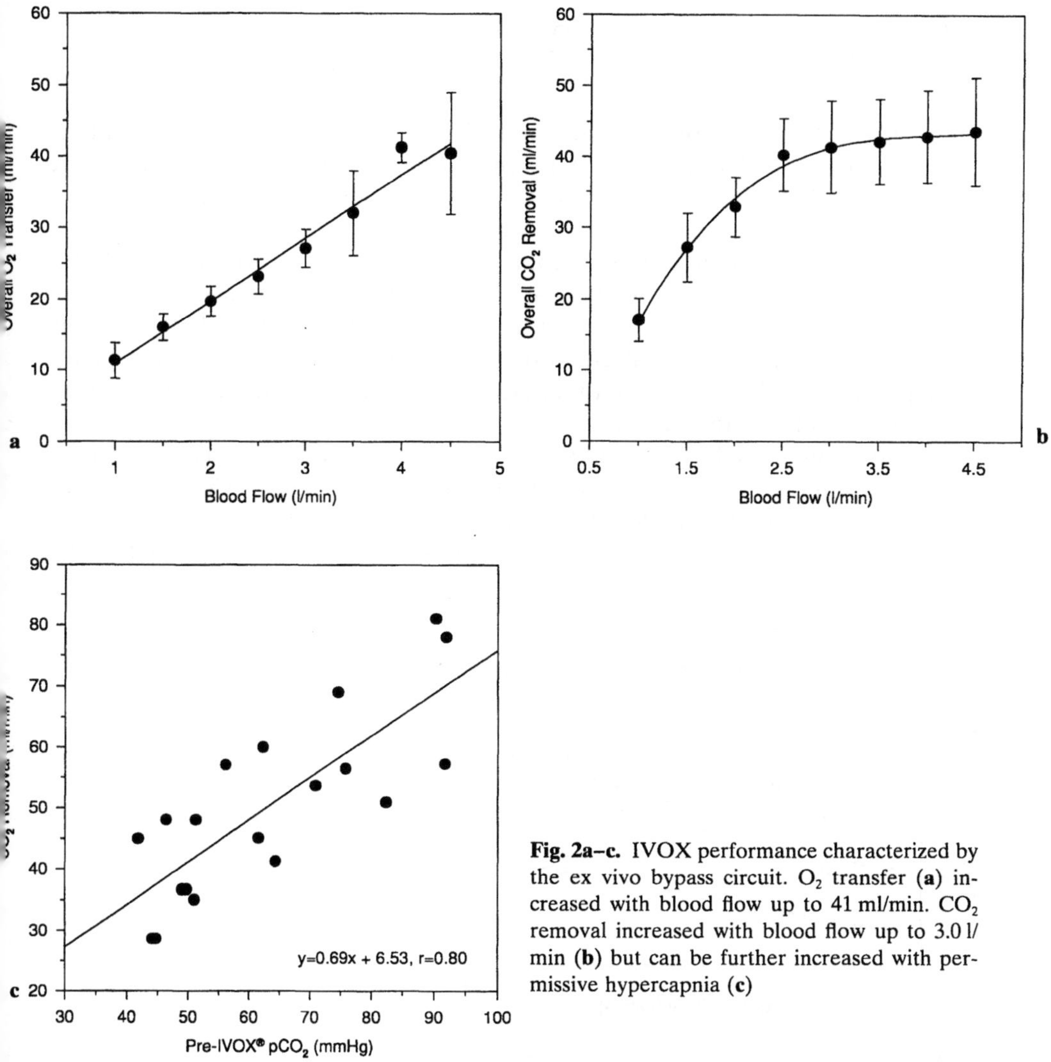


**Fig. 2a–c.** IVOX performance characterized by the ex vivo bypass circuit. $O_2$ transfer (**a**) increased with blood flow up to 41 ml/min. $CO_2$ removal increased with blood flow up to 3.0 l/min (**b**) but can be further increased with permissive hypercapnia (**c**)

units. The performance of the entire device can be simply deduced from the analysis of this unit structure. This modeling approach is similar to the Krogh cylinder model used previously to quantitate gas transport in vascular capillaries surrounded by tissue [29].

Model equations are obtained by writing mass balance equations for $O_2$ and $CO_2$ in the gas, membrane, and blood phases. Blood is treated as a homogeneous fluid over a sample volume in which blood-gas reactions are assumed to occur instantaneously [30]. Empirical dissociation curves are used to relate partial pressures of $O_2$ and $CO_2$ with their respective content in whole blood. Blood and gas velocities are assumed to be fully developed, laminar, at steady state, parallel to the fiber axis, and independent of mass transfer. Species continuity equations may be represented as:

$$\left(\frac{\partial[C_i]^j}{\partial t}\right)+(-1)^k V_z^j(r)\left(\frac{\partial[C_i]^j}{\partial z}\right)=\frac{D_i^j}{r}\frac{\partial}{\partial r}\left(r\frac{\partial[C_i]^r}{\partial r}\right)+D_i^{jz}\left(\frac{\partial^2[C_i]^j}{\partial z^2}\right)$$

where $[C_i]^j$ is the molar concentration of the $i^{th}$ species ($O_2$ or $CO_2$) in the $j^{th}$ phase (gas, membrane, or blood), r and z are the radial and axial coordinates, $D_i^j$ and $D_i^{jz}$ are the radial and axial diffusivities of $i^{th}$ species in the $j^{th}$ phase in the radial and axial directions, respectively, and $V_z^j$ is the molar averaged axial velocity in phase j. Boundary conditions of continuity of wall transfers are imposed at the gas-membrane interface as well as at the membrane-blood interface. Radial symmetry is assumed on the gas side at the center of the fiber. The diffusion-convention partial differential equations for both $O_2$ and $CO_2$, in each of the three phases, are discretized and numerically solved using an alternating direction implicit finite difference procedure.

The computed results obtained with the mathematical model are very similar to those obtained in the ex vivo bypass model (Fig. 3). Figure 3 shows the effect of changing blood and gas flow on $CO_2$ removal. For all cases, countercurrent flow of blood versus gas flow results in a higher rate of $CO_2$ removal. There is a

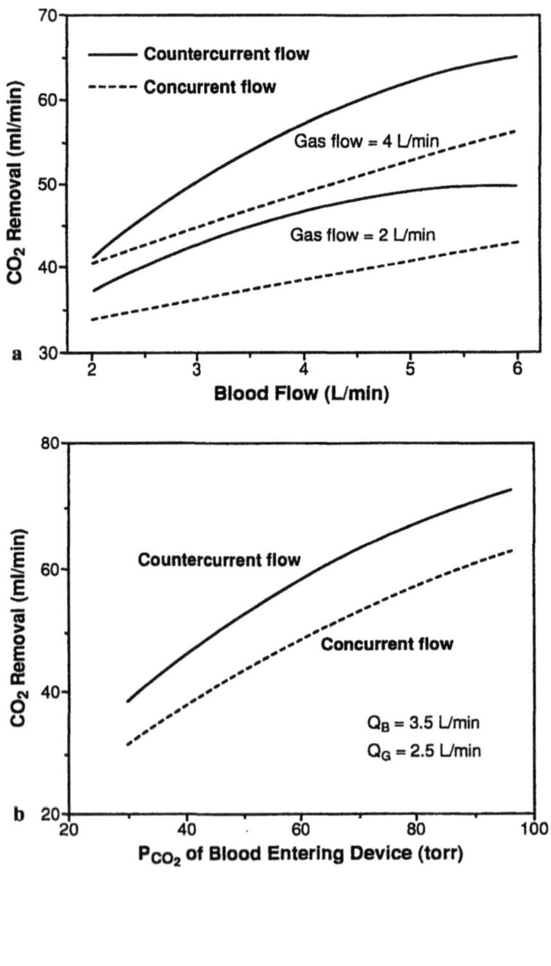


**Fig. 3a,b.** Mathematical modeling of IVOX gas exchange. $CO_2$ removal can be increased by higher blood flow, countercurrent blood flow, or higher gas flow (**a**) and increased blood $pCO_2$ levels (**b**)

substantial increase in $CO_2$ excretion with increases in blood flow. Higher gas flows result in a reduced back pressure of $CO_2$ in the gas phase, thereby augmenting $CO_2$ removal. In addition, as the $pCO_2$ of blood arriving at the device is allowed to rise, there is a near-linear increase in the rate of $CO_2$ removal by the device, due to increased blood-to-gas driving force for $CO_2$ diffusion. This result serves as the theoretical basis for the application of IVOX with permissive hypercapnia.

Additional results using this model indicate that most of the mass transfer resistance to $O_2$ uptake and $CO_2$ removal is in the blood phase and could be diminished by enhanced mixing of blood in the vena cava. While an increase in fiber surface area could significantly enhance gas transfer, increased resistance to venous return would result. Newer generations of IVOX designed to increase blood mixing may significantly enhance the efficiency of IVOX gas exchange.

## Design Improvements of IVOX

Design changes have recently been proposed to improve the gas exchange capabilities of IVOX. New prototype IVOX designs (IVOX IIa and IIb; Table 5) include increased fiber number, decreased fiber length, decreased fiber diameter, and increased crimping to possibly enhance gas exchange. A prospective randomized study was conducted in 17 sheep with smoke inhalation injury treated with the conventional IVOX (IVOX I, $n = 8$) and new prototype IVOX (IVOX IIa, $n = 4$ and IVOX IIb, $n = 5$) [31]. IVOX IIa or IIb did not adversely influence hemodynamics or hemoglobin concentration. No significant differences between groups were noted for insertion technique, thrombosis, emboli, or bleeding complications.

The mean oxygen transfer throughout the 72-h study period was $59 \pm 4$ ml/min for IIa and $57 \pm 7$ ml/min for IIb, both significant improvements over IVOX I. There was no significant difference between the two new prototypes. The new IVOX significantly improved $CO_2$ removal up to 60–70 ml/min for IIa and 70–80 ml/min for IIb, 60% and 80%, respectively, over that of IVOX I. As before, the $CO_2$ removal by the new IVOX prototypes is also directly proportional to the partial pressure of $CO_2$ in the blood [17, 18]. $CO_2$ removal can be plotted as a linear relationship ($y = mx + b$) of arterial $pCO_2$, yielding a measure of the

**Table 5.** Design properties of different prototypes of IVOX (size 7)

| | IVOX I | IVOX IIa | IVOX IIb |
|---|---|---|---|
| Surface area ($m^2$) | 0.21 | 0.23 | 0.26 |
| No. of fibers | 589 | 1400 | 1400 |
| Fiber length (mm) | 28 | 31.5 | 35 |
| Fiber crimp size (mm) | 4.76 | 4.76 | 3.17 |
| Internal fiber diameter (μm) | 200 | 120 | 120 |
| External fiber diameter (μm) | 246 | 167 | 167 |

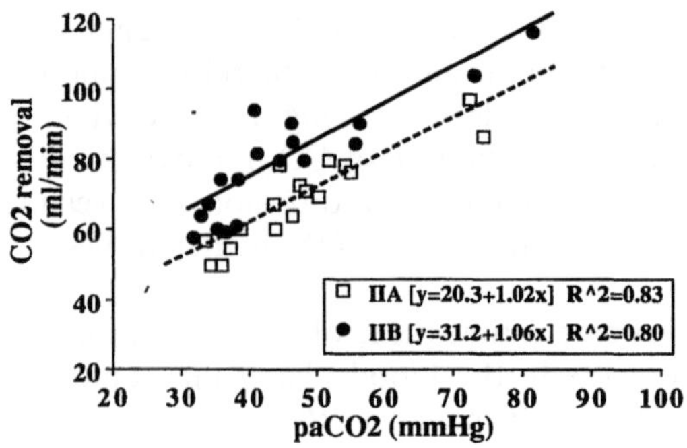


**Fig. 4.** $CO_2$ removal of IVOX prototypes IIa and IIb. Both prototypes show a linear relationship between $CO_2$ removal and blood $pCO_2$ levels.

efficiency of gas transfer by prototype IIa or IIb (for IVOX IIa, y = 1.02x + 20.3, with $r^2 = 0.834$, and for IVOX IIb, y = 1.06x + 31.2, with $r^2 = 0.799$) (Fig. 4). The $CO_2$ transfer efficiency expressed as the average ratio of $CO_2$ removal for given arterial $pCO_2$ levels is 1:1 for IVOX I, but it was 1.63 ± 0.02:1 for IVOX IIa and 1.81 ± 0.03:1 for IVOX IIb, representing a 60–80% increase [31, 32].

The design changes implemented in the IVOX prototypes IIa and IIb have resulted in significantly enhanced gas exchange, particularly $CO_2$ removal. $CO_2$ elimination from a membrane lung is dependent on three main factors: (a) the pressure gradient for $CO_2$ diffusion (relative difference in concentrations of $CO_2$ between the blood and membrane lung ventilating gas), (b) flow rate of the sweep gas, and (c) membrane diffusion capacity. The membrane diffusion capacity is, in turn, a function of: (a) surface area, (b) membrane permeability for $CO_2$, and (c) membrane thickness. As $CO_2$ is a readily diffusible gas at a given pressure gradient (45–50 mmHg – the difference in $pCO_2$ between venous blood during normocapnia and the sweep gas), $CO_2$ transfer is dependent mainly upon the surface area. By increasing the number of fibers despite decreased fiber length and diameter, the surface area of the new prototypes increased by approximately 10% in IIa and 20% in IIb. The increased $CO_2$ removal characteristics of the new devices are probably the direct result of the increased surface area, because the membrane permeability and thickness are identical for each prototype. With the flow rate of the sweep gas limited by the diameter of fibers, the new IVOX IIa and IIb prototypes incorporated more fibers at a smaller diameter to increase membrane surface area at the expense of increased sweep-gas flow resistance. As a result, despite the larger overall area of the hollow fibers, the added resistance decreases the gas flow by 30–40% from IVOX I. Damage or malfunction of the fibers that diminishes overall surface area will also decrease $CO_2$ transfer. IVOX prototypes with fiber breakage upon insertion and subsequent blood accumulation within the fibers and potting of the IVOX experienced a precipitous drop in $CO_2$ exchange.

Being a more diffusion-limited gas, $O_2$ transfer across a membrane lung is dependent on membrane diffusion capacity and blood path thickness, blood flow rate, and oxygen gradient across the membrane. Because the membrane and surface coating, blood flow rate, and oxygen gradient are the same for the IVOX prototypes, the membrane diffusion capacity is influenced by surface area and blood path thickness. As previously noted, the IIb has 10% greater surface area than does the IIa. By increasing the crimping, IIb was designed to effectively decrease the blood path thickness and increase the rate at which $O_2$ diffuses through the blood phase, since increasing the crimping of the IVOX fibers serves to increase turbulence at the blood/membrane interface and minimize the blood-phase resistance to the transfer of $O_2$ and $CO_2$ across the IVOX membrane.

Despite these technical differences, the two IVOX II prototypes demonstrate similar $O_2$ transfer. In addition, the prototype devices do not exhibit as much enhancement in $O_2$ transfer performance over IVOX I as they do in $CO_2$ exchange. This must be attributed partly to the inaccuracy of the current method of measuring $O_2$ transfer in the in vivo model – multiplying the hemoglobin level and cardiac output in large units by the small changes in mixed venous $O_2$ saturation between IVOX-on and IVOX-off, and the results are almost invariably affected by changes in the animals' physiological status (compensation in respiratory efforts, instability of metabolism, shunting into the superior or inferior vena cava or through the lungs, etc.) between the periods of IVOX-on and IVOX-off [33]. A more accurate measurement of $O_2$ exchange using mass spectrum analysis of the IVOX inflow and outflow gas concentrations, or in an ex vivo bypass circuit described earlier, may show a more significant difference in $O_2$ exchange, not only between IVOX I and II prototypes, but also between IIa and IIb.

Another potential improvement in design is active mixing of the blood in contact with IVOX. Since IVOX is a diffusion-limited device with most of the mass transfer resistance in the boundary layer of the blood phase (as predicted by the mathematical model), the efficiency can be enhanced by increased mixing of the blood in the vena cava. An "intra-aortic" balloon was inserted adjacent to IVOX to test the hypothesis of improved gas exchange by active mixing of the blood, and an increase of up to 35% of $CO_2$ removal and 49% in $O_2$ transfer was seen [34] (Fig. 5). Hattler and Reeder et al. [35, 36], working on related gas exchange devices, adopted an integrated and more complete convective mixing of the blood shown by fluorescent image-tracking velcimetry in the vena cava by a pulsatile balloon incorporated within the fibers and achieved a 100% increase in vitro and a >50% increase in vivo in $O_2$ transfer compared with the results obtained with same device at the static state.

Vaslef et al. [37] developed a different type of intravascular lung assist device by potting the membrane fibers into subunits of rosette-like layers, allowing the membrane surface area to increase up to 0.4–0.6 $m^2$ and blood flow across the fibers without increasing the overall size for intravascular placement. Although the device achieved up to 100 ml/min of both $O_2$ and $CO_2$ exchange in their in vitro studies, the blood pressure gradient needed to overcome the resistance of the device and achieve this gas exchange was too high (23–105 mmHg). If placed in the vena cava the device would certainly cause venacaval obstruction to blood flow and hemodynamic instability. Further attempts were made by the same group [38] to arrange the fibers in a helical or screw-like form so the device can be rotated to increase mixing and produce a pumping action for the blood. $O_2$

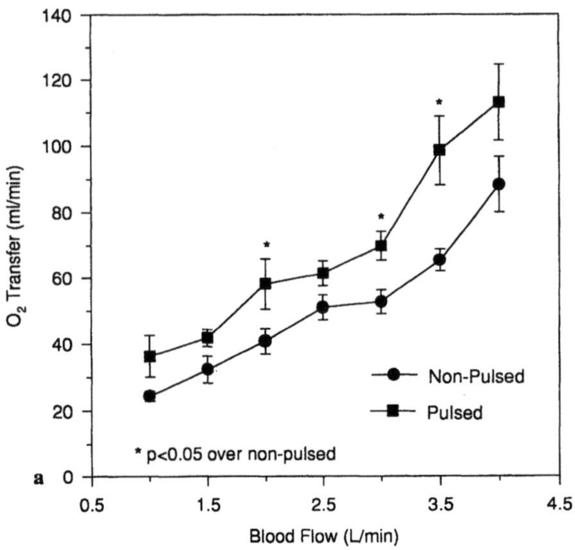


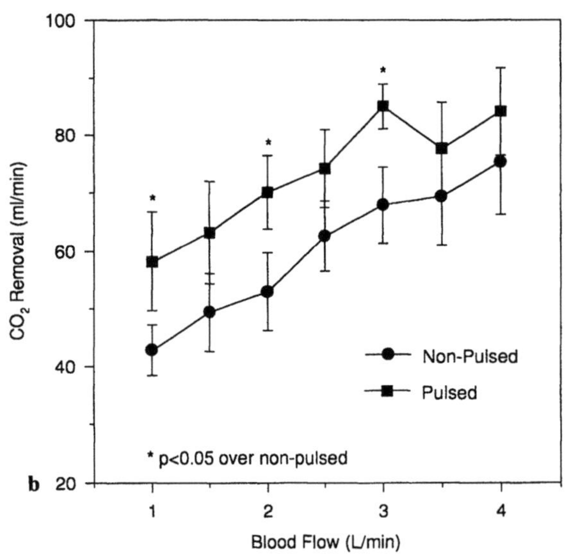


**Fig. 5a,b.** Increase in $O_2$ transfer (**a**) and $CO_2$ removal (**b**) by IVOX with transradial mixing of blood in the ex vivo bypass circuit

transfer by the device (surface area = 0.18 m²) increased 1–5 times as the rotational speed increased compared with a static state, and was able to reach as much as 100 ml/min while rotated at extremely high speed (500 rpm). In vivo experimental studies will be needed before the feasibility of such aggressive mixing is demonstrated in animals or patients. None of the above devices has been studied in a well-established acute respiratory failure animal model, or in patients with severe respiratory failure.

## Permissive Hypercapnia – the Management Technique

In the initial design, the IVOX was capable of removing approximately 40 ml/min, approximately 30% of $CO_2$ production in sheep [15]. This amount of $CO_2$ removal, although significant, proved to be of limited clinical value. However, it is observed that as mixed venous $pCO_2$ increased to 95 mmHg, as in severe patients, IVOX $CO_2$ exchange concomitantly increased from 30 to 95 ml/min [$y = (0.86580)x + 8.9888$] $r^2 = 0.804$. Data from the ex vivo veno-venous bypass also indicated a 1:1 relationship between blood $pCO_2$ and $CO_2$ removal by IVOX. These observations provide the basis of permissive hypercapnia: as blood $pCO_2$ is allowed to increase into the 60–100 mmHg range, the IVOX efficiency can double to further reduce the required ventilator support.

Permissive hypercapnia, therefore, serves a twofold purpose for the management of respiratory failure: (a) to enhance $CO_2$ excretion by the IVOX device, and (b) to minimize the minute ventilation requirements to maintain $pCO_2$ and the associated barotrauma. IVOX with permissive hypercapnia removes approximately 90 ml of $CO_2$ (50% of adult $CO_2$ production) at the blood $pCO_2$ of 90–100 mmHg, and the improved design of IVOX with permissive hypercapnia removes up to 100–120 ml/min $CO_2$ (50–60% of adult $CO_2$ production). Meanwhile, IVOX with permissive hypercapnia significantly reduced ventilatory requirements. A significant (50–70%) reduction of minute ventilation and peak inspiratory pressures was achieved in an ovine model of severe inhalation injury

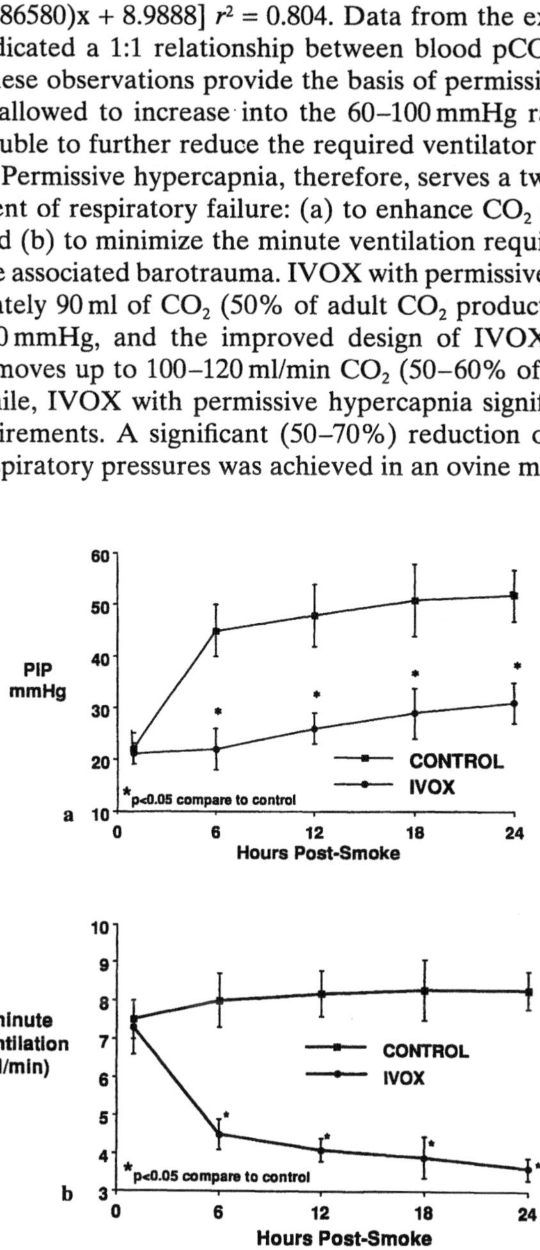


**Fig. 6a,b.** Significant reduction in peak airway pressure (**a**) and minute ventilation (**b**) was achieved with IVOX plus permissive hypercapnia in sheep with severe smoke inhalation injury

treated with IVOX with permissive hypercapnia (Fig. 6), This reduction is almost double the amount obtained with IVOX alone.

Application of permissive hypercapnia alone in patients with severe respiratory failure by Hickling et al. has been shown to be associated with a significantly lower mortality than that predicted by Apache II [39]. This reduction in patient mortality may be due to the avoidance of high airway pressure-induced lung injury that might occur to patients with conventional ventilatory treatment [4, 5, 40]. Induced gradually to minimize respiratory acidosis, even exaggerated hypercapnia (arterial $pCO_2$ up to greater than 100 mmHg) can be well tolerated [39], and hemodynamics was not significantly affected in our experience. Long-term follow-up of patients who experienced extreme hypercapnia has shown no neurological sequel [41, 42].

In conclusion, the current IVOX design can remove only 20–30% of $CO_2$ in an adult with severe respiratory failure under normocapnia conditions. For IVOX to become a more clinically applicable membrane gas exchange device, design changes to improve gas exchange efficiency are needed. Permissive hypercapnia can significantly increase the elimination of $CO_2$ by IVOX, as well as significantly reduce the ventilator-induced lung injury. IVOX with permissive hypercapnia as a management technique for acute respiratory failure can significantly decrease minute ventilation and $FiO_2$ to minimize barotrauma and oxygen toxicity and provide lung rest for patients with ARDS.

## References

1. Cox CS, Zwischenberger JB, Graves D, Raymond G (1992) Mortality from ARDS remains unchanged. Am Rev Respir Dis 145:A83
2. Cunningham AJ (1991) Acute respiratory distress syndrome – two decades later. Yale J Biol Med 64:387–402
3. Dal Nogare AR (1989) Adult respiratory distress syndrome. Am J Med Sci 298:413–430
4. Hickling KG (1990) Ventilatory management of ARDS: can it affect the outcome? Intensive Care Med 16:219–226
5. Tsuno K, Prato P, Kolobow T (1990) Acute lung injury from mechanical ventilation at moderately high airway pressures. J Appl Physiol 69:956–961
6. Parker JC, Hernandez LA, Peevy KJ (1993) Mechanisms of ventilator-induced lung injury. Crit Care Med 21:131–143
7. Biondi JW, Schulman DS, Mathay RA (1988) Effects of mechanical ventilation on right and left ventricular function. Clin Chest Med 9:55–71
8. Zwischenberger JB, Cox CS jr, Minifee PK, Traber DL, Traber LD, Flynn JT, Linares HA, Herndon DN (1993) Pathophysiology of ovine smoke inhalation injury treated with extracorporeal membrane oxygenation. Chest 103:1582–1586
9. Anderson H, III, Steimle C, Shapiro M, Delius R, Chapman R, Hirschl R, Bartlett R. (1993) Extracorporeal life support for adult cardiorespiratory failure. Surgery 114:161–173
10. Cornish JD, Heiss KF, Clark RH, Strieper MJ, Boecler B, Kesser K (1993) Efficacy of venovenous extracorporeal membrane oxygenation for neonates with respiratory and circulatory compromise. J Pediatr 122:105–109
11. Minifee PK, Zwischenberger JB, Flick GR, Navaratnam N, Linares HA, Allison PL, Herndon DN (1988) Pulmonary leukosewquestration and lung edema after severe smoke inhalation injury are not improved with extracorporeal membrane oxygenation. Surg Forum 40:251–253

12. Bartlett RH (1990) Extracorporeal life support for cardiopulmonary failure. Curr Probl Surg 27:621–705
13. Mortensen JD (1987) An intravenacaval blood gas exchange (IVCBGE) device. A preliminary report. ASAIO Trans 33:570–573
14. Mortensen JD, Berry G (1989) Conceptual and design features of a practical, clinically effective intravenous mechanical blood oxygen/carbon dioxide exchange device (IVOX). Int J Artif Organs 12:384–389
15. Cox CS jr., Zwischenberger JB, Traber LD, Traber DL, Herndon DN (1991) Use of an intravascular oxygenator/carbon dioxide removal device in an ovine smoke inhalation injury model. ASAIO Trans 37:M411–M413
16. Zwischenberger JB, Cox CS Jr (1991) A nex intravascular membrane oxygenator to augment blood gas transfer in patients with acute respiratory failure. Text Med 87:60–63
17. Zwischenberger JB, Cox CS, Graves D, Bidani A (1992) Intravascular membrane oxygenation and carbon dioxide removal – a new application for permissive hypercapnia? Thorac Cardiovasc Surg 40:115–120
18. Cox CS Jr., Zwischenberger JB, Graves DF, Niranjan SC, Bidani A (1993) Intracorporeal $CO_2$ removal and permissive hypercapnia to reduce airway pressure in acute respiratory failure. The theoretical basis for permissive hypercapnia with IVOX. ASAIO J 39:97–102
19. Conard SA, Bagley A, Bagley B, Schaap RN (1994) Major findings from the clinical trails of the intravascular oxygenator (IVOX). Artif Organs 18:846–863
20. Gentilello LM, Jurkovich GJ, Gubler KD, Anardi DM, Heiskell R (1993) The intravascular oxygenator (IVOX): preliminary results of a new means of performing extra-pulmonary gas exchange. J Trauma 35:399–404
21. High KM, Snider MT, Richard R, Russell GB, Stene JK, Campbell DB, Aufiero TX, Thieme GA (1992) Clinical trails of an intravenous oxygenator in patients with adult respiratory distress syndrome. Anesthesiology 77:856–863
22. Jurmann MJ, Demertzis S, Schaefers HJ, Wahlers T, Haverich A (1992) Intravascular oxygenation for advanced respiratory failure. ASAIO J 38:120–124
23. Kallis P, al Saady NM, Bennett ED, Treasure T (1993) Early results of intravascular oxygenation. Eur J Cardiothorac Surg 7:206–210
24. Conrad SA, Eggerstedt JM, Morris VF, Romero MD (1993) Prolonged intracorporeal support of gas exchange with an intravenacaval oxygenator. Chest 103:158–161
25. von Segesser LK, Schafner A, Stocker R, Lachat M, Speich R, Baumann PC, Turina M (1992) Extended (29 days) use of intravascular gas exchanger. Lancet 339:1536
26. Tönz M, von Segesser LK, Leskosek B, Turina M (1994) Quantitative gas transfer of an intravascular oxygenator. Ann Thorac Surg 57:146–150
27. Tao W, Zwischenberger JB, Nguyen TT, Tzouanakis AE, Matheis EJ, Trader DL, Bidani A (1994) Performance of an intravenous gas exchanger (IVOX) in a veno-venous bypass circuit. Ann Thorac Surg 57:1484–1490
28. Niranjan SC, Clark JW, San KY, Zwischenberger JB, Bidani A (1993) Analysis of factors affecting gas transfer in an intravascular blood oxygenator. J Appl Physiol 77:1716–1730
29. Krogh A (1919) The number and distribution of capillaries in muscles with calculations of the oxygen pressure head necessary for supplying the tissue. J Physiol 52:409–415.
30. Bidani A (1991) Analysis of abnormalities of capillary $CO_2$ exchange in vivo. J Appl Physiol 70:1686–1699
31. Nguyen TT, Zwischenberger JB, Tao W, Traber DL, Herndon DN, Duncan CC, Bush P, Bidani A (1993) Significant enhancement of carbon dioxide removal by a new prototype IVOX. ASAIO J 39:M719–M724
32. Cox CS, Jr., Zwischenberger JB, Kurusz M (1991) Development and current status of a new intracorporeal oxygenator. Perfusion 6:291–296
33. Mortensen JD (1991) Augmentation of blood gas transfer by means of an intravascular blood gas exchanger (IVOX). In: Marini JJ, Roussos C (eds) Ventilatory failure. Springer, Berlin Heidelberg New York, pp 318–346

34. Tao W, Schroeder T, Nguyen PJ, Bidani A, Bradford DW, Traber DL, (1994) Zwischenberger JB. Improved gas exchange performance of the intravascular oxygenator by active blood mixing. ASAIO J 40:M527–M532
35. Hattler BG, Johnson PC, Sawzik PJ, Shaffer FD, Klain M, Lund LW, Reeder GD, Walters FR, Goode JS, Borovetz HS (1992) Respiratory dialysis. A new concept in pulmonary support. ASAIO J 38:M322–M325
36. Reeder GD, Hattler BG, Rawleigh J, Walters FR, Sawzik PJ, Lund LW, Klain M, Goode JS, Borovetz HS (1993) Current progress in the development of an intravenous membrance oxygenator. ASAIO J 39:M461–M465
37. Vaslef SN, MOckros LF, Anderson RW (1989) Development of an intravascular lung assist device. ASAIO Trans 35:660–664
38. Makarewicz AJ, Mockros LF, Anderson RW (1993) A pumping intravascular artificial lung with active mixing. ASAIO Abstr 22:68
39. Hickling KG, Henderson SJ, Jackson R (1990) Low mortality associated with low-volume pressure limited ventilation with permissive hypercapnia in severe adult repiratory distress syndrome. Intensive Care Med 16:372–377
40. Dreyfuss D, Soler P, Basset G, Saumon G (1988) High inflation pressure pulmonary edema. Am Rev Respir Dis 137:1159–1164
41. Potkin RT, Swenson ER (1992) Resuscitation from severe acute hypercapnia. Determinants of tolerance and survival. Chest 102:1742–1745
42. Goldstein B, Shannon DC, Todres ID (1990) Supercarbia in children: clinical course and outcome. Crit Care Med 18:166–168

# Part VIII
# Horizons and Future Trends

# Horizons

F. UNGER

It is fascinating to be active and to watch how the exciting field of assisted circulation has evolved over the last 20 years, a field I have been personally involved in since 1972. The general anticipation was especially very high in 1975, a time when the first clinical implantations of assist devices took place. A real break through was expected soon. The feeling was the same in 1986, when I performed my first clinical bridge in Europe, using the Ellipsoid Heart. It was anticipated that the clinical feasibility of the total artificial heart and of assist devices would come much earlier. Today the total artificial heart is no longer an object of discussion. At present the prerequesites for a long-term use of assist devices are given; the technology of the devices in clinical use is so advanced that a long-term use seems to be reality. Another breakthrough that is nearly on the horizon might break all expectations in treating failing hearts. Gene technology may turn out to provide a new effective strategy for avoiding atherosclerosis and treating cardiac failure. It will make possible implantation via a catheter in impaired heart myocysts, which can then develop within the ventricle and result in new muscle mass.

The future becomes reality much faster than we can imagine. Despite all high-powered investigations and experimental research, cardiac assist devices are clinical techniques to overcome heart failure. Intra-aortic balloon pumping is indicated in postcardiotomy failure syndrome and in pump failure after acute myocardial infarction. For postcardiotomy failure syndrome, nonpulsatile assist devices are sufficient to overcome the first critical period. Implantable pulsatile assist devices are indicated as a bridge or for chronic use in patients with end-stage cardiac failure as a result of different forms of cardiomyopathy. Further implantations will show if it is possible, under certain circumstances, for a failing heart to recover.

# Horizons

D.A. Cooley

As we prepare to enter the twenty-first century, no aspect of cardiovascular surgery has more of a futuristic aura than mechanical cardiac assistance. What changes and challenges will the new century bring to this field? Before attempting to characterize the next few decades, I will briefly review the history of mechanical circulatory support systems. By coincidence, much of this history has spanned my own career as a heart surgeon.

Modern cardiac surgery dates back to World War II, when operations undertaken for battlefield trauma proved that, contrary to widespread opinion, the heart could withstand surgical manipulation. During the next few decades, no specialty witnessed greater miracles. With the advent of the heart-lung machine in 1953, surgeons were finally able to stop the heart, open it, and repair intricate defects. At the same time, new diagnostic breakthroughs enhanced our ability to detect specific cardiac diseases. By the mid 1960s, heart surgeons were riding the crest of a seemingly endless wave of progress. A host of conditions, including acquired valvular disorders, cardiac arrhythmias, and even coronary artery disease, became amenable to the scalpel. These breakthroughs culminated in 1967, when Dr. Christiaan Barnard, in Cape Town, South Africa, performed the first human heart transplant. During the ensuing 2-year period, this procedure was widely duplicated. At the Texas Heart Institute, we performed the first successful cardiac transplant in the United States. Despite initial enthusiasm for heart transplantation, the medical community quickly became disenchanted when recipients began to succumb to tissue rejection. Between 1970 and 1980, only a handful of surgeons continued to perform heart transplants.

In response to disillusionment with heart transplantation, investigators redoubled their efforts to create a mechanical circulatory support system that would sustain the failing heart on either a short- or a long-term basis. These efforts centered around (a) ventricular assist devices, which would work in tandem with the natural heart, and (b) the total artificial heart, which would replace the natural organ altogether. From the beginning, this research has been a cooperative, multidisciplinary endeavor. One important breakthrough came in the early 1960s, with the advent of the intra-aortic balloon pump, which was developed by Moulopoulos's group and introduced clinically by Kantrowitz's team. This simple device remains extremely effective in salvaging patients with potentially reversible left ventricular impairment.

Since its founding, the Texas Heart Institute has been at the forefront of research into mechanical assist devices. In 1969 and 1981, we performed the earliest clinical implantations of an artificial heart; on both occasions, the device sustained the patient until heart transplantation could be performed. Moreover, in 1978, we became the first to use a left ventricular assist device (LVAD) for staged cardiac transplantation in a human being. Through the success of these procedures, we proved that both the LVAD and the artificial heart could serve as bridges to transplantation.

In the early 1980s, new methods of diagnosing and treating tissue rejection finally allowed cardiac transplantation to become a widely accepted option for patients with end-stage heart disease. Nevertheless, the number of candidates continues to exceed the number of donors, and many of these patients require some form of mechanical support until a suitable donor organ can be found. Owing to progress in materials and designs, the 1980s saw a new generation of cardiac assist devices capable of providing left-, right-, and biventricular support. These devices have proved highly effective as both short- and long-term bridges to transplantation.

In addition, investigators have continued their attempts to produce a workable total artificial heart. In late 1982, the Jarvik-7 model, a pneumatically driven pump intended as a permanent heart substitute, was implanted in a patient who survived for 112 days. Between late 1982 and mid 1985, William DeVries implanted this device in four additional patients in the United States, one of whom survived for 620 days. Like other artificial hearts, however, the Jarvik-7 was plagued by blood-clotting and thromboembolic complications. Because of these problems, the United States government declared a ban on implantation of the total artificial heart as a permanent cardiac substitute, although centers in other countries have continued clinical investigations. In the United States, artificial hearts have recently been reapproved as bridges to transplantation. The experience gained in these cases may bring the dream of permanent mechanical replacement closer to fruition.

Before permanent implantation of a total artificial heart is justified for routine use, however, researchers must find a way to combat the potentially lethal complications of hemorrhage, thromboembolism, infection, and stroke. Moreover, the ideal energy source has not yet been defined. Investigators have, however, made significant progress recently in the development of electrical power sources. Although these problems will take some time to overcome, a reliable, permanent total artificial heart should eventually be an option for patients throughout the world.

The latest advance toward long-term mechanical assistance is the Heartmate, a left ventricular assist device that may ultimately become an alternative to transplantation. Clinical trials of a portable, battery-operated Heartmate are now underway at our institution. So far, this pump has avoided many of the complications that have plagued other mechanical assist devices. As a result, I believe the immediate future lies in this direction, rather than in transplantation. With a long-term mechanical assist device, patients would not have to endure a prolonged waiting period; they would not have to be on a lifelong regimen of immunosuppressive therapy; and they would have the psychological comfort of keeping their natural heart.

Critics of modern medicine have their doubts about the wisdom of using extraordinary measures to prolong life indefinitely, particularly for patients who have no further hope of enjoying a meaningful existence. Many experts believe that the funds devoted to these efforts would be better used to provide basic health care for a broader segment of the population. I cannot agree with those who denounce high-tech medicine per se. In fact, patients supported by assist devices in our hospital alone save about $2900 per day when their charges are compared with those of patients awaiting a transplant in the ICU. I do agree, however, that in order to have more equitable health care, we – as a society – may be forced to modify our idea of what constitutes necessary treatment, particularly in the face of impending "natural" death.

Of course, in reducing overall mortality and the need for sophisticated devices, prevention is the simplest approach and the one that benefits the largest number of persons. In the exciting new field of molecular epidemiology, researchers are using genes and biologic markers to determine why certain individuals are vulnerable to heart disease. Within the next few decades, DNA recombinant techniques may help control heart disease by removing harmful genes or by introducing therapeutic ones. However, we can be sure that mechanical cardiac assistance will continue to save lives and intrigue medical researchers for years to come.

I congratulate Dr. Unger for producing this outstanding volume, which will prove a valuable guide to state-of-the-art circulatory support systems as we enter the twenty-first century.

# Horizons for Cardiac Prostheses

Y. Orime and Y. Nosé

## Introduction

There are various types of clinical cases requiring circulatory support, ranging from short-term to long-term or permanent. Based upon the clinical experiences, currently available cardiac prostheses are classified in Fig. 1 according to the duration of support [1, 2]. In general, nonpulsatile pumps can cover the spectrum of support duration, ranging from short-term to typically up to 1 month (it is possibly to extend it up to 3 months with current technology and use of multiple devices), while pulsatile devices are suitable to support a broader spectrum, ranging from 3 months to permanent use (Fig. 1). As for bridge to heart transplantation, it is necessary to utilize a cardiac prosthesis capable of supporting circulation for at least 2 weeks to 6 months (Fig. 1).

## Pulsatile Cardiac Prostheses

Various types of pulsatile cardiac prostheses, such as a ventricular assist device (VAD) and a total artificial heart (TAH), have been developed by various groups during the past 35 years, since Drs. Kolff and Akutsu implanted their device in a dog in 1957 [3]. Some of those devices were proven to be clinically effective for ventricular support, postcardiotomy cardiac support and as a bridge to transplantation [4–9]. According to the registry report, all these pulsatile devices demonstrated that the lives of one quarter of postcardiotomy cardiac failure patients were salvaged by these devices and one half of bridge-to-transplant patients were alive after heart transplantation [10]. With the combination of great enthusiasm on the part of the development team and skill on the part of the clinical team, these pulsatile cardiac prostheses are highly effective tools in the management of patients with refractory cardiac failure despite aggressive medical therapy.

However, at the present time we cannot always select a device appropriate to the patient's condition because of the limited availability of devices under the strict regulation of the Food and Drug Administration (FDA) in the USA [11]. Actually, in almost all institutes and hospitals, the choice of a cardiac prosthesis for a patient depends not only on the clinical indication and support duration, but also on device availability and the expenses for the clinical team. The clinically available devices under the Investigational Device Exemption (IDE) approval

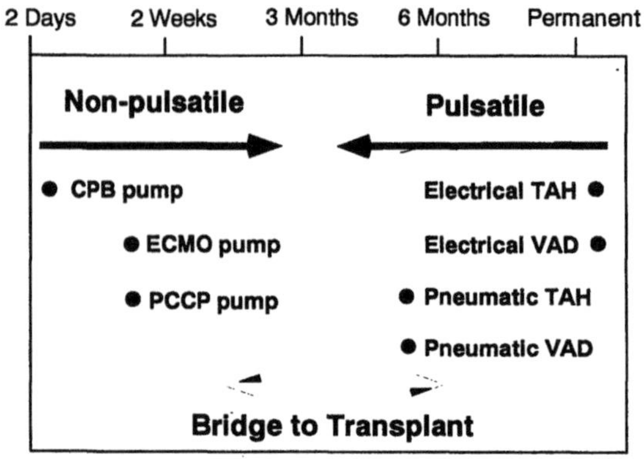


**Fig. 1.** Duration and type of circulatory support used, derived from clinical needs. *PCCF*, Postcardiotomy cardiac failure

are limited to 15–20 centers, and only a few of those centers have approval for more than one device [12]. In addition, these clinically available pulsatile devices, which are currently the only means of long-term circulatory support, are large, complex, and expensive [13]. Although they are able to provide over 1 year of support, these devices are extremely complex and cost approximately $50 000 for each unit [14]. Thus, the currently available pulsatile cardiac prostheses are not applicable for use in a large population due to regulatory and financial limitations.

## Nonpulsatile Cardiac Prostheses

Meanwhile, for years, roller pumps were the only pumps used for cardiopulmonary bypass (CPB). However, in recent years several types of commercially available centrifugal pumps have been employed; hence the term "second-generation cardiopulmonary bypass pumps" [13]. The centrifugal pump is far superior to the roller pump. Its merits are many, but, to name a few, it is easy to set up accurately and requires much less priming volume because of its small size; it is easily moved to any position in the operating room or can be transported to another area while suppporting the patient's life; and it causes very little trauma to the blood cells [13, 15].

Recently, several types of commercially available centrifugal pumps have been widely used not only for cardiopulmonary bypass, but also for postcardiotomy support [16–20]. According to the registry report, almost 70% of postcardiotomy cardiogenic shock patients were supported by centrifugal pumps [10]. Results are almost identical to those with pulsatile pumps. Nowadays, because of their low cost and simple control, centrifugal pumps are becoming more popular than the pulsatile VADs and TAHs.

Unfortunately, the life expectancy of the currently available centrifugal pumps is officially limited to 2 days, mainly because of thrombus formation and blood leakage around the shaft [19]. At present, there are no centrifugal pumps and axial flow pumps suitable for long-term usage. Therefore, it is necessary to make nonpulsatile cardiac prostheses more safe, practical, reliable, durable, and implantable. From a clinical point of view, a nonpulsatile pump which can operate for 3 months is desired when bridge to transplantation is considered (Fig. 1).

As many people recognize, the nonpusatile pump is less expensive, smaller, simpler, and easier to handle and it does not need complex control logic. Thus, it is obvious that most clinicians would use a nonpulsatile pump, if it could operate for a long period (more than 3 months) without thrombus formation and critical hemolysis. If this dream comes true, nonpulsatile pumps will be able to take the place of pulsatile pumps and operate for long-term circulatory support. Is it a dream? No, it is a very real possibility in the near future.

## Baylor Cardiac Prostheses

In order to realize this dream, our team has been ambitiously developing various types of cardiac prostheses. Since October 1989, when one of the authors (Y.N.) came to the Department of Surgery at Baylor College of Medicine as Professor of Surgery, our projects have advanced remarkably. At the beginning of this "re-start" there were only four members (two medical doctors and two engineers) in our laboratory. Through these members' contributions, many new projects have been developed. At present, we have 20 full-time members in the Surgical Research Laboratory, including ten faculties and ten technical staff members, together with six part-time faculties [21]. In our laboratory, six types of blood pumps (three nonpulsatile pumps and three pulsatile pumps) have been developed [21].

### The Baylor-Nikkiso Pump

The Baylor-Nikkiso pump (Fig. 2), a compact and atraumatic centrifugal pump, is available for clinical use as a second-generation cardiopulmonary bypass pump. The pump housing and impeller are made of polycarbonate. This pump has a magnetically coupled system with a V-ring seal separating the blood chamber and magnet chamber. The impeller has six straight veins and six small washout holes which reduce the thrombus formation behind the impeller [22, 23]. This pump already has been approved for clinical use as a cardiopulmonary bypass pump in Japan, and currently has the FDA 5–10K approval in the USA. It is an atraumatic pump, indicating the lowest hemolysis (index of hemolysis: 0.001) in comparison to other commercially available centrifugal pumps [15, 23].

In order to extend the life of the Baylor-Nikkiso pump, we incorporated a purging chamber behind the V-ring seal. Using saline for purging, in vivo tests demonstrated this modified pump to be effective in preventing thrombus formations around the shaft [24]. This purging-type pump can run for 2 weeks as postcardiotomy circulatory support, ECMO (extracorporeal membrane oxygenation), and bridge to transplantation.

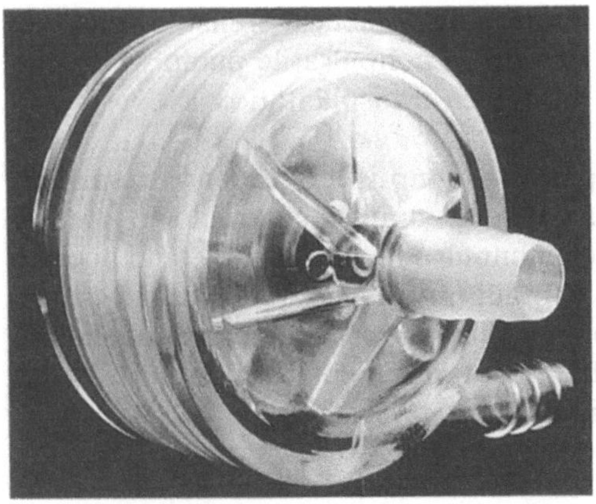

**Fig. 2.** The Baylor-Nikkiso centrifugal pump

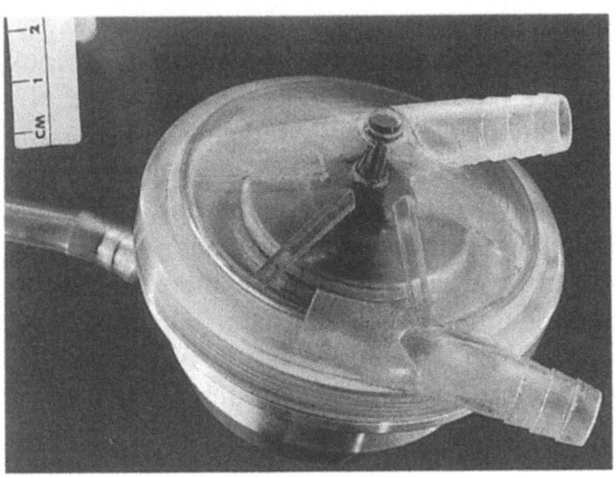


**Fig. 3.** The Baylor-Kyocera gyro pump (C1E30 type)

## The Baylor-Kyocera Gyro Pump

In order to extend the life of the centrifugal pump further, it is necessary to eliminate the shaft for the pump. To eliminate the shaft, a gyroscopic principle was introduced to the Baylor-Kyocera gyro pump (Fig. 3).

This pump was developed aiming for 1-month or longer operation. The gyro pump is conceived as a one-piece rotor-impeller, supported by the gyroscopic principle. One pivot bearing supports the bottom, while the top of the rotor-impeller may be supported by various methods [25–27]. The inlet bearing supports of this sealless compact centrifugal pump were successfully eliminated, demonstrating good performance, low hemolysis, and antithrombogenicity for more than 2 weeks in an initial in vivo study [28]. This model will meet the requirement of a long-term centrifugal VAD. Currently, a sealless and shaftless free impeller model is under development for an implantable VAD, aiming for up to 3 months' application.

## The Baylor-NASA Axial Flow Pump

A cooperative effort between Baylor and NASA/Johnson Space Center is under way to develop an implantable axial flow pump for LVAD, with Dr. M.E. DeBakey as the principal investigator (Fig. 4). This pump is intended as an assist device for either pulmonary or systemic circulatory support for more than 3 months' duration. The stator of the motor is incorporated in the flow tube; magnets are incorporated in the impeller [29]. Its size (75 mm in length and 25 mm in diameter) and weight (53 g) make it ideal for use as an implantable device for a wider patient population including women and children [29]. The total displacement volume of this pump is 15 cc. Against 100 mmHg of total head, this pump provides a flow of 6–8 l/min, indicating that it is suitable for left heart assistance [29, 30].

In order to establish an optimal pump design with minimum hemolysis, six pump parameters were evaluated systematically using 83 units of fresh bovine blood. Currently, the best index of hemolysis achieved is 0.018 g/100 l, which is lower than that with a Nimbus axial pump [31]. Initial 2-day in vivo feasibility studies in calves are under way to evaluate the antithrombogenic nature of this pump [30].

## The Baylor Total Artificial Heart (TAH)

The Baylor TAH is a one-piece totally implantable electromechanical TAH system (Fig. 5). In order to have a good anatomical fit, the pump was miniaturized (97 mm outer diameter, 83 mm center thickness, 620 g total weight, and 510 cc displacement volume). The anatomical compatibility of this pump was verified in the human pericardial space of 26 orthotopic heart recipients [32]. The pump can be easily and simply controlled by a left master alternate (LMA) mode, using Hall-effect position sensors [33]. A biolized coated surface of dry gelatin has a good biocompatibility [34]. Because of the large-orifice inflow valve and passive fill mode, this TAH shows extremely high sensitivity to a low preload [35]. At the

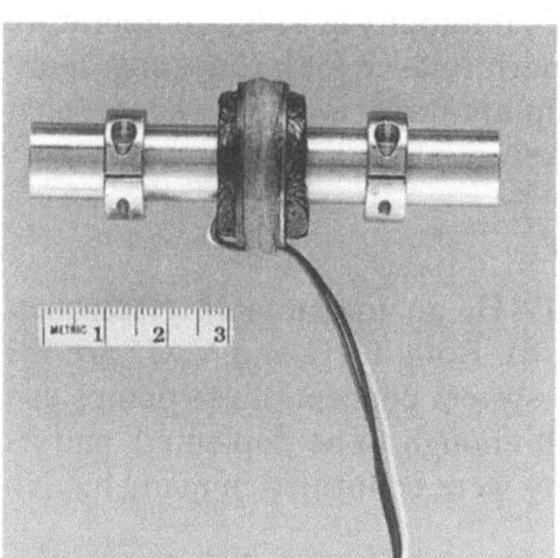


**Fig. 4.** The Baylor-NASA axial flow pump

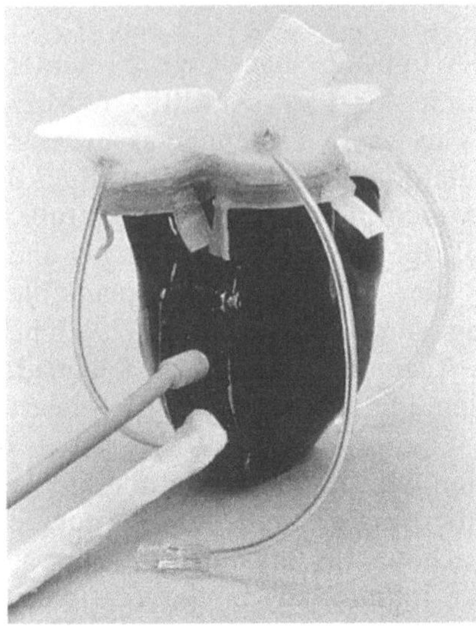

**Fig. 5.** The Baylor total artificial heart

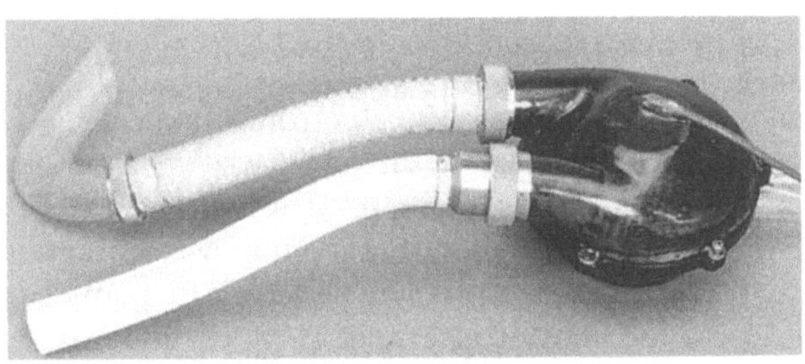

**Fig. 6.** The Baylor ventricular assist device

same time, afterload sensitivity is very low. Therefore, we do not need afterload control logic and use only preload sensitive control.

This TAH has a reproducible high performance with good quality assurance. Additionally, the pump demonstrated long-term durability in a high-temperature environment, indicating a stable and reliable performance [36]. Currently, more in-depth flow visualization studies of this pump are under way to validate long-term thrombus-free design [37].

## The Baylor Ventricular Assist Device (VAD)

Using many universal components of the TAH, an implantable electromechanical VAD has also been developed (Fig. 6). Both TAH and VAD are for permanent use. Because of the multi-purpose system concept, these pumps can be easily fabricated [2, 35]. This VAD is small enough to be implanted, and its good hemodynamic performance and reliability were confirmed in many in vivo studies [38].

According to the results of thermal management tests, this pump has proved to be safe and has an effective thermal dissipation [39]. Currently, a multi-

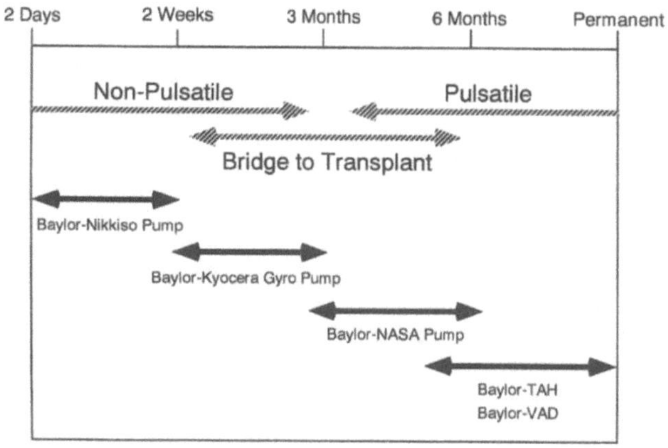


**Fig. 7.** Support duration of Baylor cardiac prostheses

purpose miniature electromechanical energy system has been developed for both TAH and VAD [40].

### Muscle-driven Pump

Using the same driving mechanism of the TAH and VAD, a muscle-driven pump has been also developed, as a permanent pulsatile device. It is the authors' opinion that the above-mentioned six different cardiac prostheses being developed at Baylor College of Medicine will be able to provide support from 2 days to several years (Fig. 7) [21].

## Conclusion

Recently, several implantable nonpulsatile pumps have demonstrated their possible features as long-term systems with good antithrombogenicity [41, 42]. Thus, the authors strongly believe that inexpensive and simple implantable nonpulsatile pumps will be used primarily as bridge-to-transplantation devices and as long-term ventricular assist devices for functional and therapeutic application before the twenty-first century. Our axial flow pump may be one such long-term device. On the other hand, an implantable pulsatile TAH and VAD will be applicable only as permanent devices.

## References

1. Nosé Y (1992) Is a pulsatile cardiac prosthesis a dying dinosaur? Artif Organs 16:233–234
2. Shiono M, Takatani S, Sasaki T, Orime Y, Swenson CA, Minato N, Ohara Y, Noon GP, Nosé Y, DeBakey ME (1992) Baylor multipurpose circulatory support system for short- to long-term use. Trans Am Soc Artif Intern Organs 38:M301–M305
3. Akutsun T, Kolff WJ (1957) Pneumatic substitutes for veins and hearts. Trans Am Soc Artif Intern Organs 4:230–235
4. Pennington DG, MacBride LR, Swartz MT (1989) Use of the Pierce-Donachy ventricular assist device in patients with cardiogenic shock after cardiac operations. Ann Thorac Surg 47:130–135

5. Farrar DJ, Lawson JH, Litwak P, Cederwall G (1990) Thoratec VAD system as a bridge to heart transplantation. J Heart Transplant 9:415–423
6. Champsaur G, Ninet J, Vigneron M, Cochet P Neidecker J, Boissonnat P (1990) Use of the Abiomed BVS System 5000 as a bridge to cardiac transplantation. J Thorac Cardiovasc Surg 100:122–128
7. Copeland JC, Smith RG, Cleavinger M, Icenogle TB, Sethi G, Rosado L (1991) Bridge to transplantation indications for Symbion TAH, Symbiom LVAD and Novacor LVAS. In: Akutsu T, Koyanagi H (eds) Artificial heart, vol 3. Springer, Berlin Heidelberg New York, pp 303–308
8. MacCarthy PM, Portner PM, Tobler HG, Starns VA, Ramasamy N, Oyer PE (1991) Clinical experience with the Novacor ventricular assist system: bridge to transplantation and the transition to permanent application. J Thorac Cardiovasc Surg 102:578–587
9. Frazier OH, Rose EA, Macmanus Q, Burton NA, Lefrak EA, Poirier VL, Dasse KA (1992) Multicenter clinical evaluation of the HeartaMate 1000 IP left ventricular assist device. Ann Thorac Surg 53:1080–1090
10. Oaks TE, Pae WE, Miller CA, Pierce WS (1991) Combined registry for the clinical use of mechanical ventricular assist pumps and the total artificial heart in conjunction with heart transplantation: fifth official report – 1990. J Heart Lung Transplant 10:621–625
11. Magovern JA, Pierce WS (1990) Mechanical circulatory assistance before heart transplantation. In: Baumgartner WA (ed) Heart transplantation. Saunders, Philadelphia, pp 73–85
12. Rowles JR, Mortimer BJ, Olsen DB (1993) Ventricular assist and total artificial heart devices for clinical use in 1993. ASAIO Trans 39:840–855
13. Nosé Y (1989) The need for a second-generation pump oxygenator. Artif Organs 13:89–90
14. Damm G, Mizuguchi K, Aber G, Bacak J, Akkerman J, Bozeman R, Svejkovsky P, Takatani S, Nosé Y, Noon PG, DeBakey ME (1994) Axial flow ventricular assist device: system performance considerations. Artif Organs 18 (in press)
15. Orime Y, Takatani S, Sasaki T, Aizawa T, Ohara Y, Naito K, Glueck J, Noon GP, Nosé Y, DeBakey ME (1994) Cardiopulmonary bypass with Nikkiso and BioMedicus centrifugal pumps. Artif Organs 18 (in press)
16. Magovern GJ, Park SB, Maher TD (1985) Use of the centrifugal pump without anticoagulants for postoperative left ventricular assist. World Surg 9:25–30
17. Drinkwater DC, Laks H (1988) Clinical experience with centrifugal pump ventricular support at UCLA Medical Center. Trans Am Soc Artif Intern Organs 43:505–508
18. Noon GP, Sekela ME, Glueck J, Coleman CL, Feldman L (1990) Comparison of Delphin and BioMedicus pumps. Trans Am Soc Artif Intern Organs 36:M616–M619
19. Noon GP (1991) Bio-Medicus ventricular assistance. Ann Thorac Surg 52:180–181
20. Golding LAR (1992) Biomedicus centrifugal pump for mechanical cardiac support. In: Sezai Y (ed) Artificial heart. The development of Biometion in the 21st century. Saunders, Tokyo, pp 248–252
21. Orime Y (1994) Baylor contributions to artificial organs. Artif Organs 18 (in press)
22. Jikuya T, Sasaki T, Aizawa T, Shiono M, Glueck JA, Smith CP, Feldman L, Sakuma I, Sekela ME, Noda T, Takatani S, Noon GP, Nosé Y, DeBakey ME (1992) Development of an atraumatic small centrifugal pump for second-generation cardiopulmonary bypass. Artif Organs 16:599–606
23. Sasaki T, Jikuya T, Aizawa T, Shiono M, Sakuma I, Takatani S, Glueck J, Noon GP, Nosé Y, DeBakey ME (1992) A compact centrifugal pump for cardiopulmonary bypass. Artif Organs 16:592–598
24. Naito K, Miyazoe Y, Aizawa T, Mizuguchi K, Tasai K, Ohara Y, Orime Y, Glueck J, Takatani S, Noon GP, Nosé Y (1993) Development of Baylor-Nikkiso centrifugal pump with purging system for circulatory support. Artif Organs 17:614–618
25. Minato N, Sakuma I, Sasaki T, Shiono M, Ohara Y, Takatani S, Noon GP, Nosé Y, DeBakey ME (1993) A seal-less centrifugal pump (Baylor Gyro Pump) for the application to long-term circulatory support. Artif Organs 17:36–42
26. Sakuma I, Minato N, Ohara Y, Sasaki T, Orime Y, Shiono M, Damm G, Swenson C, Glueck J, Takatani S, Noon GP, Nosé Y (1993) Development of a scalless motor-driven centrifugal blood pump (Baylor Gyro Pump). In: Akutsu T, Koyanagi H (eds) Artificial heart, 4. Springer, Berlin Heidelberg New York, pp 301–303

27. Ohara Y, Sakuma I, Makinouchi K, Damm G, Glueck J, Mizuguchi K, Naito K, Tasai K, Orime Y, Takatani S, Noon GP, Nosé Y (1993) Baylor Gyro pump: a completely sealless centrifugal pump aiming for long-term circulatory support. Artif Organs 17:599–604
28. Ohara Y, Makinouchi K, Orime Y, Tasai K, Naito K, Mizuguchi K, Shimono T, Damm G, Glueck J, Takatani S, Noon GP, Nosé Y (1994) An ultimate, compact, seal-less centrifugal ventricular assist device: Baylor C-Gyro pump. Artif Organs 18 (in press)
29. Damm G, Mizuguchi K, Bozeman R, Akkerman J, Aber G, Svejkovsky P, Takatani S, Nosé Y, Noon GP, DeBakey ME (1993) In vitro performance of the Baylor/NASA axial flow pump. Artif Organs 17:609–613
30. Damm G, Mizuguchi K, Aber G, Bacak J, Akkerman J, Bozeman R, Svejkovsky P, Takatani S, Nosé Y, Noon GP, DeBakey ME (1994) Axial flow ventricular assist device: system performance considerations. Artif Organs 18 (in press)
31. Mizuguchi K, Damm G, Bozeman R, Akkerman J, Aber G, Svejkovsky P, Bacak J, Orime Y, Takatani S, Nosé Y, Noon GP, DeBakey ME (1994) Development of the Baylor/NASA axial flow ventricular assist device: in vitro performance and systematic hemolysis test results. Artif Organs 18 (in press)
32. Shiono M, Shah A, Sasaki T, Takatani S, Sekela M, Noon GP, Young J, Nosé Y, DeBakey ME (1991) Anatomical fit study for development for one-piece total artificial heart. Trans Am Soc Artif Intern Organs 37:M254–255
33. Takatani S, Shiono M, Sasaki T, Orime Y, Sakuma I, Noon GP, Nosé Y, DeBakey ME (1993) Left and right pump output control in one-piece electromechanical total artificial heart. Artif Organs 17:176–184
34. Takatani S, Shiono M, Sasaki T, Sakuma I, Glueck J, Noon GP, Nosé Y, DeBakey ME (1992) Development of totally implantable electromechanical total artificial heart: Baylor TAH. Artif Organs 16:398–406
35. Orime Y, Takatani S, Shino M, Sasaki T, Minato N, Ohara Y, Swenson C, Noon GP, DeBakey ME, Nosé Y (1992) Versatile one-piece total artificial heart for bridge to transplantation and/or permanent heart replacement. Artif Organs 16:606–613
36. Orime Y, Takatani S, Tasai K, Ohara Y, Naito K, Mizuguchi K, Makinouchi K, Damm G, Glueck J, Summers D, Noon GP, DeBakey ME, Nosé Y (1993) The Baylor-ABI electromechanical total artificial heart: accelerated endurance test. Trans Am Soc Artif Intern Organs 39:M172–176
37. Orime Y, Takatani S, Tasai K, Ohara Y, Naito K, Mizuguchi K, Makinouchi K, Rosenow SE, Glueck J, Noon GP, DeBakey ME, Nosé Y (1994) Flow visualization in the Baylor total artificial heart. Artif Organs 18 (in press)
38. Sasaki T, Takatani S, Shiono M, Sakuma I, Glueck J, Noon GP, Nosé Y, DeBakey ME (1992) Development of totally implantable electromechanical artificial heart systems: Baylor ventricular assist system. Artif Organs 16:407–413
39. Tasai K, Takatani S, Orime Y, Damm G, Ohara Y, Naito K, Makinouchi K, Mizuguchi K, Matsuda Y, Shimono T, Glueck J, Noon GP, Nosé Y (1994) Successful thermal management of a totally implantable ventricular assist system. Artif Organs 18:•• (in press)
40. Takatani S, Orime Y, Tasai K, Ohara Y, Naito K, Mizuguchi K, Makinouchi K, Damm G, Ling J, Noon GP, Nosé Y (1994) Totally implantable TAH and VAD with multipurpose miniature electromechanical energy system. Artif Organs 18:•• (in press)
41. Butler KC, Maher TR, Kormos RL, Griffith BP, Litwak P, Konishi H, Yamazaki K, Antaki JF, Borovetz HS (1993) Development of an implantable axial flow blood pump. The proceedings; AAMI/NHLBI Cardiovascular Science and Technology Conference, p 159
42. Goldstein AH, Pacella JJ, Lazzara RR, Reddy R, Cattivera G, Magovern GJ Clark RE (1993) Four-month survival with an implanted centrifugal ventricular assist device. The proceedings; AAMI/NHLBI Cardiovascular Science and Technology Conference, p 188

# Horizons

J. T. Watson

In 1988, the National Heart, Lung, and Blood Institute (NHLBI) inaugurated research and related development on electrically powered, implantable total artificial heart systems. This program was based on the principles established and experience gained with ventricular assist devices and on the knowledge gained from investigator-initiated artificial heart research at the University of Utah, Penn State University, and the Cleveland Clinic Foundation.

Progress in this program has been rapid. Prototype semicomplete systems designed for a 5-year lifetime have been fabricated and tested. Controller tests in the laboratory on "mock" circulatory loops have verified control algorithms, and animal tests have confirmed performance. Fabrication is completely traceable and failures are analyzed for corrective actions. Animal tests of 160 days have been reported. Miniaturization, customization, and integration of all components are incomplete and not yet under full quality control.

However, this program was not without controversy, and in 1989 the NHLBI commissioned the Institute of Medicine (IOM) to direct an independent study of artificial heart research and report to the nation. In 1991, the IOM released the results of a 2-year study of the NHLBI's Artificial Heart Program. The IOM was chartered in 1970 by the National Academy of Sciences to enlist distinguished members of the appropriate professions in the examination of policy matters pertaining to the health of the United States public. The report, titled "The Artificial Heart: Prototypes, Policies, and Patients," is available through the National Academy Press, 1991.

The IOM committee concluded that research and related development should continue on the implantable artificial heart and ventricular assist devices. They noted that while there had been considerable progress in treating heart failure, cardiac transplantation remained the treatment of choice for patients with end-stage heart disease. Though cardiac transplantation is successful, the number of candidates far exceeds the donor pool, and no alternatives to this situation are on the horizon. Their analysis suggested that by the year 2010, 10 000–20 000 patients would benefit from an implantable artificial heart and that perhaps 25 000–60 000 patients would profit from an implantable ventricular assist device.

While there was enthusiasm for continued research, the committee raised several issues of concern about cost-effectiveness, appropriate use, and distributive justice. They concluded that this was an appropriate use of public research funding and recommended that the NHLBI maintain its leadership role in developing this technology and planning for the orderly introduction into clinical use.

The NHLBI Advisory Council concurred with the IOM report and conceptually approved a new initiative to design and test the first generation of implantable, electrically powered artificial hearts. An open and competitive solicitation was released to the research community. Over a 1-year period six proposals were peer reviewed by nonfederal experts and also by NHLBI staff. Awards were made to three partnership teams of academic and industrial investigators. The overall objective of this two-phase program is to demonstrate through bench and animal studies that implantable artificial heart systems are ready for human trials.

During phase I (1994–1996) of the program the investigators will complete the design of 5-year-life systems, demonstrate manufacturability, and do short-term performance testing in animals and 3-month in vitro testing of hermetically sealed TAH systems. The quality-control program of each center will be audited to see that it conforms to international standards. The progress of these three programs will be assessed by peer review and the most meritorious will be continued on to phase II.

Phase II will consist of formal testing of system reliability in vitro and in vivo testing in animals (1996–2000). In vitro testing and analysis will involve a sufficient number of TAH systems to establish a reliability of 80% with a 80% confidence level. The in vivo evaluation will be directed towards a series of animal tests demonstrating 40 animal-months of safe and effective performance. These tests will serve as supporting data for an investigational device exemption (IDE) from the Food and Drug Administration (FDA) as a prelude to clinical trials.

It is recognized that real-time reliability tests for 5 years are not feasible; therefore, the device-readiness testing is planned for at least 2 years. In phase II, the investigators will perform separate analysis and accelerated testing of components to provide reasonable assurance of projected 5-year reliability. For the future, device-reliability testing would benefit from novel research that allows short-term tests (months) to accurately predict long-term (years) safety and efficacy.

To address the nontechnical concerns raised by the IOM report, the NHLBI is sponsoring a workshop on the artificial heart: "Planning for Evolving Technologies". The workshop participants will discuss the clinical need for mechanical circulatory support, cost-effectiveness considerations in selecting advanced technologies to support, access to evolving technologies (including ethical and economic considerations), and policy aspects of selecting evolving technologies. The results of the workshop will be reported in 1994.

The clinical program to evaluate the Baxter-Novacor electrically powered ventricular assist systems (VAS) in patients with end-stage heart disease was phased out in 1992. This program began in 1989, with the Novacor system having successfully completed the rigorous 2-year reliability-testing protocols. During these tests one system experienced an early component failure, which, following the improvement of the acceptance procedure, was restarted, and all 12 systems completed the test protocol with no failures. Novacor then become the production center to provide 30 medical-grade systems for implantation in 20 patients and 10 systems for test and backup in case of device failure. In the following years, three clinical centers were selected, at Pittsburgh, St. Louis, and Stanford. A randomized trial was planned from a registry of eligible patients, some of whom would receive medical therapy while others would undergo cardiac transplantation. The Data Coordinating Center developed the manual of operations, which includes all protocols and data-reporting forms.

In 1991 it became clear that the production center was experiencing a special set of problems involving the availability of electronic components incorporated into the original design in the early 1980s. Based on the uncertainty surrounding the need to redesign the system and revalidate its reliability, Baxter-Novacor and the NHLBI came to a mutual agreement to phase out the federally funded program. Baxter-Novacor indicated that it would proceed with newer technology and eventually support a clinical trial of an implantable VAS without federal support.

While no clinical outcomes are available with completely implantable devices, the results with vented pneumatic and electrically powered systems are very encouraging. The Abiomed extracorporeal ventricular assist system received FDA marketing approval, based on a clinical study of 55 patients. The system has been used in 420 patients either with ventricular dysfunction following cardiac surgery or as a bridge to cardiac transplant.

The Thermo-Cardiosystems, Inc. (TCI) implantable pneumatic system has passed FDA peer review of its study of 162 patients. One-hundred sixteen patients were treated with the device, which utilizes a textured surface encouraging the formation of a neointima. Forty-six patients who were device eligible but received medical therapy or a cardiac transplant served as controls for the clinical trial. The incidence of thromboembolic complications was 3%, and they seemed to be generally related to pre-existent conditions. Overall, the 1-year survival was significantly better for implant patients than for the controls who underwent conventional cardiac transplantation.

The timing is propitious to move ahead to modern concepts and technologies that could be incorporated into new designs for implantable ventricular assist systems. Clinical experience in the bridge-to-cardiac-transplant series has provided insight into the safety and benefit of these devices. There is potential for further downsizing and simplification of designs with a 5-year lifetime. Other methods of pump activation, including thermal and biological energy conversion, have not yet been adequately explored for developing truly long-life systems of 10-to 20-year capability.

Biocompatibility and biomaterials research should be encouraged. Existing biomaterials continue to function well in short-term clinical trials. However, two issues limit the potential application of these circulatory support systems: adverse events and the availability of biomaterials. The adverse events will be minimized by continued, sustained laboratory and clinical research. The withdrawal of certain biomaterials from human use has resulted from a number of factors, including the trade-off between business income and risk. The latter issue will eventually be resolved with extended research and dialogue on regulation and liability.

Heart failure research is elucidating new medical management approaches. Modern biology is identifying candidate genes that may play a role in the development of heart failure. Circulatory support devices furnish a unique technique for studying the physiology and the natural history of advanced cardiac disease. These approaches will be additive and likely synergistic in expanding our knowledge of heart disease.

The promise of assisted circulation continues to be revealed as research takes incremental steps towards successful clinical use of implantable systems. The innovation process is long and has uncertainties that are yet to be revealed. One can only be convinced that there is a convergence between assisted circulation, our understanding of heart failure, and modern biology. A successful outcome will surely reduce death and disability from heart disease and may contribute new information to prevent this malady.

# Horizons

J. Ochsner

The use of circulatory assist devices has enjoyed certain periods of enthusiasm, only to be followed by dissatisfaction. On the other hand, there has also been disappointment in the initial use of specific devices, followed by gratification with increased experience.

The principal functions for mechanical circulatory assist devices are (a) to afford circulatory support and (b) to aid in myocardial recovery. In providing circulatory support, vital organs are adequately perfused to reverse organ dysfunction produced by the failing heart and thus prevent irrecoverable damage. To aid in myocardial recovery, circulatory assist unloads the ventricle, allowing equalization of myocardial metabolic supply and demand. Thus, mechanical assist devices are used as a bridge to transplantation and as a bridge to myocardial recovery.

Today there are two basic types of ventricular assistauce, mechanical and biological. Many mechanical assist systems are currently in clinical use and many others are undergoing experimental evaluation. The various principles utilized are intra-aortic balloon counterpulsation, roller pump (either occlusive or nonocclusive), centrifugal pump, axial-flow pump, pneumatically driven ventricles, and electrically driven ventricles. The biological systems are heterotopic cardiac transplants, cardiomyoplasty, and skeletal muscle ventricles.

We saw a progressive increase in the use of mechanical ventricular support from 1983 until 1988; since that peak period there has been a progressive decline in their use, but with a fall much less rapid than the earlier rise in their use. According to the combined registry of the ASAIO and ISHLT in 1993 for clinical use of mechanical ventricular assist pumps and total artificial hearts, there are over 18 000 patients who have sustained some form of mechanical ventricular support.

The adverse effects of ventricular assist devices include bleeding, hemolysis, infection, organ dysfunction, and thromboembolism; these continue, but to a lesser degree, with trial and experience. As an example, after many years of attempting to provide a smooth nonthrombogenic surface, it has been shown that a roughened surface allows pseudointimal proliferation and prevention of thrombosis and embolism. Thus, with time we should expect further advances with new knowledge until many of the dreaded complications we now fear disappear. As with most scientific endeavors, one must postulate: "What man can perceive, man can achieve," the ultimate being an implantable total mechanical heart with an internal power source.

Despite the tremendous advances made and what appears to be a definite positive shift toward the acceptance of mechanical assist devices, allow me to play the devil's advocate and mention certain aspects that may hinder, prevent, or even displace the advance of mechanical assist devices; allow me also to project why these adversities may not be sound.

Transplantation has become widely accepted as a treatment for end-stage heart disease; therefore, there may be less need or urgency for the development of a total artificial heart. However, because the demand for donor organs far exceeds supply, a substantial number of transplant candidates will die awaiting a donor organ; hence, there will be a greater need for temporary mechanical circulatory support to bridge these patients to transplantation. We have seen this become a reality as our own cardiac transplant candidate list grows.

The development and improvement of surgical procedures for coronary artery revascularization has been used to postpone transplants and thus limit the various mechanical assist devices. Approximately 5% of all patients referred to our institution for transplantation are able to be helped with extensive methods of myocardial revascularization. The newer diagnostic methods of determining hibernating vs. irreversible myocardium has enhanced our ability to properly select these patients. Likewise, new and improved pharmacological agents have also been able to better manage the failing myocardium and thereby limit the use of mechanical assist devices. Other procedures that have been helpful in postponing transplantation and avoiding mechanical assistance have been the use of cardiomyoplasty and surgery for arrhythmia, particularly the use of implantable defibrillators. However, for many of the above-mentioned patients an end-stage heart is merely postponed, and hence they eventually fall into the pool for cardiac transplantation and the possible need for a mechanical assist device.

The mandate of health reform is probably the single most important challenge to mechanical assist devices. The publicized low yield of productive patients following implantation of a mechanical assist device may severely limit their use in the future. The intervention by government to control cost is real. The tremendous cost of mechanical assist devices is related to many factors, including the device itself, the extended length of time in an intensive care unit, and the numerous sophisticated diagnostic and therapeutic modalities used during the hospital stay, while the patient's condition is being stabilized and he or she is awaiting a suitable organ. When one looks at the competition for funds available to manage health care, it is obvious that a greater emphasis will be placed on prevention of disease than on attempts to cure terminal illness, in particular the failing heart of the elderly. However, our society is such that life is regarded as the most precious gift, and emotional attitudes are such that a price for life, regardless of age, cannot be established. There is no doubt that there will be a need for careful selection of patients for mechanical assistance and transplantation, statistical analysis of the results of past and present efforts, and continued research to improve results.

There is growing support for an increase in research funds and in efforts to improve the donor supply system via xenografts. Their use as either temporary or permanent replacements would have a monumental impact on society if the astronomical problems of rejection can be controlled.

I foresee a race between the development of acceptable ventricular assist devices and changing psychological attitudes toward limitation of life in reference to quality of life and cost-effectiveness. There will be a need for public confidence and for the support of both government and industry to win this race. It is obvious to all that mechanical systems have some advantages over heart transplants, in that they have off-the-shelf availability and can be applied for a large number of end-stage heart disease patients; however, if and when total artificial hearts become implantable, the relationship of them to cardiac transplantation will be dictated by the state of the art, donor availability, and the long-term results of both techniques.

# Horizons

V.O. Björk

Thanks to the untiring, ongoing research, there is a step-by-step, slow but steady improvement of the handling of cardiovascular diseases. The most outstanding advance has lately been in the field of intracardiac diagnosis. Forty years ago, I introduced complete left heart catheterization utilizing an 18-cm-long needle above the 9th rib, three finger breadths to the right of the median line, and, after entering the left atrium, I pushed a catheter through the needle, the left atrium, the left ventricle, and out into the aorta. On withdrawal I got all the pressures on the left side of the heart. The first open heart operation in Europe, by Crafoord in 1954, was for a left atrial myxoma, diagnosed with this method when I injected the contrast medium directly into the left atrium through the needle and clearly outlined the tumor. Today, I am impressed by the noninvasive echo-Doppler technique visualizing intracardiac shunts and valvular insufficiency and estimating the valvular gradients.

Assisted circulation with limited duration as a bridge to transplantation is today an accepted procedure. The implanted artificial heart has also been used for several months in preparation for a heart transplantation. But the question is whether a total artificial heart will be available for definitive implantation earlier than the possibility of using heterografts from specially bred animals; it may take 50 or 100 years.

In the span of the 50 years I have been active in thoracic surgery I have seen that there is no future without research. It took me 30 years to verify why it is necessary to use anticoagulation for mechanical heart valves. The porosity of the suture rings are around 500 μm inviting a fibrous covering thick enough to need the invasion of blood vessels to survive. Without anticoagulation there is a risk for the organized thrombus over the suture ring to protrude in over the polished surface, where it can be cut off by the valve occluder and cause emboli, as well as interfere with the free movement of the occluder.

If, instead, the surface adjacent to the suture ring is covered with a microporous multilayer, where the particles are as small as 20 μm, the covering which we find in every case will continue over the microporous surface in such a thin layer of only 100 μm that it will survive on the nutrition arriving directly from the blood. Then no vessels will enter and during 3 months of anticoagulation a smooth endothelialized surface will develop. Then, during a 5-year period, this thin covering will stay at the same thickness and, due to the multilayer, have an excellent fixation. It will not need any anticoagulation after the first 3 months.

Following these principles, 12 children and young women with sinus rythm had their severely diseased mitral valves exchanged to partially microporous-surfaced Björk-Shiley Monostrut mitral valves and have been followed up for 6–8 years without anticoagulation and without thromboembolic complications. Four of the young women had, during these years, given birth to a total of seven children.

This is naturally only a small detail in the technical development. But this detail is very important for patients who need a valve replacement and cannot receive long-term anticoagulation. The same principle may be utilized at the connection with an artificial heart.

With the accumulation of many small technical details the artificial heart will one day be a practical alternative in the treatment of advanced heart disease. I remember when I spent most of 1946 in the basement of the Pathology Department of Sabbatsberg Hospital in Stockholm, working hard to get the spinning disc oxygenator to function together with a milk machine as a pump for open heart surgery on dogs. Before I finally was successful, an older general surgeon said to me: "You are wasting your time; this idea of open heart surgery can never be a practical surgical procedure!"

We should never give up, but without research there is no future.

# Horizons

J. WADA and W.R. ADE

*Le but que je me suis toujours proposé*
*et que j'ai la satisfaction d'avoir atteint,*
*autant que cela a été en moi, c'est de découvrir des faits*
*et de poser ou de faire naître des questions nouvelles.*
*Ces dernières, parcourant ensuite, au milieu de la discusion,*
*comme toujours, leur évolution scientifique,*
*ont pour effet de provoquer un mouvement de travaux éminemment utile*
*aux progrès de la science.*
Claude Bernard

*Natura non nisi parendo vincitur.*
Francis Bacon

## Introduction

Twenty-five years have passed since Cooley implanted the first total artificial heart with four Wada valves in 1969[2]. Those years have seen a revolution in computer technology with the miniaturization of components and the sophistication of integrated circuits and, in the United States, have brought demands for environmental stress screening according to military standard procedures. This need for military standard processes and components may give competitive advantages to researchers in other countries, but it will definitely help to protect against component failure under long-term conditions.

## Assist Devices

Now a promising, totally implantable pulsatile assist device is nearly ready for general use [3]. Nonpulsatile devices of impressive simplicity have been developed by several groups and may revolutionize the field of assisted circulation by the year 2000. They have an overall efficiency of about 30% in comparison to 20% for pulsatile devices, and they avoid the irritation of neighboring structures and the resulting complications such as reduced lung filling, heat production, coagulation, and infection which are seen with the pneumatically driven devices. These nonpulsatile devices are especially suitable as assist devices after cardiotomy and myocardial infarction and as bridges to transplantation. Implantation for more than 2 months has been reported. Pulsatile devices may achieve a 20% higher blood flow, but this is of advantage for only about 6 weeks. After that, even with nonpulsatile devices, idiopulsation of about 40 pulses/min with pressure amplitudes of up to 6.7 kPa (50 mmHg) has been reported.

Hemopumps will have a great future as a most economical means of cardiac assist, not necessitating major surgery for implantation, simplifying postoperative management, and involving minimal risks of thromboembolism, hemorrhage and infective complications [4].

Our team envisages a pump oxygenator/implantable artificial heart using hemopumps which will place perfusion into the hands of the anesthesiologist, a qualified physician [1]. These portable devices will soon replace their "battleship-like" predecessors with huge priming volumes. As in many cases the patient's own lung is the best oxygenator, the pump will be separable, to be implanted if the patient cannot be weaned from cardiopulmonary bypass.

## Total Artificial Heart (TAH)

### Nonpulsatile Devices

As the discrepancy in the numbers of hearts available for transplantation and of patients who suffer from terminal heart failure cannot be bridged, the final solution will have to be a totally implantable artificial heart. When problems with blood leakage and shaft freeze have been overcome, the electromechanical devices which Hahn calls "the future in cardiac replacement" [5] will give these patients some additional years of life. Ingenious methods for solving these problems, such as an external pump, infusing fluid at a constant rate to wash the V-ring area, have been reported [7]. Also automatic controllers which determine desired flow based on an estimation of atrial filling, using a fuzzy logic algorithm have been developed [9]. Nonpulsatile devices should be available by the end of the century and quality of life will be a major parameter for risk/benefit assessment.

### Pulsatile Devices

The pulsatile devices will continue to present challenges to their constructors even into the twenty-first century. Lapeyre provides strong arguments for combining both ventricles in a single functional unit in which the right ventricle resembles the structural properties of its natural paragon and the spatial orientation of the valves is maintained, thus avoiding compression or torsion of the inferior vena cava and its connected veins [6]. Among the classic pneumatic devices, Unger's Ellipsoidheart stands out by virtue of its reasonably small size [10]. At the second annual meeting of the World Artificial Organ, Immunology and Transplantation Society (WAITS), which was organized after many colleagues voiced the opinion that only a closer cooperation between surgeons, engineers, and basic scientists would be able to cope with the complexity of transplantation-related scientific and social issues, Nosé reported on an electromechanical, totally implantable, total artificial heart system [8]. Several groups in the United States, Europe, and Japan have developed prototypes, but fluctuations in funding and registration authorities throwing wrenches into the wheels of research make the prognosis unsure, despite the fact that every year brilliant new designs appear. Only a very few ever reach the stage of animal testing.

In 1996, we will be commemorating the hundredth anniversary of the day when the first sufficiently documented surgical procedure on the heart was carried out by Rehn in Frankfurt. From his endeavor to the development of theoretical models of circulation which allowed calculations of central and peripheral pulse curves, more than 50 years passed. At the sixth annual meeting of the International Society of Cardiothoracic Surgeons in Nagoya, vortical blood flow, which can be described by a system of successively interrelated asymmetric funnels, and concentric spiral separation of microparticles in the blood flow were reported [11]. In designing optimal devices for assisting or taking up the function of the heart, these findings will have to be reflected. This advanced understanding of circulation and the development of new materials and genial ideas such as the endothelialization of surfaces with fat cells from the recipient's peritoneum, as suggested by Donald Schmidt, will finally bring the day when surgeons face the question of transplantation or TAH implantation. We hope that pioneers like R. Hetzer, W.J. Kolff, and F. Unger will be able to see the day when their dreams actually become a reality.

## References


1. Ade WR, Hino T, Kaizuka H, Wada J (1992) Autoregulated extra- and intracorporeal pump system for perfusion. Int Surg 77:108–110
2. Cooley DA, Liotta D, Hallman GL, Bloodwell RD, Leachman RD, Milan JD (1969) Orthotopic cardiac prosthesis for two-staged cardiac replacement. Am J Cardiol 24:723–730
3. Daniel MA, Lee J, LaForge DH, Chen H, Billich J, Miller PJ, Ramasamy N, Strauss LR, Jassawalla JS, Portner PM (1991) Clinical evaluation of the Novacor totally implantable ventricular assist system. Current status. ASAIO Trans 37:M423–M425
4. Burnett CM, Vega JD, Radovancevic B, Lonquist JL, Birovljev S, Sweeney MS, Duncan JM, Frazier OH (1990) Improved survival after hemopump insertion in patients experiencing postcardiotomy cardiogenic shock during cardiopulmonary bypass. ASAIO Trans 36:M626–M629
5. Hahn C-J, Pierce WS, Olsen DB, Butler K, Kung RTV (1993) Long-term biventricular assist. Ann Thorac Surg 55:227–232
6. Lapeyre D (1990) Points critiques qui restent à résoudre pour que le cœur artificiel puisse entrer dans l'arsenal thérapeutique de routine. Ann Chir 44:168–181
7. Naito K, Miyazoe Y, Matsuda Y et al. (1993) Development of a compact centrifugal pump with purging system for circulatory support. First Congress of the International Society for Rotary Blood Pumps, Mie Prefecture, 16–17 Oct 1993
8. Nosé Y (1993) An electromechanical totally implantable total artificial heart system. First Congress of the Turkish Transplantation Society and Second Annual Meeting of the World Artificial Organ, Immunology and Transplantation Society, Ankara, 20–23 Oct 1993
9. Schima H, Schmidt C, Maar H, Trubel W, Losert U, Wolner H (1993) A two-stage controller for rotary blood pumps with fuzzy pattern recognition. First Congress of the International Society for Rotary Blood Pumps, Mie Prefecture, 16–17 Oct 1993
10. Unger F, Albes J (1990) Limitierende Faktoren beim Einsatz des Kunstherzens. Wien Med Wochenschr 140:290–293
11. Zakharov VN (1994) Structural analysis of moving blood from the viewpoint of new principles of circulation mechanics. J Cardiovasc Surg 35:19–25

# Future Directions in Assisted Circulation

R.S. Litwak and R.M. Koffsky

Prediction of the future is always a hazardous undertaking and brings to mind a remark attributed to the thirteenth-century Castilian king, Alfonso X, when the Ptolemaic astronomical concepts had been explained: "If the Lord Almighty had consulted me, I should have recommended something simpler!"

Through the rewarding collaboration of investigators and industrial groups, the past two decades have witnessed the successful development of ventricular assist devices (VADs), which have been impressive in supporting patients in postcardiotomy low cardiac output, potentially salvageable patients in shock complicating acute myocardial infarction, and hemodynamically unstable patients awaiting cardiac transplantation. Positioned in extracorporeal, paracorporeal, or implanted loci, most of them capable of not only single but also biventricular support, the VADs have progressed from the early nonpulsatile roller pump, through the centrifugal pump, to the "contemporary era," in which virtually all VADs, tethered to an external power console or pumping system, employ pulsatile pumping methodology. A relatively recent development has been the introduction of a catheter-tip centrifugal pump which is passed across a normal aortic valve into the left ventricle. Capable of effectively sustaining circulatory stability for periods of days to months, we have seen progression of "temporary" VAD technology to the development of several implantable pulsatile left ventricular (LV) support systems (Novacor and Thermo Cardiosystems LVADs, specifically designed for long-term use. The specter of life-threatening complications associated with VADs (particularly coagulopathy-related bleeding, thromboembolism, neurologic dysfunction, and infection) must be viewed with appreciation of the fact that one fourth to one third of the desperately ill patients placed on temporary VAD support are hospital survivors solely because of their efficacy.

What future directions can one envision in improving assisted circulation systems? What can we *hope* to accomplish in the next decade and, in realistic terms, what can we *expect* to accomplish? While the ideal approach to seeking the optimal design of such systems would be continued intensive study, leading to ultimate control or elimination of the molecular and biophysical distortions which are etiologic to VAD complications, attainment of this Holy Grail will be many years in coming. Pierre Galletti, in reflecting upon the speed of artificial organ development, has observed that progress – while constant – has not proceeded at a faster pace than when the field first emerged four decades ago [1]. For example, it is doubtful that our understanding of what would constitute a stable thromboresistant *environment* has been meaningfully clarified, despite more than two decades of intensive study.

Although we can *expect* small but significant technological advances to be made in the next decade, we can but *hope* to see meaningful progress in the development of highly thromboresistant and durable biomaterials suitable for use as pump bladders, diaphragms, and other VAD components. In addition to *hoping* to see improved methods of long-term passivation of flexing and other blood-contacting surfaces, we may *hope* to see methods developed in which VAD components traversing the skin would be treated with long-lasting antibacterial and possibly antiviral agents to reduce the potential for infection.

Realistically, however, the outlook is not favorable for attainment of major VAD improvements, for reasons which have been eloquently expressed by Olsen, Kolff and Poirier [2–4]. Briefly stated, development of new technology has been – and continues to be – constricted not only by the chronic problem of limited funding, but, particularly in the United States, by lengthy and sharply restrictive governmental regulatory practices and a highly litigious environment as well. Several major suppliers of biomaterials have recently limited their involvement in or completely withdrawn from VAD development in light of these negative factors. Indeed, although unstated, it is apparent that the recent corporate decision by the Baxter Healthcare Corporation to obtain European approval promptly for the Novacor Implantable Portable LVAS in the long-term management of severe LV dysfunction was sharply influenced by the delays and restrictions imposed by USA regulatory agencies and the seemingly constant threat of litigation. As a consequence of the broadening Novacor Implantable Portable LVAS clinical experience, we can *expect* quite rapid technological improvement of transcutaneous power methodology, device size, configuration, determination of component reliability, and further characterization of candidates for LVAS implantation.

A *hope* that has become an *expectation* has been the continuing development of pacemaker-triggered latissimus dorsi (LD) cardiomyoplasty (CMP) to manage chronic LV dysfunction [5, 6]. Currently, FDA-approved phase-III clinical trials are being conducted in the United States involving patients randomized to either CMP or medical management. One of the issues that appears to have been resolved was the frequent lack of objective evidence of improved cardiac function after CMP in the presence of unquestioned clinical reduction of cardiac failure. This apparent ambiguity has been clarified by recent experience in a sheep LV infarction model, which has documented reduction of the LV pressure–volume area after CMP. Additionally, Emax, an index of ventricular contractility, increased after CMP but did not change with the pacemaker either activated or off. Thus, the primary mechanism responsible for the effectiveness of CMP appears to be an "active" support or constraint of the damaged myocardium by the LD and the prevention of further ventricular dilatation. While augmentation of LV systolic function can occur with CMP, it is a secondary mechanism of action [7].

The road ahead will be difficult. Despite the fact that we have clinically effective – albeit imperfect – VADs, significant technological problems remain to be solved. In this regard, Galletti has anticipated future possibilities: "A quantum leap forward will likely await an imaginative and largely unpredictable set of discoveries . . ." [8]. Moreover, substantial economic and regulatory barriers and societal needs and demands–all defined by governmental fiat – will have a significant adverse impact on continued VAD and artificial heart development. Despite these difficulties, as Poirier has urged, ". . . we are not done. We must continue. We must push forward" [4].

## References

1. Galletti PM (1993) Organ replacement by man-made devices. J Cardiothorac Vasc Anesth 7: 624–628
2. Olsen DB (1992) ASAIO presidential address: artificial organs of the future. ASAIO Trans 38:M134–M138
3. Kolff WJ (1993) The dawn of counterpulsation: muscle and pneumatic powered LVADs. ASAIO Trans 39:825–827
4. Poirier VL (1993) The quest for a solution: We must continue. We must push forward. The 16th Hastings lecture. ASAIO Trans 39:856–863
5. Carpentier A, Chachques JC (1985) Myocardial substitution with a stimulated skeletal muscle: first successful clinical case. Lancet 1:1267
6. Magovern GJ, Christlieb IY, Kao RL (1991) The Allegheny Hospital experience. In: Carpentier A, Chachques JC, Grandjean PA (eds). Cardiomyoplasty. Futura, Mount Kisco, pp 159–170
7. Nakajima H, Niinami H, Hooper TL et al. (1994) Cardiomyplasty: probable mechanism of effectiveness using the pressure–volume relationship. Ann Thorac Surg 57:407–415
8. Galletti PM (1993) Cardiopulmonary bypass: a historical perspective. Artif Organs 17:675–686

# Further Development of Extracorporeal Life Support

C.N. Steimle and R.H. Bartlett

## Introduction

Extracorporeal life support (ECLS) is a means of providing prolonged extracorporeal cardiopulmonary bypass to patients with acute, reversible cardiac or respiratory failure unresponsive to conventional medical management. This intervention has traditionally been deemed extracorporeal membrane oxygenation (ECMO), but the current mnemonic "ECLS" more appropriately expresses the fact that this modality encompasses functions other than oxygenation, including cardiac support, renal support, and carbon dioxide removal.

The origins of extracorporeal life support lie in the pioneering work of John Gibbon in the 1930s, when he developed the first heart-lung machine [1]. The ability to externally oxygenate and pump blood led to the evolution of cardiac surgery in the 1950s. The initial heart-lung machines utilized direct contact between the blood and oxygen in order to achieve adequate oxygenation and removal of carbon dioxide. Bypass was initially limited to no more than 6 h in duration because the direct blood-gas interface resulted in progressive hemolysis, thrombocytopenia, and plasma protein denaturation. The development of gas-permeable membranes in the 1960s allowed the construction of membrane oxygenators and permitted prolonged bypass without these complications [2–4]. These developments led to the application of extracorporeal circulation to the nonoperative setting for the purpose of providing oxygenation to patients with severe respiratory failure.

The first successful case of prolonged extracorporeal support in a human subject was reported by Hill in 1972 [5], with several other successful cases following [6, 7]. The initial enthusiasm for extracorporeal support in severe adult respiratory failure led to a prospective randomized trial, funded by the National Institutes of Health (NIH), to assess the efficacy of this intervention. This study, which was conducted from 1975 to 1979, showed no significant difference between patients managed with ECLS (9.5%) and those receiving conventional ventilator therapy (8.3%) [8, 9]. This lack of proven efficacy led to discontinuation of most US efforts at adult ECLS; instead, attention was redirected toward neonatal extracorporeal support.

Neonatal respiratory failure is ideal for the application of ECLS, because all the usual causes of neonatal respiratory failure have in common an abnormal postnatal shunting of blood, known as persistent fetal circulation (PFC). PFC is a temporary, reversible phenomenon and therefore represents an ideal setting for ECLS management. If the infant could be supported until the PFC resolved, and if the infant could be adequately oxygenated and ventilated without barotrauma during the acute disease process, salvage of these infants would be possible. In 1976, Bartlett reported the first successful case of neonatal ECLS [10]. Since then, two prospective studies have confirmed the efficacy of ECLS in the management of neonatal respiratory failure [11, 12]. ECLS has become the accepted therapy for neonates with severe respiratory failure who fail attempts at conventional ventilation. To date, over 8000 neonatal patients have been treated with ECLS worldwide, with a survival rate of 82% (ELSO registry data).

While US efforts were focused on the use of ECLS in neonates, Gattinoni and Pesenti continued to explore the use of ECLS in adult patients. Review of the original NIH trial data indicated that the entrance criteria for that study were too stringent, and most patients who were enrolled probably had permanent and irreversible lung injury, caused either by the disease process itself or by prolonged aggressive ventilatory support. Gattinoni's group in Milan continued to pursue the possibilities for extracorporeal support in adults by focusing on the use of ECLS for carbon dioxide removal. He postulated that the major problem in patients with ARDS was lack of adequate ventilation and that oxygenation could be accomplished by inflation and airway oxygenation alone. If membrane lungs with large surface areas could be employed, venovenous access could be used to provide carbon dioxide exchange. Venovenous bypass would allow normal pulmonary blood flow, which may aid in lung healing and help prevent microthrombosis. Gattinoni also performed CT scan evaluations of patients with ARDS and found that these patients had significant overdistension of the most normal alveoli [13]. He concluded that, in patients with ARDS, the functional residual capacity was severely decreased, and use of high tidal volumes would result in overdistension injury to the remaining alveoli, with resulting fibrosis. By utilizing extracorporeal support, the need for high airway pressures and high $FiO_2$ would be eliminated, thereby diminishing the airway injury. Following these principles, Gattinoni's group began to utilize venovenous ECCOR (extracorporeal $CO_2$ removal) in a variety of adult patients who were selected by the same criteria used for the NIH ECMO study. Patients were managed with apneic oxygenation and extracorporeal $CO_2$ removal. In 1986, Gattinoni's group reported a 49% survival in 43 patients [14]. These results were corroborated by a variety of other investigators over the next 3 years [15]. Based upon these improved results, interest in ECLS for adults was rekindled in other European centers and in the US.

## Selection of Patients

Clinical application of extracorporeal life support is based upon the ability to select appropriate patients who have failed conventional means of management and who have a high mortality risk. For patients with pulmonary failure, the mortality is estimated by measuring the extent of pulmonary dysfunction and the level of ventilator support required to sustain gas exchange.

## Neonates

In the neonate with severe respiratory failure, persistent pulmonary hypertension of the newborn (PPHN) is the major pathophysiologic mechanism, regardless of the underlying disease process. In these infants, disease processes causing hypoxia, hypercarbia, and acidosis lead to pulmonary vasospasm, with resulting pulmonary hypertension and right-to-left shunting across a patent ductus arteriosus or patent foramen ovale. Despite increasing levels of inspired oxygen, the shunting of blood causes a vicious cycle of progressively worsening hypoxia, hypercarbia, and acidosis, which in turn causes even more shunting. In the majority of infants, treatment with paralysis, mechanical ventilation, induced respiratory alkalosis, and pharmacologic pulmonary vasodilation is successful in breaking this cycle. However, 2–5% of infants fail to respond to these treatments, and ECLS has been shown to be effective in this situation.

A set of criteria for predicting a 90%-mortality group was utilized in the prospective, randomized ECLS neonatal trial to select patients for ECLS [11]. Although these criteria were useful at the time, they are outdated and impractical for general use. In our center, we currently use the oxygenation index (OI) as a method of determining which infants have a high mortality risk. The OI is computed by the following formula:

$$OI = \text{mean airway pressure} \times (FiO_2 \times 100)/PaO_2$$

In our neonatal intensive care unit, an OI consistently greater than 25 defines a 50%-mortality group; OI over 40 defines 80% mortality. We therefore consider a neonate to be a possible candidate for ECLS if the OI is consistently over 25. If improvement does not occur or if the OI reaches 40, ECLS is initiated.

Certain criteria are utilized to exclude neonates from support with ECLS if there is no reasonable chance of meaningful recovery. Infants with estimated gestational age (EGA) under 35 weeks were initially excluded, since this group had a very high rate of intracranial hemorrhage and resulting mortality [16]. Improvements in technical and management aspects of neonatal ECLS have led to extension of the indications to include infants of 32 weeks EGA and 1.5 kg birth weight; survival and rate of intracranial hemorrhage have been shown to be improved over those in previous reports [17, 18]. Infants with severe preexisting intracranial hemorrhage are excluded, though neonates with grade-I hemorrhages have been successfully managed on ECLS. Profound neurologic impairment, congenital anomalies or conditions not compatible with a meaningful life, and irreversible lung disease such as severe BPD are also contraindications to use of ECLS. Mechanical ventilation for more than 7 days is a relative contraindication because of the high rate of irreversible lung injury in this group. Major cardiac anomalies which are not amenable to surgical repair also constitute contraindications to use of ECLS in the neonate.

## Children and Adults

As in the neonate, extracorporeal life support is indicated for use in children and adults when the patient has acute, severe, potentially lethal respiratory failure which is unresponsive to conventional management but is resulting from a primary condition which is reversible. Selection criteria used for the NIH adult ECMO trial are still generally used for children and adults, since these criteria define patients with very high mortality rates [19–21]. In brief, these criteria are a transpulmonary shunt of greater than 30% despite optimal ventilator settings and pharmacologic management, and a static compliance of less than 0.5 cc/cm $H_2O$/kg. These selection criteria are more reproducible than minor variations in blood oxygenation which occur in the course of treatment of patients with respiratory failure.

Identification of patients with reversible lung disease is significantly more difficult in children and adults than in neonates. Unlike in neonates, where virtually all causes of PPHN are reversible, the diseases which cause respiratory failure in children and adults lead to interstitial inflammation, which in turn causes fibrosis, bacterial infection, and necrosis. The extent of fibrosis seen seems to relate both to the severity and duration of interstitial inflammation and to the duration of high airway pressure from mechanical ventilators. Our group's experience is that adult patients who have received more than 5 days of conventional mechanical ventilation prior to initiation of ECLS have a significantly lower survival rate than those with 5 days or fewer (65% vs. 27%). Based upon these findings, we consider a course of greater than 5 days of mechanical ventilatory support to represent a relative contraindication for initiation of ECLS in adults. Although a similar principle would seem to apply to children, no specific criterion has yet been established for this group. Other exclusion criteria are: age greater than 60 years, presence of irreversible systemic disease (such as cancer), or contraindication to anticoagulation.

## Methods of Extracorporeal Life Support

Patients are cannulated for bypass utilizing either venovenous or venoarterial modes. Cannulation is accomplished in the intensive care unit with the assistance of an operative team. In adults, venoarterial bypass can be performed through the neck, with cannulation of the right internal jugular vein and placement of a cannula into the right atrium for venous drainage; arterial reinfusion is preferably via the right common carotid artery into the aortic arch. Another option for venoarterial bypass in adults is through the femoral vessels. A third choice is cannulation of the axillary artery with placement of a cannula in the aortic arch; in this case the venous drainage cannula is generally inserted through the internal jugular vein. Finally, venoarterial bypass can be achieved by direct cannulation of the right atrial appendage and aortic arch via sternotomy; this option is generally utilized only in patients being placed on ECLS immediately after cardiac surgery. Venovenous bypass in adults is usually performed with cannulas in the right internal jugular vein for venous drainage and in the femoral vein for reinfusion. The development of percutaneous catheterization kits has enabled venovenous bypass to be performed without the need for cutdowns, thereby diminishing sites of potentially troublesome bleeding in these anticoagulated patients. Percutaneous cannulas are available in sizes up to 21 French; this will allow flows up to 4–4.5 l/min, which are adequate for all but the largest adult patients. In infants, venoarterial bypass is almost always performed via the internal jugular vein and common carotid artery, since the femoral vessels are too small to allow adequate cannulas for support. A two-lumen 14-F venovenous cannula is available for use in neonates who require primarily respiratory support; this cannula can be used in infants up to 5 kg. For infants and children >5 kg but less than about 3 years of age, venoarterial bypass is the only reasonable option, since the femoral vessels are too small to allow a cannula of adequate size for reinfusion and no larger two-lumen cannula is available.

The choice of venovenous or venoarterial modes for bypass is made based upon a number of factors. For patients requiring cardiac support, venoarterial bypass is required in order to support cardiac function. Venoarterial bypass is also utilized in older infants and small children who cannot be reasonably cannulated for venovenous support. For most patients with primarily respiratory failure, however, venovenous bypass is preferred for a variety of reasons. Venovenous bypass provides normal pulmonary blood flow, which may aid in lung healing and in prevention of microthrombi in the lungs. It also minimizes the risks of microemboli in the bypass circuit, since reinfusion is into the venous system. In addition, with venovenous bypass arterial cannulation is not required, so the real or theoretical risks of occluding an artery with a cannula are eliminated.

## Circuits for ECLS

The ECLS circuit is built from polyvinyl chloride (PVC) tubing 1/4 to 3/8 inch in diameter, with standard polycarbonate connectors. Blood is drained from the venous cannula with a gravity siphon to an expandable silicone rubber bladder with a microswitch, which controls a double-occlusion roller pump. When the pump outflow exceeds venous drainage, the bladder collapses, the microswitch senses the change in volume, and power to the pump is interrupted. Venous drainage continues with the pump stopped; this restores volume to the bladder, which is again sensed by the microswitch, and pump power is restored. This servoregulation of pump flow prevents excessive suction from being applied to the venous line with the resultant cavitation of dissolved gases, hemolysis, and blood vessel injury. From the roller pump, blood travels to a membrane or hollow-fiber oxygenator which provides the gas exchange. Blood then travels to a heat exchanger, which rewarms it before it is returned to the patient. A variety of monitoring devices are employed to manage the circuit. An inline fiberoptic monitor is placed in the venous drainage line to monitor mixed venous oxygen saturation. Inlet and outlet pressures are monitored before and after the membrane lungs.

Before the patient is connected to the ECLS circuit, the circuit is flushed with $CO_2$ and then primed with crystalloid and albumin. pH, calcium level, and temperature are carefully regulated. In infants, children, and some adults, the circuit is primed with blood to prevent serious hemodilution.

## Management of the Patient on Extracorporeal Life Support

After the vessels have been exposed for cannulation, the patient is systemically heparinized (100 U/kg). Once the cannulas are in place, extracorporeal support is initiated. The patient is then placed on low "rest" ventilator settings to prevent further lung injury from high airway pressures and to prevent harmful effects of high oxygen concentrations. Typical ventilator settings for infants are: pressure limit 20 cm $H_2O$, positive end-expiratory pressure (PEEP) 4 cm $H_2O$, respiratory rate 10/min, and $Fio_2$ 30%. In adults, pressure-controlled ventilation is generally used, and common settings are: pressure control 30 cm $H_2O$, PEEP 10 cm $H_2O$, respiratory rate 10/min, $FiO_2$ 30%, and I:E = 1:1. All efforts are made to keep peak airway pressures below 40 cm $H_2O$. Vasoactive drugs are generally discontinued, although patients on venovenous bypass may require some ongoing vasoactive drugs. Use of sedative and paralyzing drugs is minimized, although they may be required initially to limit systemic tissue oxygen consumption.

For patients on venoarterial bypass, blood is drained from the right atrium and diverted to an ECLS circuit. A servoregulated roller pump, membrane lung, and heat exchanger are utilized to oxygenate, rewarm, and return the blood into the patient's aortic arch. For venovenous bypass, the blood is drained from the right atrium but returned to the venous side. Blood flow is maintained at a level sufficient to keep the mixed venous oxygen saturation at 75%, as measured by the fiberoptic cannula in the venous drainage line. in patients on venoarterial bypass, this will generally result in arterial oxygen saturations over 90%. In patients on venovenous bypass, the systemic oxygen saturation will generally be lower, because there will be some mixing of the oxygenated blood being returned to the patient with the deoxygenated blood being returned from the body. Oxygenation of the patient is adjusted by altering the extracorporeal flow rate. In addition, oxygenation is maximized by maintaining the patient's hematocrit at 45–50% in order to optimize oxygen carrying capacity. Carbon dioxide levels are maintained at 35–45 mmHg; adjustments in the $PaCO_2$ are made by adjusting the flow of sweep gas across the membrane lung. In neonates, even very low sweep flows sometimes remove too much $CO_2$ from the patient; in these cases, carbogen is used to keep the patient's $CO_2$ in the acceptable range.

While patients are on extracorporeal life support, heparin is infused continuously to maintain a whole-blood activated clotting time (ACT) between 160 and 200 s (normal being approximately 100–120 s). As mentioned above, the hematocrit is maintained at 45–50% in order to maximize oxygen delivery to tissues. Platelets are transfused as necessary to keep platelet counts of at least 50 000; if patients develop signs of bleeding, higher platelet levels are maintained.

Many patients are quite edematous when ECLS is begun, and aggressive diuresis is instituted in order to return the patients to or below their dry weight.

If diuretics alone are inadequate to achieve this goal, a hemofilter is placed in the circuit to assist in removal of excess fluid. Patients are given very little crystalloid fluid.

Proper nutrition is essential in the recovery of these patients. Total parenteral nutrition is instituted immediately. In older children and adults, tube feedings are begun whenever feasible in order to achieve the beneficial effects of enteral feeding for prevention of bacterial translocation and maintenance of gut mucosa.

## Weaning the Patient from Extracorporeal Life Support

As native lung function returns, the need for ECLS decreases, and patients are able to be maintained on lower flow levels while still maintaining adequate blood gases and mixed venous oxygen saturations. The CXR, which often demonstrates opacification shortly after ECLS is begun, gradually shows increasing aeration. When these signs of improvement occur, the patients are trialed off ECLS by placing them on acceptable ventilator settings (low peak airway pressure, $FiO_2 \leq 60\%$) and stopping the flow through the circuit for a period of time. When the patient is able to tolerate 1–3 h off ECLS without difficulty, ECLS is discontinued. The average time on ECLS is about 4 days in neonates; older children and adults commonly spend 10–14 days on ECLS, and there have been survivors with ECLS runs of more than 30 days.

## Discontinuation of Extracorporeal Life Support

In some cases, patients will fail to demonstrate clinical improvement despite prolonged courses of ECLS. Defining patients whose pulmonary injury is not recoverable represents a difficult challenge. In children and adults, lack of recoverability is generally manifested as fibrosis of the lung. Identifying the extent of such fibrosis is somewhat difficult, however. Open lung biopsy can be useful for this purpose, but the accompanying bleeding complications are often severe, so our group has discontinued this practice. However, during the time that we did perform open lung biopsy to assess for fibrosis, we found that increasing pulmonary artery pressures which are unresponsive to changes in the patient's fluid status and to changes in arterial $pCO_2$ correlate significantly with the onset of fibrosis in the lung. Patients whose pulmonary artery systolic pressure persistently exceeded 2/3 of the systemic systolic pressure were all found to have evidence of severe fibrosis on open lung biopsy or at autopsy. Therefore, our current practice is to discontinue ECLS if the pulmonary artery pressures reach this level, since this indicates an irrecoverable state. The other major indication for discontinuation of ECLS is because the patient sustains a complication, such as irreversible brain damage, lethal multisystem organ failure, or uncontrollable bleeding.

## Complications of Extracorporeal Life Support

A number of complications have been known to occur in patients on ECLS. These fall into three categories: bleeding complications, mechanical complications, and sequelae of hypoxemia. Bleeding is the most common complication because of the need for systemic heparinization and because of the platelet consumption and dysfunction associated with prolonged bypass. Bleeding most commonly occurs as intracranial bleeding (especially in neonates), surgical site bleeding, or GI bleeding. Bleeding complications are generally managed by lowering of the ACT, increase in platelet count, and transfusion of clotting factors. Surgical site bleeding is managed with operative intervention. Occasionally patients must be removed from ECLS because of severe, uncontrolled bleeding; if these patients can be maintained for 12–24 h off the ECLS circuit and the bleeding is controlled, they can generally be successfully returned to ECLS without further difficulty.

Major mechanical complications are fortunately uncommon. Minor complications, such as oxygenator failure requiring change, are generally handled without difficulty. More serious problems, such as tubing rupture or pump failure, occur in less than 3% of cases. Constant diligence on the part of the ECLS specialist and recurrent training and drills for all team members help keep the mortality from these complications low.

Other complications of ECLS include seizures, especially in neonates. Renal failure occurs in about 2% of cases and is generally reversible. Multisystem organ failure can occur when the patient fails to recover lung function despite prolonged ECLS support. These complications are all felt to result from the systemic hypoxemia which led to the need for ECLS.

## Future Directions – Mechanical

Mechanical device research for ECLS currently takes a number of different directions. One focus lies in making the components of the system less prone to complications, thereby making ECLS even safer. For instance, the use of percutaneous catheters has already decreased the incidence of operative site bleeding in ECLS patients; as these catheters become available in larger sizes, more patients will be able to receive this method of cannulation. As two-lumen venovenous cannulas become available for adults and children, a single cannula will be sufficient to support the patient on venovenous bypass.

Probably the most important ongoing advances are in the development of nonthrombogenic prosthetic surfaces which can allow ECLS to be performed without systemic anticoagulation. At present, both Medtronic/Carmeda [22] and Bentley Laboratories [23] have developed surface coatings which permit the use of oxygenators and PVC tubing without systemic anticoagulation in the laboratory setting. Trials of oxygenators and tubing with these coatings have begun and show promise in allowing reduction in the amount of anticoagulation required [24], although it has not yet been shown that the currently available products will allow anticoagulation to be entirely discontinued. Other studies have shown that there is decreased blood usage when heparin-bonded circuits are employed [25]. Further laboratory efforts, focusing on the use of a combination of heparin, plaminogen activator, and prostacyclin analog all bound to the prosthetic surface, will be more likely to yield a surface coating which will allow prolonged extracorporeal circulation without risk of clot formation even if no systemic anticoagulation is used. This development would make it more feasible to perform ECLS in trauma patients and in those who develop heart or lung failure during cardiac surgery.

Another avenue of research lies in the development of pump systems. Both the servoregulated roller pump and centrifugal pumps have risks involved in their use. A passively filling, mechanically servoregulated pump is currently being developed in order to overcome many of these disadvantages [26, 27]. Ultimately, this type of pump could be linked into a computer system to allow ongoing automatic adjustments to maintain systemic oxygen delivery at adequate levels despite a variety of clinical conditions.

## Future Directions – Clinical

ECLS is already being used in a few centers as a rapid response in selected cases of cardiac arrest. In addition, as nonthrombogenic systems become available, the use of ECLS in postsurgical cardiac patients, especially children, will be more feasible. The use of ECLS as a "bridge to transplant" for those awaiting a heart or lung transplant remains controversial, since the ethical considerations of providing such severely ill candidates with transplants in the face of significant shortages of donor organs are multiple. However, ECLS is clearly a useful tool in the management of thoracic transplant recipients who experience rejection or initial failure to function.

## Conclusions

The development of ECLS reflects the persistence of a small group of investigators who would not be dissuaded by initial failures. In the 1960s, all efforts at ECLS in human subjects were marked by failure. In the 1970s, successful ECLS was shown to be possible, but the initial NIH trial suggested that the technology was of no clinical benefit. In the 1980s, ongoing refinements and improved management made ECLS the treatment of choice for critically ill neonates with respiratory failure; in addition, ECLS was shown to be of benefit in certain groups of children and adults with cardiac or respiratory insufficiency. The challenge of the 1990s is to further refine the mechanical devices and improve understanding of physiologic processes occurring during ECLS in order to make ECLS feasible and safe for groups of patients who currently have no reasonable chance for survival.

# References


1. Gibbon JH Jr (1937) Artificial maintenance of circulation during experimental occlusion of pulmonary artery. Arch Surg 34:1105–1131
2. Kolobow T, Bowman RL (1963) Construction and evaluation of an alveolar membrane artificial heart-lung. ASAIO Trans 9:238–243
3. Lee WH, Krumhaar D, Fonkalsrud EW et al. (1961) Denaturation of plasma proteins as a cause of morbidity and death after intracardiac operations. Surgery 50:29–39
4. Dobell ARC, Mirti M, Galva R et al. (1965) Biologic evaluation of blood after prolonged recirculation through film and membrane oxygenators. Ann Surg 161:617–622
5. Hill JD, O'Brien TG, Murray JJ et al. (1972) Prolonged extracorporeal oxygenation for acute post-traumatic respiratory failure (shock-lung syndrome): use of the Bramson membrane lung. N Engl J Med 286:629–634
6. Zapol W, Pontoppidan H, McCullough N et al. (1972) Clinical membrane lung support for acute respiratory insufficiency. Trans Am Soc Artif Intern Organs 18:553–560
7. Bartlett RH, Gazzaniga AB, Fong SW et al. (1974) Prolonged extracorporeal cardiopulmonary support in man. J Thorac Cardiovasc Surg 68:918–932
8. Zapol WM, Snider MT, Hill JD et al. (1979) Extracorporeal membrane oxygenation in severe acute respiratory failure: a randomized prospective study. J Am Med Assoc 242:2193–2196
9. United States Department of Health, Public Health Services, National Institutes of Health (1979) Extracorporeal support for respiratory insufficiency; a collaborative study. United States Department of Health, Bethesda (RFP-NHLI-73-20)
10. Bartlett, RH, Gazzaniga AB, Jeffries MR et al. (1976) Extracorporeal membrane oxygenation (ECMO) cardiopulmonary support in infancy. ASAIO Trans 22:80–93
11. Bartlett RH, Roloff DW, Cornell RG et al. (1985) Extracorporeal circulation in neonatal respiratory failure: a prospective randomized study. Pediatrics 76:479–487
12. O'Rourke PP, Crone RK, Vacanti JP et al. (1989) Extracorporeal membrane oxygenation and conventional medical therapy in neonates with persistent pulmonary hypertension of the newborn: a prospective randomized study. Pediatrics 84:957–963
13. Gattinoni L, Pesenti A, Avalli L, Rossi F, Bombino M (1987) Pressure-volume curve of total respiratory system in acute respiratory failure: CT scan study. Am Rev Respir Dis 136:730–736
14. Gattinoni L, Pesenti A, Mascheroni D et al. (1986) Low-frequency positive-pressure ventilation with extracorporeal $CO_2$ removal in severe acute respiratory failure. J Am Med Assoc 256:881–885
15. Gille JP (ed) (1989) Neonatal and adult respiratory failure: mechanisms and treatment. Elsevier, Paris
16. Cilley RE, Zwischenberger JB, Andrews AF et al. (1986) Intracranial hemorrhage during extracorporeal membrane oxygenation in neonates. Pediatrics 78:699–704
17. Hirschl RB, Schumacher RE, Snedecor SN, Bui KC, Bartlett RH (1993) The efficacy of extracorporeal life support in premature and low birth weight newborns. J Pediatr Surg 28:1336–1341
18. Schumacher RE (1993) Extracorporeal membrane oxygenation: will this therapy continue to be as efficacious in the future? Pediatr Clin North Am 40:1005–1022
19. Bartlett RH, Morris AH, Fairley HB et al. (1986) A prospective study of acute hypoxic respiratory failure. Chest 5:684–689
20. Rollins R, Morris A, Mortensen C, Cipriano P (1986) Arterial hypoxemia in 1985 predicts a mortality identical to that in 1975. Clin Res 34:79A
21. Zapol WM, Frikker MJ, Pontoppidan H, Wilson RS, Lynch KE (1991) The adult respiratory distress syndrome at Massachusetts General Hospital: etiology, progression, and survival rates 1978–1988. In: Zapol WM, Lemaire F (ed) Adult respiratory distress syndrome. Dekker, New York, pp 367–380
22. Mottaghy K, Oedekoven B, Poppel K et al. (1989) Heparin-free long-term extracorporeal circulation using bioactive surfaces. ASAIO Trans 35:635
23. Toomasian JM, Hsu L-C, Hirschl RB et al. (1988) Evaluation of Duraflo II heparin coating in prolonged extracorporeal membrane oxygenation. ASAIO Trans 34:410–414

24. Rossaint R, Slama K, Lewandowski K et al. (1992) Major thoracic surgery during long-term extracorporeal lung assist for treatment of severe adult respiratory distress syndrome. Eur J Cardiothorac Surg 6:43–45
25. Pesenti A, Gattinoni L, Bombino M (1993) Long-term extracorporeal respiratory support: 20 years of progress. Intensive Crit Care Digest 12(2):15–18
26. Durandy Y, Chevalier JY, Lecompte Y (1990) Single-cannula venovenous bypass for respiratory membrane lung support. J Thorac Cardiovasc Surg 99:404–409
27. Montoya JP, Merz SI, Bartlett RH (1992) Laboratory experience with a novel, non-occlusive, pressure-regulated peristaltic blood pump. ASAIO Trans 38:M406–M411

# Recent Progress Using the Anstadt Cup for Direct Mechanical Ventricular Actuation*

M.P. Anstadt, R. Anthony Perez-Tamayo, J.E. Lowe, and G.L. Anstadt

## Introduction

The non-blood contacting biventricular assist device that has come to be known as DMVA (Direct Mechanical Ventricular Actuation), or the Anstadt Cup, was first conceptualized in 1945. In this year, Dr. George L. Anstadt, upon witnessing the death of his father from cardiogenic shock following a myocardial infarction, was inspired by an illustration in Life magazine of an iron lung. He envisioned a cardiac assist device that would be applied atraumatically through a low pressure suction, and actuate the ventricles both in systole and diastole by the application of external positive and negative pressures (Fig. 1). Dr. Anstadt undertook the initial experiments in DMVA at the USAF School of Aerospace Medicine, San Antonio, Texas from 1960 to 1962 [1].

Recent progress has focused on the use of the Anstadt cup in the following settings

1. Resuscitation (typically less than 48 hours)
2. Post-cardiotomy (typically less than 7 days)
3. Extended Support (greater than 1 week)

## Resuscitation

Initial investigation of the Anstadt cup's potential for use in resuscitation compared DMVA to support generated by standard CPR/ACLS protocols [2]. Studies in animals and humans examining hemodynamics, myocardial perfusion, renal function, ease of defibrillation, and survival, repeatedly demonstrated the superiority of DMVA over open and closed chest cardiac massage for resuscitation. These studies have also shown that direct mechanical actuation of the ventricles does not cause significant myocardial injury. Histologic examination of hearts supported in arrest with DMVA generally showed only a thin, non-constricting, fibrinous epicardial layer [3].

Recent advances in cannulation techniques allowing percutaneous application have led to increasing use of cardiopulmonary bypass circuits (CPB) for resusci-

*Supported in part by NIH grants R01-HL48618, F32-HL08705, and NSF grant CDR8622201

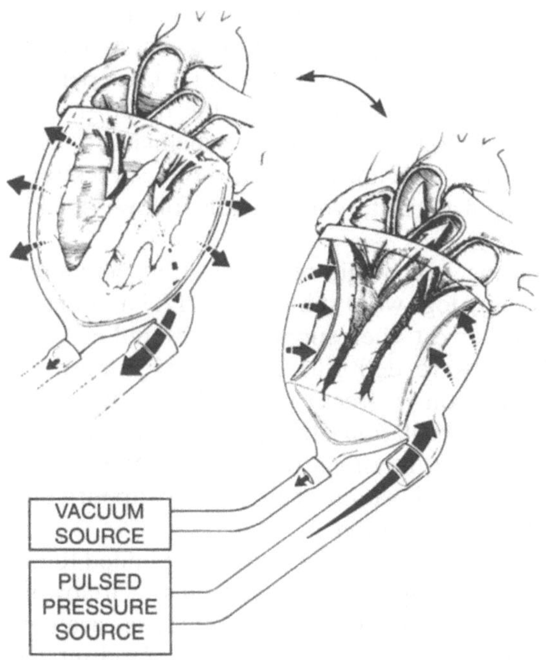


**Fig. 1.** The Anstadt Cup, or Direct Mechanical Ventricular Actuation (DMVA). The soft, compliant diaphragm is bonded to the more rigid housing at the base and apex of the cup. Positive pressure and vacuum are alternated through a drive port, compressing the heart (systole), and assisting ventricular filling (diastole). A low-grade, continuous vacuum through the apex line is used to apply the device atraumatically

tation [4–6]. Therefore, DMVA was compared to the only other mechanical circulatory support system available for resuscitative support, CPB. Compared to CPB, DMVA provides physiologic, pulsatile hemodynamics, free from the complications of blood contact. Moreover, clinical feasibility studies have shown that DMVA can be applied in under two minutes, more rapidly than can CPB [2]. In a model of VF arrest, DMVA and CPB both generated hemodynamics and gross organ perfusion similar to control values [7]. DMVA delivered greater flows to the renal cortex, in a more normal autoregulatory pattern. This finding correlated with the observation of better preserved renal function in DMVA animals. Unlike DMVA, CPB support resulted in abnormal patterns of regional myocardial perfusion, significantly increasing flow to the LV epicardium, septum, and RV regions. A subsequent study showed significantly better myocardial high energy phosphate content in DMVA supported hearts compared to CPB. Hearts supported by DMVA also showed significantly greater tolerance to ischemia [8].

The improved ease and frequency of defibrillation seen in laboratory and clinical resuscitation studies are most likely due to DMVA's ability to restore normal hemodynamics and coronary circulation upon application. Recent investigations have examined other ways in which DMVA could be used as a tool to lower defibrillation thresholds and improve chances of recovery of rhythm [9, 10]. In these studies, the cup was applied to a fibrillating heart and temporarily driven to a sustained compression of the heart. This compression lowered defibrillation thresholds, probably as a result of decreased cardiac blood volume and/or altered ventricular geometry.

Once DMVA's ability to support the circulation and preserve myocardial function was established, the effect of DMVA support on the organ system most sensitive to perfusion deficits was examined. It is well known that brief periods of circulatory arrest (5–10 minutes) can irreversibly damage the brain. In contrast, the heart can tolerate significantly longer periods of ischemia with subsequent recovery. This difference leads to the clinical scenario of a successfully resuscitated but severely brain-damaged patient, whose death follows quickly and inevitably.

In the first of two studies comparing neurologic recovery after circulatory support using CPB and the Anstadt cup, dogs were subjected to 12.5 minutes of electrically induced, normothermic VF arrest, then supported with either CPB, or DMVA for 60 minutes [7]. Hearts were defibrillated after 15 minutes of reperfusion in both groups. Fibrillation refractory to three successive countershocks was treated by similar defibrillation attempts every 15 minutes. After an hour, support was withdrawn and incisions were closed. Ventilatory support was continued for three hours after cessation of circulatory support, and animals were extubated six hours after resuscitation.

Neurologic function was assessed periodically by a veterinarian blinded to the animals resuscitative therapy, using a scoring system based on the following objective criteria: corneal reflex, respiratory effort, pupillary response, swallow, visual perception, pain response, touch response, voice response, food intake, sternal recumbency, standing, and walking. A separate neurologic assessment, based on visual impairments, gait defects, indifference to food, and any seizure activity, determined persistent deficits after 7 days of recovery. After seven days, the animals underwent magnetic resonance imaging (MRI) of their brains. Eight days after resuscitation, allowing sufficient time for maturation of hippocampal lesions [11], animals were sacrificed, and their brains sectioned for histopathologic analysis of regions most frequently injured on MRI images, including hippocampus, caudate nucleus, cerebellum, and watershed areas of the frontal and parietal cortex.

Despite similar flows throughout the period of support, DMVA generated significantly greater mean arterial pressures (MAP) than did CPB at 5 and 15 minutes of reperfusion. As support progressed, this disparity in MAP diminished below significance. DMVA pulse pressures, however, consistently exceeded those during CPB by five- to tenfold. Arterial blood gas values were similar between groups, with the exception of pH values, which normalized more rapidly during CPB in the first 15 minutes. Thereafter, pH remained similar between groups.

Serial neurologic scores showed significantly faster return of function in DMVA supported animals (Fig. 2). Although mean scores remained higher in the DMVA group than the CPB group, the differences were not significant after 24 hours. This trend towards superior neurologic function was also reflected in the deficit scores at 7 days, though the difference in median deficit scores did not reach statistical significance.

MRI detected gross brain lesions in 1/6 DMVA animals compared with 3/7 CPB subjects, most commonly in the region of the caudate, followed in frequency

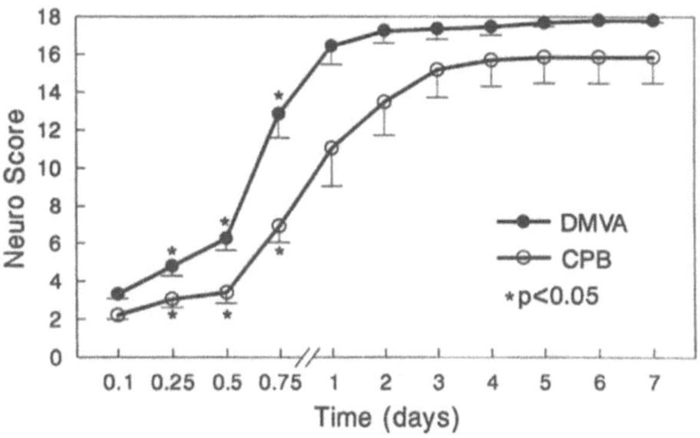


**Fig. 2.** Mean neurologic scores ± SEM after resuscitation with DMVA or CPB. The rate of neurologic recovery was significantly greater after DMVA. $p = 0.018$, group effect; * indicates significant differences ($p < 0.05$) within group recovery rates (within group effect)

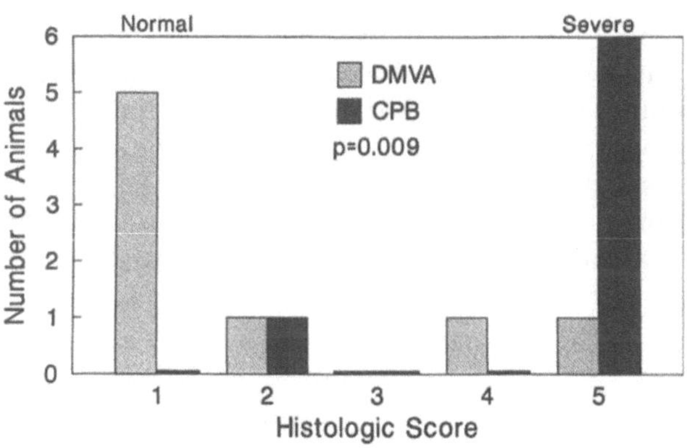


**Fig. 3.** Bar graph showing the distribution of CA1 histologic scores of the hippocampus in dogs after either DMVA or CPB for resuscitation. Only DMVA resulted in normal-appearing CA1 regions (grade 1). Six of seven hippocampi showed complete loss of pyramidal neurons (grade 5) after CPB (DMVA versus CPB, categorical analysis)

by the hippocampus, pons/midbrain junction, and the cerebellum. Microscopic evaluation of these areas provided the most convincing evidence for the benefits of DMVA resuscitation. The hippocampus was assessed because of the high vulnerability of the CA1 pyramidal neurons to ischemic injury. CA1 pyramidal neuronal damage was detected in 10 of 15 brains, generally manifesting in an all-or-none fashion. Both the frequency and severity of injury were significantly greater after CPB (Fig. 3). The incidence of histologic lesions in the caudate sections was also significantly greater after CPB, a trend seen also in examination of the cerebral cortex watershed areas. This study suggests that recovery of neurologic function after resuscitation from cardiac arrest using the Anstadt cup is superior to that after CPB resuscitation, and that the principal source of this difference is DMVA's ability to re-establish normal hemodynamics earlier than CPB [7].

A second study was designed to elucidate the metabolic and hemodynamic phenomena surrounding cerebral reperfusion during the first hour of support [12]. This study also sought to determine what degree of DMVA's advantage over CPB stems from the pulsatile nature of its flow, as opposed to its freedom from the well-described complications of blood contacting surfaces. Dogs were placed under general anesthesia and instrumented for arterial and central venous pressure monitoring, as well as for injection of radiolabeled-microspheres for perfusion measurement. In addition, a catheter was advanced into the sagittal sinus through a burr-hole in the posterior cranium, allowing assessment of cerebral oxygen consumption. Circulatory support was initiated after a 15 minute normothermic VF arrest and continued for 60 minutes. In one group, total circulatory support was provided by the Anstadt cup. In the other, continuous flow through the systemic circulation was provided by a modified left atrial-to-aortic CPB circuit. In order to remove the confounding influence of blood-contact due to membrane oxygenation in the CPB group, the right ventricle was supported by DMVA, driving blood through the pulmonary circuit. As in the outcome study, reperfusion was initiated in both DMVA and CPB groups after identical periods of VF, eliminating the advantage of DMVA's rapid application.

Cerebral blood flow did not differ significantly between groups, despite a trend toward relative hyperemia in the CPB group at 15 minutes. A significantly greater proportion of the total cardiac output was directed to the cerebral circulation in DMVA animals at 3 minutes reperfusion. Most notably, cerebral oxygen consumption in the DMVA group was twice that of CPB at 3 minutes, the difference narrowing below statistical significance at 15 and 60 minutes (Fig. 4). The difference in $O_2$ consumption at 3 minutes reperfusion was associated with greater gray-to-white matter flow ratios and less AV shunting across cerebral

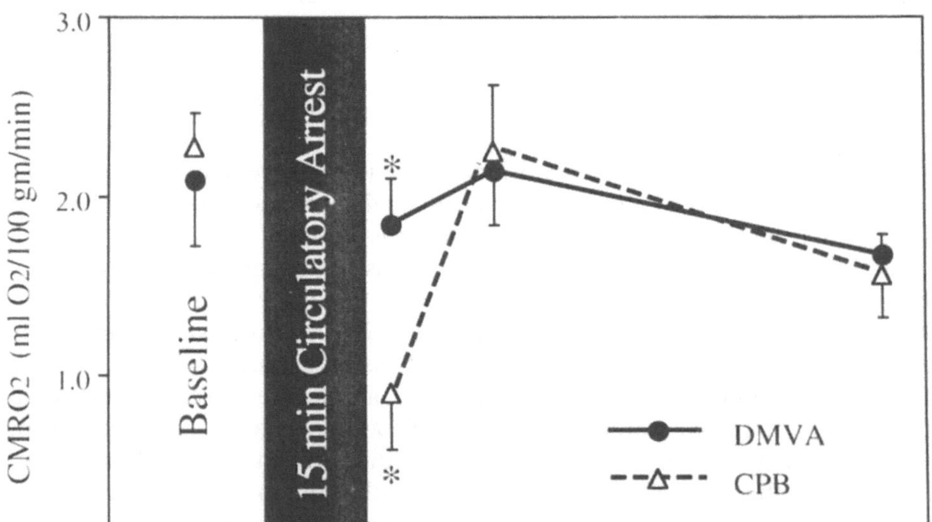


**Fig. 4.** Oxygen consumption (*$CMRO_2$*) derived from the frontal cortex of dogs during prearrest (*baseline*) conditions and during reperfusion after a 15 minute circulatory attest. *DMVA* resulted in a statistically significant increase in *$CMRO_2$* during early reperfusion. Values were similar between groups at all other time points (mean values ± standard error of the mean). (*$p < 0.05$ for DMVA versus CPB by nonpaired Student's *t* test)

beds in DMVA supported animals. The difference in $O_2$ consumption also explains the greater levels of ATP in cerebral tissues in DMVA vs. CPB supported animals (5.2 ± 0.3 vs. 2.9 ± 0.5 μm/g dry wt, $p = 0.02$), and lower levels of malondialdehyde, a marker of reperfusion injury (8.2 ± 0.5 vs. 12 ± 2.3 nm/g dry wt, $p = 0.07$) [13].

Compared to the only other mechanical alternative for resuscitative support (CPB), DMVA restores normal hemodynamics earlier, during the crucial first minutes of reperfusion, and may preserve autoregulation to a greater extent. The early return to normal hemodynamics is correlated with improved cerebral metabolism, which in turn translates to a lower frequency of histopathologically confirmed damage, and superior clinical neurological outcomes.

The American Heart Association (AHA) publishes the authoritative text for advanced cardiac life support (ACLS), and gathers statistics on the success of the recommended techniques. Closed-chest compressions are at the core of CPR and ACLS for the asystolic heart. While closed chest cardiac massage can sustain life, the flow it provides is insufficient to meet oxygen demands of vital organs, especially the brain and the heart. The metabolic consequences of this ever accumulating oxygen debt make defibrillation increasingly difficult, and are thought to potentiate reperfusion injury if circulation is restored. It is no surprise, therefore, that the AHA estimates that only 15% of *hospitalized* patients survive after CPR.

ACLS can increase chance of survival to 30% in a select group of patients. These patients fall into a "best case" scenario of early CPR (two minutes after collapse), very early defibrillation (four minutes) and early ACLS (eight minutes). Obviously, this scenario is extremely rare. A more likely scenario of early CPR (two minutes) and early defibrillation (seven minutes) decreases chance of survival to 20%. More likely still, early CPR (two minutes) followed by delayed defibrillation (ten minutes), reduces chance of survival to 2–8%. Out-of-hospital victims receiving late CPR and delayed defibrillation (ten minutes) have a 0–2% survival [14].

The problem of cardiac arrest refractory to ACLS has increasingly been addressed by the application of modified CPB circuits. As of 1994, a national volunteer registry has recorded more than 200 cases of CPB resuscitative support [4]. Twenty-one percent of these patients were successfully resuscitated with short-term survival. The principle obstacles to improving survival statistics using these techniques are the 10–20 minutes required to institute percutaneous CPB, the flow restrictions of percutaneous cannulae, the blood contact of membrane oxygenation, and the non-pulsatile flow CPB generates.

DMVA offers unique solutions to the problems facing ACLS, while avoiding the disadvantages of CPB. Unlike open-, closed-chest cardiac massage, or CPB, DMVA immediately restores normal pulsatile hemodynamics, preserving autoregulation and organ function. DMVA can increase the likelihood of defibrillation by early reperfusion, and by forcing the heart into a geometry favorable for defibrillation. Earlier reperfusion and earlier defibrillation result in an increased chance of survival. Earlier reperfusion could be furnished by CPB or DMVA, but unlike CPB, DMVA can be rapidly instituted in under two minutes, and has no blood contacting surfaces. In the light of the research presented above, the AHA has recognized the potential importance of the Anstadt cup as an adjunct to standard CPR, and concludes the section on mechanical aids for CPR in the most recent ACLS textbook with a brief description of DMVA [14].

## Post-cardiotomy Support

Several anecdotal reports from the early 1970's described remarkable success for DMVA support in the post-cardiotomy setting (see 'Clinical Experience'). These patients underwent DMVA support after coronary artery bypass grafting, for up to 3 days without injury to their grafts [15]. In order to explore DMVA's effect on coronary artery bypass grafts in a controlled fashion, animals were placed on CPB and underwent aorta-to-left anterior descending coronary artery (LAD) saphenous vein grafting after LAD ligation [16]. Animals then received either DMVA or CPB for 2 or 4 hours of total circulatory support. Cardiac perfusion was determined by radiolabeled microspheres before, during the following support. Myocardial biopsies were frozen for ATP content at the end of each experiment.

Graft patency and anastomotic integrity were identical following DMVA and CPB after 2 and 4 hours of support. Myocardial perfusion of the grafted and non-grafted regions was similar to control values at 2 and 4 hours of DMVA support

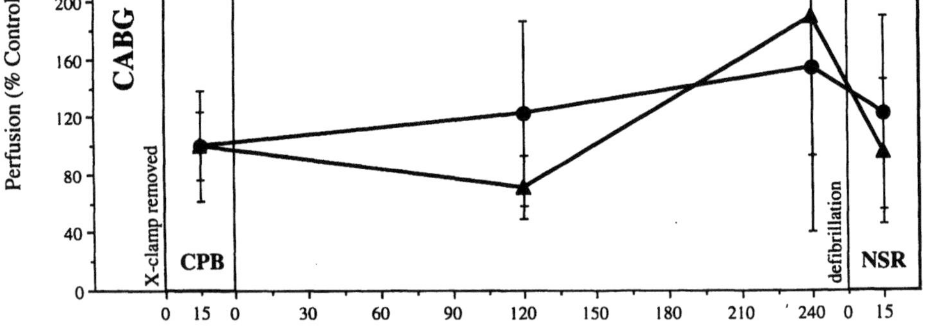


**Fig. 5.** LV endocardial perfusion in the grafted tissue bed, at 2 and 4 hours post-cardiotomy support after CABG procedure. Thirty minutes after removal of the aortic cross clamp, *DMVA* or *CPB* was employed for 4 hrs. of support during VF. Myocardial perfusion of the grafted and non-grafted regions was similar to control values at 2 and 4 hours of DMVA support. Graft patency and anastomotic integrity were identical following DMVA and CPB

and was not significantly different from CPB (Fig. 5). ATP content of the LV graft bed also did not differ between DMVA and CPB after 2 and 4 hours support. However, significantly higher epinephrine doses were required to wean from CPB vs. DMVA at 2 and 4 hours of support and a greater number of DMVA animals were successfully weaned after 2 and 4 hours of support. Mean LV power was greater following 2 hours, but similar after 4 hours of DMVA vs. CPB. This study confirms the evidence that DMVA does not adversely affect graft flow or integrity, and suggests that DMVA results in comparatively better return of cardiac function than continued CPB.

Saphenous vein grafts from post-cardiotomy experiments (2 hours of DMVA vs. CPB support) were then studied in vitro to determine whether mechanical actuation had impaired the contractile function of the graft smooth muscle cells. Maximal contractile responses of 5mm graft segments to norepinephrine, bradykinin, and serotonin were similar between DMVA and CPB animals. The biomaterial-to-tissue surface interaction created during 2 hours of DMVA support does not appear to impair the functional integrity of the aortocoronary graft smooth muscle cells [17].

## Analysis of Biomaterials

As interest grew in clinical applications that might extend support beyond 7 days, it was felt necessary to ensure the greatest period of device longevity possible. After experimentation in the 1960s with then available polyurethanes and natural latex, silicone rubber was felt to have compliance characteristics optimal for direct mechanical actuation. The devices used in all previous laboratory and clinical studies described above were made of silicone rubber. Given the strain seen during DMVA support, the silicone rubber diaphragm is extremely unlikely to undergo yield deformation or fatigue. Instead, because of the nature of bonding between two layers of cured or partially cured silicone rubber, the most vulnerable area of the device is at the seams, where the diaphragm is bonded to the more rigid housing. Polyurethanes, on the other hand, allow use of solvent bonding and vacuum-molding techniques that make possible easily fabricated devices with extremely strong seams. Seams fabricated in this manner would be as strong as the material itself. Unfortunately, greater tear resistance and tensile strength, (indices of material strength) are generally accompanied by lower compliance [18]. The goal, therefore, was to achieve maximum device longevity, while preserving the diaphragm characteristics that had resulted in DMVA's non-injurious actuation of the ventricles. This goal was pursued by maximizing silicone rubber device longevity and by experimenting with devices made from Pellethane. Pellethane is one of several modern polyurethanes approved for medical use, and has been used clinically in circulatory support devices [18].

Two methods of in vitro durability testing were examined to compare devices made of different materials: mock circulation testing and empty pumping. In mock testing, devices actuated a specially developed mock circulation consisting of artificial ventricles on windkessel type afterloads [19]. In empty pumping tests, the devices were set to standard drive parameters, but without any structure to actuate. As the expansion of the diaphragm is unopposed, the diaphragmatic excursion is greater than in any other testing mode. The ventricles of the mock circulations were actuated to physiologic pressures and flows. Diaphragmatic excursion in this case is much less than in empty pumping, but has been observed to be greater than the in vivo setting. These observations have been confirmed by the durability results. Scanning electron microscopy of seam fractures has shown that both in vitro testing models, and in vivo use produce identical failure modes. Empty pumping, with its exaggerated diaphragmatic excursion, is a much harsher and accelerated test.

Silicone rubber cups are currently made by an industrial consultant (Specialty Manufacturing, Inc., Saginaw, MI), providing a controlled environment with assembly line standardization. These industrially manufactured cups have already achieved greater than 90 day endurance on empty pumping tests. It must be kept in mind that this translates to a much greater in vivo longevity. A patient, at the time of this writing, has been supported for greater than 50 days using one of these silicone rubber cups. Pellethane cups, by comparison, vacuum-molded and bonded as described above, have been virtually indestructible, lasting over 60 days on testing frames without failing.

Studies were undertaken to compare the effects of silicone rubber and pellethane cups on the myocardium [20]. Animals were supported in VF for 4 hours using either silicone rubber (SR) or Pellethane (PU) cups. Microspheres were used to determine perfusion during sinus rhythm and at 2 and 4 hours of support. After support, myocardial biopsies were assayed for high energy phosphate content. There were no significant differences between the hemodynamics (MAP, CVP, Cardiac Output) of support using SR and PU cups. Despite a trend towards hyperemic flow in the PU group, there were no significant differences in regional myocardial perfusion. Regional myocardial ATP content, however, revealed three- to sixfold greater ATP levels in SR supported hearts than in those supported with PU devices. The injury reflected in the markedly reduced ATP content of PU hearts was thought to be due to the stress-strain moduli of this material, which is typical of polyurethanes. Medical grade polyurethanes have moduli that are substantially greater than that of silicone rubber (Fig. 6) [18]. PU cups were observed to require greater, more abrupt, drive pressures to effect diaphragmatic excursions similar to those of SR devices. Unlike SR, the material characteristics of PU are temperature- and time-varying, requiring more frequent alterations of drive settings to maintain support at a given level. Compliant SR diaphragms, therefore, are thought to consistently actuate the heart according to its inherent bending modes, avoiding myocardial injury through impact or ischemia.

This is not to say that polyurethanes have been excluded as potential materials for Anstadt cup fabrication. If it were assumed that SR and PU device longevities and characteristics were to remain at current values, there may still be a use for devices made of both materials. Generating nearly identical hemodynamics, SR and PU cups could support the circulation equally well, distinguished solely by PUs greater longevity and more severe myocardial injury. Resuscitation and

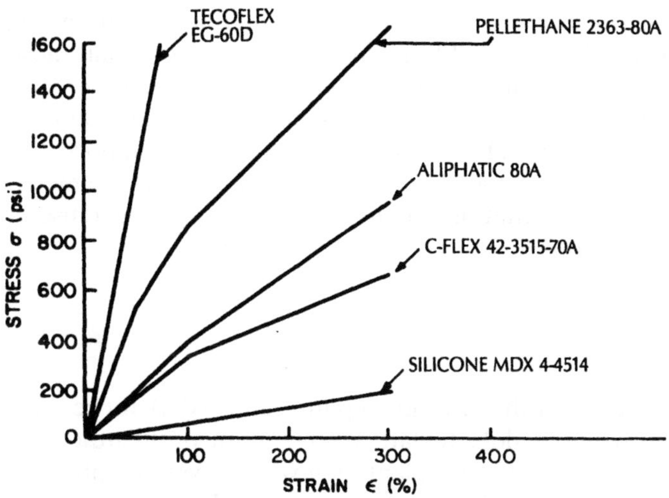


**Fig. 6.** The stress-strain relationships for representative biomedical polymers. Note the relatively high modulus of elasticity (stress-strain ratio) of Pellethane versus SR. The strain range depicted here is far greater than that required for DMVA function. Reprinted with permission from [18]

post-cardiotomy support involve time periods well within SR device durability, and place a premium on the myocardial salvage SR cups can furnish. PU cups might be better suited to extended periods of circulatory support, in circumstances where myocardial salvage was no longer felt to be an option. If the issue of myocardial salvage is deferred, an SR cup may be exchanged for a PU device when the decision is made. Experimental materials are currently being evaluated that could combine the compliance characteristics of SR with the tear resistance and seam strength of polyurethanes.

## Extended Circulatory Support

Clinical experience with DMVA (see "Clinical Experience") has extended beyond 7 days of support with long term survival [21]. In order to investigate DMVA's potential in this time frame, a large ruminant model has been developed, similar to those used to evaluate other circulatory support devices [22]. Suffolk sheep were supported in VF cardiac arrest for up to seven days without vasopressors. The subject supported for the maximal time period (7 days) was defibrillated into sinus rhythm. No CK-MB fraction was greater than 1%, suggesting that DMVA, even with prolonged application during VF, does not result in myocardial injury. As reflected by the blood urea nitrogen and creatinine levels, renal function was preserved throughout the period of support. These experiments represent the longest period any animal has been totally supported using DMVA. It must be kept in mind that VF arrest in a normal heart is the most difficult challenge for long term circulatory support using the Anstadt cup. This situation requires total circulatory support, as opposed to a weakened, myopathic heart, beating in rhythm, which merely requires augmentation. Furthermore, dilated, myopathic hearts can be actuated to greater stroke volumes than those with normal dimensions. This relationship between heart size and greater DMVA generated cardiac output is also seen in normal hearts: mature animals and species with larger hearts respond most favorably to DMVA support, and more closely reflect experience in humans. For these reasons, the bovine model will be useful to determine what limitations, if any, exist to the prolonged use of DMVA for total circulatory support.

## Clinical Experience

The earliest clinical applications of the Anstadt cup utilized DMVA for resuscitation. These took place in the middle to late 1960's, when post-cardiotomy support was in its infancy, and cardiac transplantation was not yet an option. A total of 12 patients, treated at Johns Hopkins, University of Pennsylvania, and Wilford Hall Medical Center, were supported with DMVA following cardiac arrest [2]. Despite prolonged periods of CPR (average time 3 hours) prior to device application, DMVA provided immediate hemodynamic stabilization at normal values, and was continued for 6–7 hours. Although there were no survivors, several patients regained cardiac and neurologic function to varying degrees. One patient regained normal cardiac and neurologic function before succumbing 6 days later from pre-existing renal failure.

Later experience with resuscitation was similarly handicapped by prolonged periods of ischemia prior to application of DMVA [2]. 22 patients received DMVA support in the emergency room after witnessed cardiac arrest refractory to 40 or more minutes of ACLS. In reality, the acquisition of informed consent delayed DMVA application, increasing the average period of CPR prior to support to 81 minutes. Four patients were successfully defibrillated, two of which regained cardiac function sufficient for chest closure and transfer to intensive care. Another patient awoke during DMVA, and was bridged to CPB for CABG. Though there were no survivors because of the long ischemic period, the study confirmed the hemodynamic efficacy of DMVA support, and its application in less than 2 minutes by either surgeons or emergency medicine physicians.

Initial clinical experience with post-cardiotomy support was understandably better. Unlike resuscitation, the post-cardiotomy period does not typically involve an ischemic period, though prolonged CPB is known to produce injury of a milder, though progressive character. An unknown number of patients underwent post-cardiotomy support using DMVA in the early 1970s outside of any controlled study. The reports received from this time can therefore only be considered anecdotal. DMVA was applied in at least 37 patients after coronary artery bypass grafting by three different surgeons at different institutions. There were no graft failures in any patient. Support ranged from 2–72 hours. The patient supported for 72 hours recovered, and was discharged from the hospital with long term survival [15].

Clinical experience at Duke University consists of five cases illustrating the full spectrum of cardiac assistance. The fifth patient has been supported for >50 days at the time of this writing. As his clinical history is still ongoing, it will not be detailed here.

**Case #1**

The first patient at Duke to receive DMVA was a 56 year old female suffering from an idiopathic dilated cardiomyopathy [23]. She was admitted to the intensive care unit in acute cardiogenic shock. Despite maximal inotropic support, her hemodynamic status deteriorated to pulmonary arterial (PA) pressures of 48/42 and cardiac indices at or below 1.8 liters/min/meters$^2$. Catheterization also showed 3+ mitral regurgitation. Upon application through a left anterior thoracotomy, DMVA immediately decreased PA pressures to 24/8, increased arterial pressures to 100/60, and increased cardiac index to 2.67 liters/min/meters$^2$. The time required for DMVA application was 38 minutes from incision to closure. All inotropes were discontinued in the first twelve hours after the procedure. She remained stable for 56 hours, periodically waking from mild sedation and expressing no discomfort. At 56 hours, a donor heart became available, and she underwent cannulation for CPB followed by successful transplantation. She remains alive and well over five years after her transplant. Histopathology of her native heart showed LV dilation and evidence of a right ventricular myocardial infarction, all predating DMVA application. There was no evidence of myocardial injury due to DMVA. Interestingly, DMVA functioned well despite atrioventricular valve regurgitation. It is possible that DMVA's base acted as an annuloplasty ring, closing the valve orifice and allowing valve leaflets to coapt.

**Case #2**

The early clinical experience demonstrated the increased mortality and morbidity associated with delayed application and extended CPR prior to DMVA. The second patient to receive DMVA support underscored this lesson. The patient was a 46 year old male suffering from acute cardiogenic shock after massive myocardial infarction, unresponsive to angioplasty and thrombolytic therapy [23]. Despite IABP and maximal inotropic support, hemodynamic status deteriorated to cardiac indices of approximately 1 liter/min/m$^2$. Before the DMVA device could be implanted, cardiac arrest requiring prolonged CPR occurred at a mean arterial pressure of 40 mmHg. Upon application of the cup, cardiac output increased to 4.7 liters/min (index of 2.14 liters/min/m$^2$). Arterial pressures increased to 120/80 mmHg, and PA diastolic pressure decreased from 45 to 22 mmHg. Even though he remained in fibrillation, hemodynamic status remained stable during 45 hours of support, with mean cardiac indices around 2.8 liters/min/m$^2$. Unfortunately, the patient remained neurologically unresponsive after his arrest, and was pronounced brain dead. The device was removed at 45 hours, and the patient died. Histopathologic examination of the heart after death

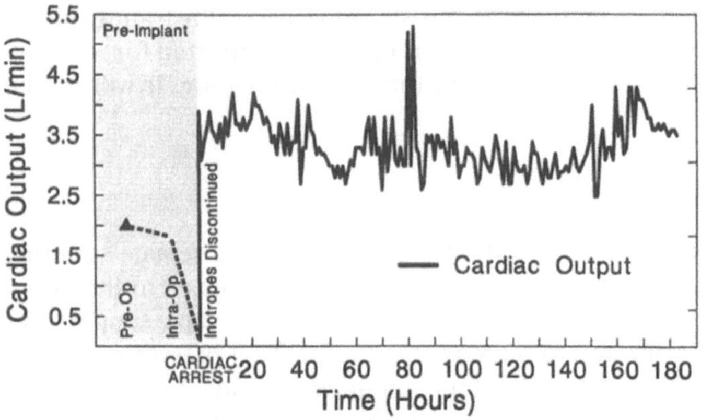


**Fig. 7.** Graph of cardiac output for Case #3. Despite maximal inotropes, cardiac output was less than 2.0 liters/min pre-operatively. Intra-operatively, the patient arrested. Upon DMVA application, normal hemodynamics were restored. Support was continued until spontaneous recovery of normal cardiac function was confirmed (total period of support, 182 hours)

showed infarction of 50% of the myocardial mass with no evidence of injury secondary to DMVA.

### Case #3

An 18 year old female in an excellent state of health developed rapidly progressive cardiogenic shock secondary to a viral cardiomyopathy [21]. Prior to application of DMVA, she required maximal inotropic support as well as ventilatory support for florid pulmonary edema in the context of arterial pressures of 60/40 mmHg, with cardiac indices less than 1.5 liters/min/m$^2$, and pulmonary artery pressures of 50/40 mmHg. The patient arrested intra-operatively. Upon application of the cup, normal hemodynamics were restored (cardiac index of 2.5 liters/min/m$^2$, arterial pressures 115/79 mmHg, PA pressures 30/15 mmHg), followed by resolution of the pulmonary edema over the first 24 hours (Fig. 7). The patient was placed on the active transplant list. She was supported for a total of 182 hours. Remarkably, on the third and fourth days of support, her heart began to show signs of independent function. Over the course of the next three days, the recovery of her native heart was monitored. At 7.5 days of support, she was taken to the operating room, and DMVA support was discontinued. Her post-operative course was uneventful, and she was discharged from the hospital after a two week stay. Over three years later, she remains in excellent health, with normal resting and exercise ejection fraction by MUGA scan.

### Case #4

The fourth patient was a 72 year old male whose coronary artery bypass grafting procedure was complicated by cerebral and myocardial embolic showers from an atheromatous and calcific aortic root [21]. Following CABG, he could not be weaned from CPB. The patient was weaned with DMVA and supported for 40 hours. Unfortunately, brain function never returned, and the device was removed, allowing the patient to expire. Autopsy revealed patent and intact bypass grafts, with no evidence of DMVA related injury to grafts or myocardium.

## Conclusion

DMVA is a unique non blood contacting, biventricular cardiac assist device capable of total circulatory support. Apart from its rapid and technically undemanding application, the essence of DMVA's success is its proximity to the natural state. Blood is received and propelled by the same surfaces as in normal contraction, through the same valves, into the same arteries. Providing hemodynamic pressure and flow traces nearly indistinguishable from the normal physiologic state, its advantage over less natural forms of support (open-, closed-chest CPR, CPB) is perhaps not so surprising. Though DMVA has been effective in the setting of valvular insufficiency, there may be some conditions where damage to the valves/arteries/tissues may preclude the application of DMVA. This remains to be investigated. Experience with the resuscitative use of DMVA leaves only a multicenter, prospective trial (currently being planned) to determine what role this device should play in the ACLS armamentarium. As confidence increases in resuscitation, further investigation in post cardiotomy and extended support will drive continued experimentation with different biomaterials to achieve greater device longevity. Extended support may include bridge to transplant (as in Duke Case #1), bridge to bridge, and bridge to recovery (as in Duke Case #3). The Anstadt Cup's role in this arena remains to be determined.

## References

1. Lowe JE, Anstadt MP (1992) Correspondence: Direct Mechanical Ventricular Actuation, Response to SK Khanna. Ann Thorac Surg 55(1):198–199
2. Anstadt MP, Anstadt GL, Lowe JE (1991) Direct Mechanical Ventricular Actuation: A Review. Resuscitation 21(1):7–23
3. Coogan SP, Casey HW, Skinner DB, Anstadt GL (1969) Direct Mechanical Ventricular Assistance: Acute and Long-Term Effects in the Dog. Arch Pathol 87:423–431
4. Hill JG, Bruhn PS, Cohen SE, Gallagher MW, Manart F, Moore CA, Seifert PE, Askari P, Banchieri C (1992) Emergent Applications of Cardiopulmonary Support: A Multi-institutional Experience. Ann Thorac Surg 54:699–704
5. Dembitsky WP, Moreno-Cabral RJ, Adamson RM, Daily PO (1993) Emergency Resuscitation Using Portable Extracorporeal Membrane Oxygenation. Ann Thorac Surg 55: 304–309
6. Moritz A, Wolner E (1993) Circulatory Support with Shock Due to Acute Myocardial Infarction. Ann Thorac Surg 55:238–244
7. Anstadt MP, Stonnington MJ, Tedder M, Crain BJ, Brothers MF, Hilleren DJ, Rahija RJ, Menius JA, Lowe JE (1991) Pulsatile Reperfusion After Cardiac Arrest Improves Neurologic Outcome. Ann Surg 214(4):478–490

8. Anstadt MP, Taber JE, Hendry PJ, Plunkett MD, Tedder M, Menius JA, Lowe JE (1991) Myocardial Tolerance to Ischemia After Resuscitation: Direct Mechanical Ventricular Actuation Versus Cardiopulmonary Bypass. ASAIO Trans 37:M518–M519
9. Idriss SF, Anstadt MP, Anstadt GL, Ideker RE (1993) Cardiac Compression Improves Defibrillation Efficacy. Circulation (Suppl I) 88(4):I-593
10. Idriss SF, Anstadt MP, Anstadt GL, Ideker RE (1995) The Effect of Cardiac Compression on Defibrillation Efficacy and the Upper Limit of Vulnerability. The Journal of Cardiovascular Electrophysiology (In Press)
11. Brierly JB, Graham DI (1984) Hypoxia and Vascular Disorders of the Central Nervous System. In: Adams J, Corsellis J, Duchen L (eds) Greenfield's neuro-pathology. Edward Arnold, London, pp 125–107
12. Anstadt MP, Tedder M, Hegde SS, Perez-Tamayo RA, Crain BJ, Ha VL, Abdelaleem S, White WD, Lowe JE (1993) Pulsatile Reperfusion Improves Cerebral Blood Flow Compared to Nonpulsatile Reperfusion Following Cardiac Arrest. Ann Thorac Surg 56(3):453–461
13. Anstadt MP, Tedder M, Banit DM, Crain BJ, Perez-Tamayo RA, Abdel-aleem S, Lowe JE, (1993) Pulsatile Flow Attenuates Cerebral Reperfusion Injury. Circulation (Suppl I) 88(4):I-170
14. American Heart Association (1994) Advanced Cardiac Life Support Textbook
15. Lambert CJ (1992) Clinical Experience with Direct Mechanical Ventricular Actuation at Baylor University, Dallas, Texas
16. Anstadt MP, Perez-Tamayo RA, Banit DM, Walthall HP, Chen FA, Abdel-aleem S, Reimer KA, Lowe JE (1994) Direct Mechanical Ventricular Actuation vs Continued Cardiopulmonary Bypass for Postcardiotomy Circulatory Support Following CABG. 30th Annual Meeting of the Society of Thoracic Surgeons
17. Anstadt MP, Perez-Tamayo RA, Davies MG, Hagen P-O, Walthall HP, St. Louis J, Hendrickson SC, Aleem SA, Anstadt GL, Lowe JE (1995) Aortocoronary Saphenous Vein Graft Function After Mechanical Cardiac Massage. ASAIO J (Suppl) 41(1):19
18. Sharma CP, Szycher M (1991) Blood Compatible Materials and Devices: Perspectives Toward the 21st Century. Technomic Publishing, Lancaster
19. Perez-Tamayo RA, Anstadt MP, Walthall HP, St. Louis J, Wurzel D, Anstadt GL, Lowe JE (1993) In Vitro Analysis of Cardiac Actuation. The 39th Annual Meeting of ASAIO, Abstract Book 22(40)
20. Anstadt MP, Perez-Tamayo RA, Banit DM, Walthall HP, Cothran JRL, Aleem SA, Anstadt GL, Jones PL, Lowe JE (1994) Myocardial Tolerance to Mechanical Actuation is Affected by Biomaterial Characteristics. ASAIO J 40:M329–M334
21. Lowe JE, Anstadt GL, Unpublished Case Reports
22. Perez-Tamayo RA, Anstadt MP, Cothran RL, Lowe M, St. Louis J, Anstadt GL, Lowe JE (1995) Extended Total Circulatory Support Using Direct Mechanical Ventricular Actuation. ASAIO J (In Press)
23. Lowe JE, Anstadt MP, Van Trigt P, Smith PK, Hendry PJ, Plunkett MD, Anstadt GL (1991) First Successful Bridge to Cardiac Transplantation Using Direct Mechanical Ventricular Actuation. Ann Thorac Surg 52(6):1237–1245

# Subject Index

# Springer-Verlag and the Environment

We at Springer-Verlag firmly believe that an international science publisher has a special obligation to the environment, and our corporate policies consistently reflect this conviction.

We also expect our business partners – paper mills, printers, packaging manufacturers, etc. – to commit themselves to using environmentally friendly materials and production processes.

The paper in this book is made from low- or no-chlorine pulp and is acid free, in conformance with international standards for paper permanency.

MIX
Papier aus verantwortungsvollen Quellen
Paper from responsible sources
FSC® C105338

If you have any concerns about our products, you can contact us on
**ProductSafety@springernature.com**

In case Publisher is established outside the EU, the EU authorized representative is:
**Springer Nature Customer Service Center GmbH**
**Europaplatz 3, 69115 Heidelberg, Germany**

Printed by Libri Plureos GmbH
in Hamburg, Germany